Superb Praise for
JUST LIKE A WOMAN

"*Just Like a Woman* is an extraordinary book about the unique biology of women. It provides up-to-the-minute scientific information that's accurate and balanced, yet engaging to read. A fantastic book!"
—*Miriam Nelson, Ph.D., director, Center for Health Promotion and Physical Activity at the School of Nutrition, Tufts University, and author of* Strong Women Stay Young

"A superb achievement—Dianne Hales has challenged accepted 'wisdom' and presented alternative ways of looking at gender in the light of the exciting emergence of 'gender science.' This book is at the cutting edge and should be widely read." —*Carol C. Nadelson, M.D., clinical professor of psychiatry, Harvard Medical School and past president, American Psychiatric Association*

"A book on women which is both factual and moving—a rare combination! A masterful book—from both a scientific and a literary perspective, this is a unique contribution to our understanding of the psychology of women." —*Vivien Burt, M.D., Ph.D., director, Women's Life Center, Neuropsychiatric Institute, UCLA School of Medicine*

"I could not put this spectacular book down. Dianne Hales synthesizes scientific information in an informative and easily readable way. *Just Like a Woman* should help to revolutionize the way women are viewed in the world." —*Beverly Whipple, Ph.D., R.N., F.A.A.N, professor, Rutgers, the State University of New Jersey, and president, American Association of Sex Educators, Counselors and Therapists*

"This lively account of the newest developments in gender-specific medicine should be obligatory reading for every woman who has felt confused, patronized, and/or misunderstood in her doctor's office. . . . A resource for patient and physician alike." —*Marianne Legato, M.D., director, Partnership for Women's Health, Columbia University*

"Hales uses the results of medical and psychological studies as well as anecdotes to make a confident case for women and men as divergent evolutionary, biological, and emotional creations. . . . By pulling together current knowledge on the subject, [she] has provided an engrossing snapshot of today's complicated gender landscape." —*Library Journal*

JUST LIKE A
WOMAN

*How Gender Science Is Redefining
What Makes Us Female*

DIANNE HALES

BANTAM BOOKS

New York Toronto London Sydney Auckland

This edition contains the complete text
of the original hardcover edition.
NOT ONE WORD HAS BEEN OMITTED.

JUST LIKE A WOMAN

PUBLISHING HISTORY

Bantam hardcover edition published March 1999
Bantam trade paperback edition / June 2000

PRINTED IN THE UNITED STATES OF AMERICA

BVG   10 9 8 7 6 5 4 3 2 1

To the women—
mother, daughter, friends, colleagues, mentors—
who have taught me what an honor it is
to be called woman

C O N T E N T S

P R E F A C E

At the turn of the nineteenth century, a new item of furniture made its way into fashionable dressing rooms throughout Europe: a long mirror of cheval glass that could be tilted to allow a woman to behold herself from head to toe. It was known as a "psyche."

Did this term indicate a new awareness of the totality of a woman—the many connections linking her body and mind, her inner *and* outer dimensions? "Oh, no," a historian tells me. "Women still looked at themselves the way everyone always did—from the outside in." For countless centuries, philosophers, scholars, poets, playwrights, educators, physicians, and politicians did indeed base their notions about women on observations that were rarely more than skin deep. It's no wonder they got it so wrong.

Man was the sole measure of all things human. And so, at least to a male beholder's eye, woman seemed biologically blighted, "a fair defect of nature," as the poet Milton observed. Some early scientists relegated women to a category somewhere above monkeys yet below men. Before the eighteenth century, medical opinion saw the female body as a lesser variation on the male model, with analogous reproductive organs turned about and tucked inside. In the Enlightenment, another notion took hold: of woman as the opposite of man, inexorably different (and deficient) in functions and feelings.

Of course, these were not scientists' only errors. Learned men of other times were mistaken about most things, from the position of the planets to the flatness of the earth. But long after the sun was granted its rightful place and the earth its proper shape, influential thinkers, even of the early twentieth century, clung to the notion of a woman as abnormal and inferior—in body and therefore in mind and spirit.

"Some ideas keep having to be affirmed from the ground up, over and over," the poet Adrienne Rich observed in *Of Woman Born*. "One of these is the apparently simple idea that women are as intrinsically human as men." We are indeed, yet we are not the same. Both concepts are in need of restating—and redefining. These days the new approach of gender-specific research is expanding our appreciation of all human beings by looking at what makes each sex unique. Today, for the first time ever, we are learning about women from the inside out.

This scientific revolution—as profound in its own way as the social evolution that has transformed gender roles and rules—is replacing stereotypes with deeper understanding. The differences between women and men, we can now see, are exactly that: differences, not signs of defects, damage, or disease. Women are *not* the second sex but a separate sex, female to the bone and to the very cells that make up those bones. Thanks to an explosion in research into the long-neglected fields of women's health and reproductive biology, we also know more than ever before about how the female body develops, changes, cycles, ripens, conceives, gestates, gives birth, and grows old. And we are gaining greater insight into womanly ways of creating and connecting, expressing emotion and finding spiritual and sexual fulfillment.

Even today, though, many women remain wary of their biology— with reason. Through most of history, femaleness defined and confined women's lives. Well into the twentieth century, pseudoscientific notions about female variability and vulnerability were used to justify discrimination and sexism. To escape the "body trap," some women have tried to distance themselves from the physical tethers of gender and live as if they were disembodied spirits. Others insist that whatever sex differences do exist simply don't make a difference. "Why not just talk about all the ways we're similar?" one friend asked. Respected social psychologists urged me not to include a chapter on the controversial subject of sex differences in the brain. Others advised steering clear of any mention of PMS, depression, menopause, or abortion. "Remember," a pro-choice advocate cautioned, "anything that can be used against women will be."

Such concerns are understandable. However, as someone who has spent the last quarter century reporting on women, I'm convinced that *not* asking how our bodies work, *not* finding out what makes them unique, *not* acknowledging every aspect of being female, susceptibilities as well as strengths, is a far greater disservice. While biology is no longer destiny, it remains a crucial part of our reality. In affirming our femaleness, we are not diminishing or discrediting our mental ability or essential equality. Rather, we are recognizing a fundamental source of strength and sustenance. One of the gifts of gender science and of the recent revelations in reproductive biology—beyond their practical applications in clinical medicine—is that they allow women to reclaim their bodies with true pride in their distinctiveness, their evolutionary resilience, their physiological stamina, and their remarkable capacity for renewal and lifelong growth.

The Blind Spot

Years ago, when I was researching an article on irregular heartbeats, a cardiologist thumbed through a pile of electrocardiogram tracings to show me an example of a normal pattern. "Here's one," he said, then cast it aside, mumbling, "No, that won't do. It's a woman's." To my chagrin, neither he nor I questioned the assumption that the only norm—not just for hearts, but for all of human physiology—had to be male.

In every field of scientific study, an enormous blind spot all but obscured females from serious consideration for any reason other than reproduction. This didn't begin to change until significant numbers of women began peering through microscopes, observing animal behavior, rethinking basic theories of evolution, assessing the role of female chromosomes and hormones, and studying the effects of gender on every bodily process, in health and in disease.

The first part of this book focuses on their findings. In animal behavior, as described in Chapter 2, field research has shown that females of various species play critical roles that male observers mostly missed—as sly sexual strategists, enterprising providers, and keepers of kinship bonds. In anthropology, discussed in Chapter 3, new theories have provided fresh insight into the evolution of womanly bodies, female involvement in sexual selection, and the unheralded contributions women have made to the survival and success of the human species.

Chapter 4 highlights the revelations that gender-specific research has yielded into genetics, the role of the sex chromosomes, and the importance of "female" and "male" hormones to the well-being of both women and men. It also shows how women athletes—swimming, running, skiing, and skating farther and faster than any man could a few decades ago—are redefining the potential of the female body. The emphasis shifts to clinical medicine in Chapter 5, which documents the impact of gender on longevity and on vulnerability to various diseases, and reports on what science now knows about the sex medical research so long ignored.

Life Stages

"I never think of myself as a woman," a college student tells me during a group interview. "I am a person. Period." "Right," says another young woman. "A person who gets periods."

Of all the aspects of female physiology, none has been more stigmatized than menstruation—and none more poorly understood. Rather than exploring the intricacies of this basic physiological function, researchers long excluded women from their studies, in part because their cycles might "skew the science." The one aspect of menstruation that did receive attention was premenstrual syndrome (PMS), perhaps the most controversial of female diagnoses. Yet research into PMS, which some women see as politically suspect, has yielded an unexpected payoff: important discoveries about the normal changes of the menstrual cycle and about premenstrual variations that affect the course of many common illnesses, including asthma, migraines, diabetes, and depression.

As the second section of this book reports, all the stages of a woman's biological life—menarche, menstruation, pregnancy, menopause—can affect more than her reproductive organs. Chapter 6 starts this discussion by tracing the physical and psychological development of girls from infancy through adolescence.

Chapter 7 focuses on menstruation, including a history of taboos, an explanation of molimina (normal cycling), and a discussion of positive and negative changes. Chapter 8 looks at another aspect of female biology, fertility, and the steps women have taken throughout time to control it. It explores the psychological issues related to contraception and abortion and reports on the emergence of a new commitment to "childfree" living. In Chapter 9, the emphasis is on motherhood—the quest to conceive, the psychological aspects of infertility and pregnancy, the emotional problems that can develop after delivery, and the unexpected ways in which maternity transforms a woman.

Chapter 10 takes on a topic that once was even more taboo than menstruation: the midlife passages of perimenopause and menopause, stages that, to me, represent a woman's second puberty. Just as she did in adolescence, a woman experiences a biological transformation that can affect everything from mood to sexuality to long-term physical well-being. The more she understands about what is happening and why, the better she can anticipate and adapt to the changes "the change" brings.

An Inner Quest

A new generation of female theologians, redefining spirituality from a woman's perspective, has made a distinction between "authoritative knowledge," the information gleaned from science and scholarly investigations, and "embodied knowledge," the understanding born of life experience and sensed with the heart as well as the head. For the most part, *Just Like a Woman* is based on authoritative knowledge, on data from recent research on women. But this information falls short when it comes to exploring all the ways in which women feel, sense, love, communicate, and connect to sources of spiritual strength. The final section of the book, which focuses on a woman's brain, emotions, psychiatric vulnerability, sexuality, and spirituality, reports on provocative new research in all these areas. However, it also presents the embodied knowledge of real women—of today and yesterday—to illuminate areas that science is just beginning to investigate.

Chapter 11 asks a question that has ignited controversy for centuries—whether the brain has a gender—and presents various perspectives on female intelligence, cognitive skills, and creativity. Chapter 12 explores another subject that psychological science long ignored, gender and emotion, and reveals the similarities as well as the differences in the way the sexes experience human feeling. Chapter 13 presents professional and personal views of the mental disorders most common among women, including depression, anxiety disorders, and alcohol abuse. In Chapter 14 we see how women's search for sexual and spiritual fulfillment can lead to reaffirmation of bodily joys and wisdom. The final chapter puts today's woman into the context of the new realities of her social and economic life and looks at the open-ended possibilities that await tomorrow's woman—and man.

Beyond the Stereotypes

This book challenges any one narrow view of what "woman" is like. Its purpose is to encourage women everywhere to consider, reassess, and redefine for themselves what it truly means to be female—an experience that remains, as always, both universal and unique. When I write about women, I do so realizing that no two of us are alike. Gender is only part of our identity, and each woman's life is shaped by myriad factors— among them genetic endowment, innate temperament, childhood experience, physical health, race, culture, ethnicity, sexual orientation, and economic status. Neither gender science nor women's health research has yet taken all such variables into account, so on certain topics, in particular those relating to women of color, lesbians, and women with disabilities, there is unfortunately not a great deal to report specifically.

In other areas, this book treads into territory usually regarded as politically incorrect or intensely controversial. To the greatest extent possible, I have tried to steer clear of politicizing. "What women need are facts," a congressional aide who spearheaded the political fight for more research funding for women's health remarked several years ago. "What we've gotten is ideology, which thrives in the absence of factual information." This book, I hope, will help fill that vacuum.

Men, such an important part of women's lives, also stand to benefit from the revelations of gender science. At a practical level, new insights into women's greater longevity, hardier hearts, and more vigorous immune systems may yield clinical benefits for all of us. Ultimately, I believe, the best in both sexes will shine more brightly after each casts aside the stultifying stereotypes of what the other gender is "like."

"In our civilization," the psychologist Theodor Reik once observed, "men are afraid that they will not be men enough, and women are afraid that they may be considered only women." Such assumptions shortchange us all. As the only species capable of self-comprehension, we humans cannot fully know ourselves or realize our potential unless we find out as much as we can about both halves of the human race. And women cannot fully understand or appreciate being female unless we delve beyond the surface to comprehend all the dimensions that make us who we are. Only by exploring this long-mysterious "foreign land" can we begin to claim this rich and varied territory as our own.

PART ONE

The Foreign Land

A Woman is a foreign land
Of which, though there he settle young,
A man will ne'er quite understand
The custom, politics, and tongue.

Coventry Patmore,
"The Angel in the House"

C H A P T E R   1

What Is a Woman?

I run with a wobble in my hips—just like a woman. I throw a ball underhand rather than overhand—just like a girl. I cry during sad movies and take everything personally. I also walk, talk, smile, worry, gossip, flirt, and change my mind just like a woman. Or so I've been told—in appreciation at times, in exasperation at others.

Just like a woman, I like spring blossoms, silky lingerie, babies' gummy grins, French perfume, and slow dancing. I've melted in the arms of the man I love and been swept away by the sight of my newborn child. I've twirled in gowns of black velvet and laughed long and hard in the company of good friends. Just like a woman, I can act like a lady, think like a man, and work like a dog. But what do all the ways I'm just like a woman tell you about who I really am? Not very much. "Woman" is generic; I am not.

In legends and literature, it was just like a woman to be bitch or witch, madonna or muse, angel or harlot. Eve tempted, Delilah betrayed, Medea avenged, Cleopatra seduced. Juliet loved too much, Anna Karenina hoped too little—just like a woman. Ours was the emotional sex, irrational, manipulative, deceitful, never to be trusted. Or so we were told.

Hippocrates described woman as a damp, soggy

3

creature. Aristotle declared her naturally defective, a "mutilated male." The Old Testament depicted her as unclean; the New, as a "weaker vessel" in need of male forbearance. Medieval monks damned her as a necessary evil, a "sack of dung" wrapped in seductive flesh, "a domestic danger, a delectable detriment." All were wrong.

In 1710 the British essayist Richard Steele defined woman as "a daughter, a sister, a wife, and a mother, a mere appendage of the human race." Her greatest possible aspiration was as self-sacrificing "angel of the house." She seemed capable of nothing more. An obstetrics textbook widely used in the early twentieth century declared, "A woman has a head too small for intellect but just big enough for love."

Only men—or at least a few great men—made history; women made the sons who would grow up to fight the battles, conquer the kingdoms, and perform the daring deeds that other men would record and long remember. Women, living by rules they never made in roles they never chose, remained in the shadows of time, on the margins of meaning. Until now.

To a breathtaking extent, the old rules, confining roles, and presumed biological imperatives no longer apply. These days it's just like a woman to soar into space, march off to war, manage (and make) millions, govern countries, pass laws, negotiate treaties, fly jets, transplant organs, conduct symphonies. Not only do women hold up half the sky, we hold down nearly half the jobs and head one quarter of the world's households.

From Asia to America, women are learning and earning more than any previous generation. Once barred from universities, women now receive the majority of baccalaureate degrees. In national elections, women cast the decisive votes. Whether buying televisions or trucks, we control the bulk of consumer dollars—with good reason. In almost half of American two-income homes, women earn as much as their spouses; in about a quarter, they earn more.

We have become women of independence as well as independent means. More women everywhere are delaying or deferring marriage. In Great Britain, women are waiting until an average age of 27 to wed; American brides are older (at an average of 24.5 years) than they've been in three decades. Fewer women are having babies, and those who do have fewer of them. In certain regions of Italy, Spain, and Eastern Europe, women's birth rates have fallen to an average of fewer than 1.2 children, the lowest ever recorded. Of those women who do become mothers, more remain single. In Germany, one in seven new mothers is unmarried; in Great Britain and the United States, one in three; in Sweden, one in two.

Women, occupants of bodies once believed flawed and fragile, are outliving men by about seven years. Female athletes are sprinting faster, jumping higher, and running longer distances than anyone once thought a woman possibly could. Female minds, derided for centuries as incapable of intelligence and instruction, are becoming the best-educated in history. Female hands, once deemed suitable only for rocking cradles, are wielding scalpels and gavels. Female presidents and prime ministers have taken the helm of nations as politically diverse as Great Britain, Canada, Bolivia, Poland, Israel, Pakistan, New Zealand, and the Philippines. In Sweden and Iceland, women head 40 percent of government ministries. In Great Britain, France, and Italy, a record number of women hold parliamentary seats.

In thousands of ways both subtle and significant, in a revolution so gentle it feels like evolution, the planet's 2.8 billion women are changing the world. We have moved into places where women rarely went. We are doing things only men used to do, often in ways men never tried. We have unprecedented opportunities, power, money, and autonomy—as well as the burdens they can bring. To an extent never before possible, women can live just like men. Yet most of us, even as we eagerly explore new realms of possibility, prefer to remain true to who and what we are: female in body, mind, and spirit.

Fifty years ago an American polling firm asked women and men two questions: Which sex has an easier time in life? And if you were to be born again, would you rather come back male or female? In the postwar 1940s both sexes agreed that women had an easier lot. In 1996 both said men did. But fifty years ago, despite their supposedly easy life, most women said they'd prefer to be men; no men wanted to come back as women. Men of the nineties still like being male, but women, by an overwhelming majority, said they'd choose to remain female.

In the course of talking to hundreds of women, formally and informally, about the substance of this book, I got the same response—from women who work and women who don't, from hurried mothers and harried managers, from the woman who invests my retirement funds and the woman who cuts my hair. But one made an important distinction: "I'd always want to be a woman," she said. "But I'd never want to be 'just like' one." I can understand why.

With an Italian's fine-tuned ear, the writer Paola Bono notes that being "just like a woman" misses the essential point: It doesn't address what it means, simply, to *be* a woman, but defines us in terms of someone or something else. Throughout history, the invariably male powers that were beheld women often with disdain, always with presumed superiority. In their eyes, we were pets or parasites, objects of desire or disgust, vanity's name or hell's fury, the eternal "other."

The fault, they said, lay in the very cells that make up the female body. "A woman is a pair of ovaries with a human being attached," a nineteenth-century physician observed, "whereas a man is a human being with testes attached." It was a cruel distinction—and a false one. Because it was just like a woman to have a womb, it was presumed she should not, could not, use her brain. Because it was just like a woman to give life, her own life seemed to have no other value. Because her mental and physical health seemed too precarious, she was told she could not, should not, learn to read, dare to run, hope to rule. Biology wasn't just woman's destiny; it was her definition.

In every age exceptional women defied such dictates, but it wasn't until the 1970s that the women's movement began to sweep aside barriers for women of all ages, races, and classes. In the course of these changes, a new notion took hold, at least in some quarters: that liberated women could somehow transcend biological realities—menstruate without cramps, give birth without pain or painkilling medication, sail through menopause without breaking a sweat. As many women soon discovered for themselves, this isn't so. Once again we found ourselves caught between stereotypes and reality.

When women looked to science for data on female physiology and biology, they found few answers. Ours truly has been the invisible sex, ignored in almost every area of research and scholarship. While everyone has always had notions of what it's just like a woman to be or do, hardly anyone ever set out to study, objectively and scientifically, what being female truly means. As a result, virtually every assumption about women—from the absurd to the seemingly astute—has turned out to be unproven, untested, or untrue.

In the last two decades, as women themselves began to matter more, economically and politically, long-unanswered questions have taken on new significance: What does it mean to live in a woman's body, to think with a woman's brain, drink in the world with a woman's senses, act and react with a woman's sensibility? How do milestones such as menarche, pregnancy, childbirth, and menopause shape women's lives? How do our bodies affect our minds—and vice versa? What makes us strong? What leaves us vulnerable? What gives meaning to our lives?

Finally, gender-specific research in various disciplines—from biology and anthropology to physiology and psychiatry—is providing some answers and asking ever more intriguing questions. By including women in their research samples, by establishing female norms rather than applying male standards, by exploring the full meaning of female reproductive stages, researchers have added a new lens to the microscope. Slowly the "second sex," so long defined only as the "other," has emerged as a separate sex, equal to the male but not the same.

As a medical writer covering this work, I have watched the pieces of the puzzle come together and a new image of woman as unique in body, mind, and spirit come into focus. As a woman, I behold this creature—so much more complex and compelling than the stereotyped females of the past—and I think: "Yes, *this* is who I am."

What Does It Mean to Be Female?

When the chaotic exhilaration of the first few hours after her son's birth was over, after her husband had slumped into sleep and her caregivers had retreated from the room, a friend of mine confesses that she propped up her newborn, removed the tiny knit cap from his head, and gave in to the irresistible impulse to lick his still-sticky scalp. "It was primal," she says. "You'd have thought I was a big-mama baboon."

The notion is not as far-fetched as it might seem. A DNA difference of only 1.6 percent separates humans from our closest primate cousins, the chimpanzees. Like them, we have a large brain, V-shaped jaw, opposable thumb, big toe, and the same reproductive hormones. And we both are mammals, members of the deeply maternal animal class that takes its name from the mammae, or breast glands, that nourish our young.

In the dazzlingly diverse animal kingdom, females of various species defy every stereotype about their sex. Some are solitary; many are social. Some are good mothers; others are indifferent. Some achieve high status and wield great power; others seek protection from bigger, stronger males.

Only one generality holds true: In no species on earth does the stereotyped "female"—docile, dumb, and totally dependent—exist. If she ever did, evolution, in its ruthless pruning, long ago eliminated her. The females who soar above, swim below, or roam about today's planet are survivors—robust and resilient, strong and capable. If they'd been anything less, they wouldn't still be here. Neither would we.

Yet even though we share many of the biological traits of the females of other species, the one creature on earth that a woman resembles most is a man. We are, above all else, human. Women and men walk upright as only humans do. We speak languages as only humans can. We reason and remember with the most complex organ on the planet—a human brain. We love in all the astoundingly varied ways that only humans do. We laugh at jokes as no other being does. Women and men, alone among the earth's billions of residents, write poetry, sing arias, file legal briefs, celebrate birthdays, shoot hoops, teach school, worship God, rent videos, surf the Internet, and charge by mail, phone, or fax.

In every species, however, the female is different from the male. We are no exception. This biological reality is not a curse or a blessing. "Neither women nor men can be considered superior or inferior to the other," says evolutionary psychologist David Buss, of the University of Texas, "any more than a bird's wings can be considered superior or inferior to a fish's fins or a kangaroo's legs."

A woman is as glorious a piece of work as the idealized man Shakespeare extolled in *Hamlet*—beauty of the world, paragon of animals, noble in reason, infinite in faculty, in action like an angel, in apprehension like a god. But our beauty, nobility, actions, and apprehension are, in ways both subtle and significant, uniquely female. And as the new field of gender biology has documented, so are our anatomy and physiology.

What Does It Mean to Have a
Woman's Body?

Women are, on average, 10 to 15 percent smaller than men. The bones of the female skeleton are shorter and thinner, our shoulders narrower, our rib cages shorter, our joints looser. We hold our arms closer to our bodies; our necks are longer and slimmer. We are more likely to be right-handed and less likely to be color-blind.

Our hearts beat faster, even during sleep. Our core body temperature runs higher. Women's blood carries higher levels of protective immunoglobulin and lower amounts of oxygen-rich hemoglobin. We are twice as sensitive to sound, but only half as sensitive to light as men are. Our vocal cords are shorter, our larynx 30 percent smaller. Even the mix of chemicals in female saliva is different—and changes throughout the menstrual cycle.

What difference do such differences make? By most measures of performance, very little. The abilities of the sexes, physical and mental, often overlap, and the variability within each sex can be greater than that between them. And human biology and behavior are anything but immutable. Stimulate the brain, and neurons branch out to form new connections. Arouse the senses, and hormonal levels change. Exercise the muscles, and the body becomes stronger and sleeker.

Nonetheless, for centuries, biological differences, alleged or actual, were used to justify discrimination. In the late nineteenth century, for instance, delicate women of the upper classes displayed a troubling propensity for dizzy spells and fainting. Physicians, concluding that small, ladylike lungs were intrinsically incapable of breathing deeply, cautioned against the rigors of higher education or physical exercise. Eventually one of America's first women doctors tracked down the true culprit: tight-laced whalebone corsets that squeezed a woman's waist to an unnaturally tiny eighteen inches—and cut off her oxygen supply.

Other stereotypes about women's bodies have proven equally constricting—including the more modern presumption that we are simply shorter, smaller, rounder versions of men, an assumption that can be hazardous to women's health. Certain medications (including diet pills and psychiatric drugs) tested only in men have triggered serious side effects in women, for whom they are prescribed far more often. Diagnostic tests (such as the exercise stress or treadmill test) that based "normal" readings solely on men have failed to detect early signs of heart disease in women. Certain treatments such as carotid endarterectomy, an operation to clear blockages in the blood vessels to the brain, have proved safer or more beneficial in men.

"Many physicians still aren't convinced that women and men are not biologically interchangeable and that what works in men may not work in women," says internist Marianne Legato, director of the Partnership for Women's Health at Columbia University and a pioneer in gender-specific research. Recently she asked a group of top-flight dermatologists where they got the cells they used for research on women's cosmetics. From the foreskins of newly circumcised male babies, they informed her. These researchers, who prided themselves on the rigor of their scientific investigations, simply assumed that the cells of a woman's face would react the same way to cosmetics as those from a newborn boy's penis.

Such assumptions reflect an enormous blind spot in medical science— a long-standing inability to see the sex differences that exist in virtually every organ and system of the body. Yet it is only by learning how the bodies of women as well as men function, in health and in sickness, that medicine can fully expand its understanding of all human beings.

What Are the Rhythms of a Woman's Life?

One biological reality has always shaped the lives of women: We change. Just like a man's, our temperature and blood pressure rise and fall throughout the day; our heart rate speeds up and slows down; our hormones surge and ebb. But for us, that's just for starters.

"Change is the inherent pattern in women—minute to minute, day to day, week to week, month to month," says Vivien Burt, a physiologist and psychiatrist who heads the Women's Life Center at the Neuropsychiatric Institute of the University of California, Los Angeles School of Medicine. We are by our very nature cyclic, more responsive than men to the shifts from day to night and season to season. This variability, increasingly viewed as a hallmark of health, may at least partly account for our longevity. Some now view men's much-vaunted stability as a worrisome lack of flexibility, a tendency to get stuck in physiological ruts so potentially ominous that a recent seminar for specialists in biological rhythms focused on "the toxic aperiodicity of males."

Of course, the dominant rhythm of a woman's life, the menstrual cycle, has no counterpart in the male. While men, with lives as linear as vectors, think of cycles in terms of physics, women live them. From the first gush of blood at puberty to the last premenopausal trickle, the menstrual cycle—nature's own metronome—keeps us going around in circles.

Menstruation is indeed the thing women do—all of us, regardless of creed, culture, race, or ethnicity, virgin and mother, lesbian and straight. Every month for almost forty years, our periods remind us that we are, quite literally, flesh and blood. They also epitomize another basic truth about women: We are always operating at more than one level. As a woman litigates, lectures, or lies in a lover's arms, something else is going on inside. The female body, like an endlessly busy housekeeper, is always making ready or tidying up, preparing the new or discarding the old, cleansing and renewing.

Yet no biological process has stigmatized women more than the menstrual cycle. Menstrual taboos long branded women as unwell, unworthy, unequal, unclean. Well into the twentieth century educators were contending that young women could not possibly menstruate and matriculate at the same time. Not long ago a mean-spirited menstrual joke spread through cyberspace: "If anything else bled for a week every month, we'd shoot it."

These days the "blood mysteries"—menarche, menstruation, pregnancy, menopause—that once transformed (and limited) women's lives have been transformed themselves. Modern medical science has developed ways to regulate menstrual cycles, relieve troubling symptoms, control or enhance fertility, "manage" menopause. This is new—to us as a species and as a sex—and the ramifications of such tinkering with the fundamentals of female physiology are not yet clear.

Most women, today as always, still sense the subterranean changes that are part of our female nature. Try as we may, we cannot completely ignore the blood on the tampon, the inexplicable hunger for a baby, the unsettling aftershocks of birth, the temperature spikes of menopause. We're aware, at a certain level, of "something" neither purely biological nor wholly psychological, something that affects not just how we function but how we feel, that influences us inside and out. Our female reproductive rhythms no longer constrict the steps we can take and the moves we can make, but they remain the chemical choreography of our lives.

How Are Our Bodies and Minds Connected?

When anatomists began dissecting human cadavers at Bologna in the late thirteenth century, they searched for the most ephemeral of human traits—the soul—by probing the mighty, muscular heart and the spongy, convoluted brain. Nowhere did they find any traces of the life force behind the plans, hopes, dreams, and desires that make us human. Everything—function and feeling, thoughts and emotions, passions and pleasures—connects, in women arguably even more so than in men.

Women register the impact of trauma, abuse, or loss not just intellectually or viscerally, but throughout the complex network of hormones that link our bodies to our brains. So sensitive is female physiology to psychological distress that, as recent studies have shown, girls troubled by anxiety may fail to grow to their expected height and women suffering from depression are much more likely to develop osteoporosis—almost as if worry or sadness permeates to the bone.

A woman's brain itself seems a model of connectedness. As discussed in Chapter 11, women typically use more cells in more parts of their brain than men. Even as we read, rhyme, or balance our checkbooks, it seems, we never shut down the parts of the brain that sense and feel. Could such fundamental differences in the workings of a woman's brain explain our gender's renowned empathy, compassion, and intuition? We don't yet know. As always, the generalities that derive from research on a specific group or population may not apply to any or every individual woman. And whatever predisposition nature instills, nurture—by environment and experience—modifies.

"It's not that men don't have the same feelings as women, but that they have never been allowed to show them," comments therapist Virginia Sadock of New York City. "It's only very recently that they've started to realize what they've missed out on—and they've missed out on a lot. There's a richness in the emotional life of women that I don't see in most men." I ask her if perhaps this is why men so often say—usually with that age-old air of superiority—that it's just like a woman to be emotional. "Oh, no," she tells me with a knowing smile. "They say that because they're jealous."

Especially as they age, men also might understandably come to envy another complex aspect of a woman's being: our sensuality. From the tips of our nipples to the depths of our wombs, we are primed for pleasure. Our sexual availability knows no seasons. Our sexual response requires no complex (and far from foolproof) hydraulics. And in terms of sexual satisfaction, once doesn't have to be enough; women alone are capable of orgasmic encores.

Yet female sexuality always has been suspect. Some contend it's just like a woman to tempt, tease, titillate, seduce, or sleep her way into places of privilege or power. On the other hand, it's also seemed just like a woman to be cold, frigid, rejecting, sexually unsatisfied—and unsatisfying. With so many stigmas and stereotypes, it's not surprising that, for all our deep desire and undisputed desirability, many women have yet to come to terms with their sexual selves. Even the much-hyped sexual revolution, which made it possible for a woman to have sex just like a man (that is, without commitment or, thanks to effective contraception, concern for reproductive consequences), has not changed a fundamental reality: We prefer to make love, as Bob Dylan sang, just like a woman.

What Puts Us at Risk?

"Tell me about the women you see," I've said to dozens of therapists over the years. "Why do they come to you? What do they say? Are their stories different from men's?" The counselors hesitate. They know there are no easy answers, no generalities that can encompass the complexity and diversity of the individuals they come to know so intimately.

"Free-associate," I prod. "What words come to mind when you think of your women patients?" A litany of adjectives, many contradictory, pours out: *worried, tired, overwhelmed, strong, scared, smart, stressed, angry, savvy, confused*—all of which, they quickly point out, might just as well apply to men who make their way into therapy. But there is one word that attaches far more often to women: *vulnerable*.

Through much of time, physical vulnerability was a fact of female life. Our prehistoric foremothers were physically stronger than contemporary women—by some estimates, as powerful as today's men. Even so, they were vulnerable—not just to fearsome beasts, harsh climates, physical dangers of every sort, and lethal illnesses, but to their own reproductive biology. Through most of time, giving birth meant facing the very real possibility of death.

These days we think of a woman's vulnerability quite differently—as a consequence not of biology but of psychology. Although many still assume it's just like a woman to bear life's psychological burdens, no one—female or male—negotiates life's twists and turns without some psychological bruises. However, each sex is more prone to different mental disorders, develops different symptoms at different times in life, and responds to different treatments. One problem above all others has become emblematic of female psychological susceptibility: depression.

Whether the word is used for a fleeting feeling, a lingering mood, or a serious illness, depression most often wears a female face. With few exceptions, cross-cultural studies indicate that, even in different countries, ethnic groups, and social classes, women are two to three times more likely than men to become depressed. This sex discrepancy, for unknown reasons, is greatest in Germany, where depression strikes 3.5 times more women than men, and lowest in egalitarian environments (such as college campuses) and in developing countries, where men are as prone to depression as women.

Why, in most settings, do women seem the sadder sex? There are so many theories (neurochemical, hormonal, psychological, socioeconomic, and more), so many premises (tested and not), and so many possibilities that it's unlikely that any one of them could possibly provide a complete explanation. For most women, clinical depression (one serious enough to warrant treatment) stems from a complex mix—a witch's brew, as one psychiatrist puts it—of factors that range from the neurotransmitter levels in our brains to the tidal changes of our hormones to the nuances of our closest relationships to the inequities of our economic lives.

Female reproductive biology may set the stage for vulnerability: A woman's risk of depression soars at puberty and subsides after menopause. A family history of depression or inadequate levels of mood-regulating neurotransmitters, such as serotonin, may put some women at higher risk. Others may be especially sensitive to the hormonal fluctuations that accompany menstruation, childbirth, and midlife. But psychosocial factors—loss, abuse, trauma, illness, and violence—are equally important. Poverty and a lack of options in life increase a woman's likelihood of depression; education and available contraception diminish it.

Why Learn About Women?

Even before Alexander Pope declared man "the proper study of mankind," men had made their gender the center of scholarly attention. The names of great men roar down the corridors of time. Only a few women—mostly queens and concubines—have won more than a whisper of recognition. Conventional history, as Jane Austen complains in *Northanger Abbey*, tells mainly of "the quarrels of popes and kings, with wars or pestilences in every page; the men . . . all so good for nothing, and hardly any women at all."

But women, as a new generation of female historians has shown, were always part of history—in often surprising roles. There were warriors like the British queen Boadicea, who battled the Roman invaders; great philosophers like Hildegard of Bingen, whose rediscovered musical chants are now New Age hits; renowned medieval healers like Trotula, who wrote medical texts used for centuries. Theirs are stories that history—by colossal oversight or deliberate omission—forgot to tell.

Anthropology, the study of humans, focused single-mindedly on man—the hunter, the explorer, the creator of culture. "It's not that prehistoric women weren't as active or interesting or important as males," says anthropologist Martha Ward, of the University of New Orleans. "It's just that male anthropologists never saw them." Rather than dismissing our earliest foremothers as mere backdrop, the women who have flooded into this field have recast their role as gatherers who provided the major part of a family's food supply, as nimble-fingered tool-users who fashioned the first baskets and farming implements, and as nurturing mothers whose lullabies may have predated human language.

Women also have long made significant but unheralded contributions in science, math, and technology. In the fifth century, Hypatia, a teacher and mathematician in Alexandria, wrote treatises on geometry and algebra and invented scientific instruments. An empress of China, Shi Dun, developed the first paper from the bark of mulberry trees. In 1738, at the age of twenty, Maria Gaetana Agnesi of Milan wrote a textbook of calculus and mathematical analysis considered so brilliant that the University of Bologna sent her a diploma and named her to its faculty. In eighteenth-century Bath, Caroline Herschel, who learned astronomy from her brother while serving as his housekeeper, discovered eight new comets and earned a pension from King George III—the first woman to win such support for scientific work.

The twentieth-century counterparts of these largely unknown women remain almost as obscure. Few people know—or could be expected to know—who invented such modern innovations as bulletproof vests, Macintosh computer icons, the laser optics used in CD players, or the ceramic tiles that allow the space shuttle to survive reentry into the earth's atmosphere. Yet most would be surprised to discover that these inventors are all female.

In fact, much that we're learning about women comes as a surprise—in part because we've known so little about them and in part because very real differences based in biological sex (that is, femaleness and maleness) have gotten mixed up with dubious distinctions about gender (the meaning culture attaches to sex). The absolutely fundamental sex differences between females and males are few: women menstruate, gestate, and lactate; men manufacture sperm. Differences in gender, on the other hand, vary with place and time.

Why study difference at all? The intellectual and writer Lou Andreas-Salome gave her answer a century ago: "Although the time is no doubt slowly disappearing when women believed it necessary to imitate men in any area in which they wished to prove their worth," she wrote in 1899, "we are still a long way from respecting all that is unique in women."

Her words still ring true—including her caution that if women did not "attempt to understand themselves as passionately and as profoundly as possible in those ways in which they *differ* from men—*and at first exclusively in those ways*—to that end using, scrupulously, the slightest evidence of their bodies as well as their souls, they will never know how broadly and powerfully they may blossom . . . and indeed how vast the boundaries of their world are." (The italics are hers.)

Today researchers are, passionately and profoundly, continuing to explore these boundaries. "When women ask me, 'What are you trying to do?' I say, 'I'm trying to understand who we are, and understanding is freedom,'" says neuroanatomist Marian Diamond, of the University of California, Berkeley, one of the first scientists to demonstrate sex differences in the brain. Decades after this discovery, she recalls her own exhilaration: "It was like the first time I was in Africa and saw a giraffe that wasn't in a cage. I didn't realize how different it looked. And I didn't realize how caged I'd felt by always thinking of myself as an abnormal or inferior male. I wasn't like a male at all: I was unique." And like the giraffes in Africa, she felt free.

Ultimately, the goal is not to prove either sex better or worse, stronger or weaker, smarter or dumber, but to work toward the whole, greater than its parts, that emerges when female and male join together—physically, emotionally, intellectually, spiritually, sexually. Just as yin shapes yang and day defines night, women and men are designed to complete and complement each other. The synergy that we can create together may yet lead to the greatest revelation of all: what it means to be fully human, strong, sensitive, smart, spiritual, and sensual in ways both feminine and masculine, yet not limited to either females or males.

What Does It Mean to Be Just Like a Woman?

This is a question I've asked endlessly over the course of the last few years. Men, grown wary in these politically precarious times, often dodge it. Women themselves almost always start out by saying what they think it means to men. "It's a guy's way of saying you don't cut it; you're not in the club," says a corporate vice president. "When my boss is really pleased with something I did, he'll say, 'You handled that just like a man'—meaning just like he would, which is his highest compliment."

But among women, this now is changing. Some I've interviewed—most often the distinguished women at the top of their fields who had to fight hardest and longest for opportunity—take pride in thinking, working, and succeeding just like a man. But others believe that being just like a woman is high praise indeed.

"To me, it means being like a willow tree, bending but never breaking," one woman explains. To another, it means heeling like a sailboat with every gust but always managing to steer back into the wind. A self-defined "spiritual feminist" believes that it's just like a woman to have special powers of creativity and magic, to conceive and nurture and, above all else, transform things: "blood into milk, clay into vessel, feeling into movement, wind into song, egg into child, fiber into cloth, stone into crystal, memory into image, body into worship."

A woman from Hong Kong describes herself—and other Asian women—as bullets wrapped in marshmallow, deceptively soft and sweet on the outside yet steel-tough on the inside. An Italian journalist compares being a woman to being a goalkeeper in a soccer match—eyes scanning everywhere, body poised to move in any direction, ready for any possibility. An American thinks being like a woman is not unlike driving her pickup truck: "It rides hard, so you feel every bump in the road. But for the long haul, there's nothing like it. It's tough; it doesn't break down. It can handle any kind of weather. It doesn't spin out on curves. Guys are like sports cars: On a smooth stretch of road, they whiz right by you. But if they hit one pothole, they fall apart."

In the quest to understand fully what being female means, analogies remain no substitute for actual knowledge, anchored in data and confirmed by experience. This is what gender-specific research offers. Because of its breakthrough discoveries, the ideal woman is no longer defined—as she so long was—as a man, and difference no longer is equated with deficiency. The female body, once viewed as an imperfect copy of the male model, is now seen as unique in both its strengths and susceptibilities, with its own norms for sickness and health. Female intelligence and intuition, so often derided if not denied, have gained new respect. The feminine code of caring and commitment no longer smacks of dependency but of depth.

What, then, *is* a woman? A biological creature, to be sure, but one shaped by education, opportunity, and experience. More than seven decades ago a group of young women posed the same question to Virginia Woolf. "I do not know," she responded. "I do not believe that anybody can know until she has expressed herself in all of the arts and professions open to human skills."

This is exactly what women everywhere are doing. But before we can determine for ourselves, on our own terms, what it can, could, should, might, and will mean to *be* a woman, we must learn about the bodies we occupy, the rhythms we live by, the minds we use, the emotions we experience, the relationships we cherish. This book is a beginning.

The Female of the Species

On a cloudless summer day, four women enjoy an afternoon at the seashore. The first unfurls her towel and lies facedown to soak up the sunshine. Under the shade of an oversized umbrella, the second settles into a beach chair to nurse her baby. The third unpacks sandwiches from a picnic hamper as she keeps a watchful eye on her five-year-old daughter scampering in the waves. The fourth strolls along the water's edge and then settles down to read a book, occasionally jotting a note in the margin.

At first glance these seem like perfectly ordinary women—and so they are. But look closer: The sunbather is displaying the body and limb design of a vertebrate. The nursing mother, just like the mammal she is, nourishes her newborn with breast milk. Just like a primate, the other mother provides food and protection for a child who, though mature enough to walk and talk, cannot survive on her own. It is only the fourth—reading, thinking, writing—who engages in a tour de force of uniquely human talents.

These women, like most of us, rarely think of a hidden biological dimension of our lives: our link to other species. We often assume—wrongly—that the femaleness we share with other animals has become irrelevant. What, after all, can bugs, bears, birds, or baboons teach us—finless, furless, wingless, thoroughly modern women of the twenty-first century—about what it means to be female? The answer: more than we might care to admit.

Many achievements we think of as "human," such as aerial flight and undersea navigation, other species have done first, if not better. Some have mastered skills once thought to be uniquely ours, such as tool use and cooperative hunting. And females of other species have confronted many of the hassles today's women face, including sexual harassment and unwanted pregnancy. It's not surprising. They've been around a lot longer.

Hundreds of millions of years before our earliest ancestors lifted themselves upright, other females were crawling over lava rocks, plunging into icy seas, or slithering through tropical jungles. Unknown numbers of species died out before a human's arched sole ever touched the earth, but those that endured became masters of the art of survival. Only the fittest of both sexes, those best able to adapt and reproduce, passed time's innumerable tests.

In the course of their evolutionary marathon, females became so diverse that they challenge every stereotype about their sex. Among the biggest creatures on the planet, blue whales, the female is often larger than the male. The weaker sex? In many forms of animal life—from mice to marsupials to our own species—the female outlives the male. The gentler sex? The praying mantis casually emulsifies her lover in the process of copulation. Natural-born mothers? In less than 10 percent of all species do mothers devote themselves to the care and feeding of their young; female insects, fish, and frogs often release their eggs and flit, glide, or slide on their way. The submissive sex? Females of certain species, such as rhesus monkeys, are dominant; among monogamous primates like gibbons, females and males share power and status.

Stereotypes about what it means to be a female—or just like a female—have long gotten in the way of our understanding of half the planet's inhabitants. Aristotle, impressed by the industriousness of the queen bee, assumed it had to be a male king—a misconception that persisted for centuries. Biologists observing nurturing behavior, such as the back-brooding of the giant water bug, routinely took males for females.

The grande dame of feminism, Simone de Beauvoir, writing half a century ago, considered the very word *female* derogatory, an insult rather than an identity. To her, being female meant becoming "victim of the species"—to swell with eggs or bray in heat, to submit to a dominating male or to be enslaved by perpetual pregnancy. But as we've learned since, nature's design for both sexes is far more complex.

While virtually all healthy female animals (and males) strive to perpetuate their species, reproduction is not the only story of any of their lives. Even females of the most primitive species are participants, not spectators, in the daily enterprise of living. They gather food for themselves and their young; they hunt, fish, forage, farm, explore, build homes, protect themselves from predators, and, not uncommonly, kill.

Some females pursue serial careers. A worker honeybee, for instance, serves as cell cleaner, queen's attendant, nursery aide, construction worker, guard, long-distance pilot, and food transporter. Others display a different sort of versatility. The female blue sea bass, along with a number of other fish species, can morph into a male (changing from her usual indigo blue into a "nuptial dress" of fiery orange streaked with white) and release a stream of milt to fertilize another female's clutch of eggs. If no partner is available, she can lay eggs, switch her sex, and fertilize them.

No less than males, females can be capable and cunning. A mare gallops as swiftly as a stallion; a hunting bitch sniffs down her prey with a nose as keen as her brother's; a lioness fights off an attacker as ferociously as her mate. Yet even when their lives are similar, nature fosters different strategies for each sex to use to fulfill its evolutionary mandate of pushing new life into the future. These differences—lumped together into what scientists call "sexual dimorphism"—open up new possibilities for each species, including our own.

As noted in Chapter 1, there is more animal in humans than many of us realize—a genetic similarity greater than 98 percent between us and the chimpanzees. Women, like many other females, are egg makers. We mate and mother. We compete and cooperate. We attract and attach. But we do so in ways that set our species apart.

Our ancestors diverged from apes about five to eight million years ago—relatively recently in what geologists call "deep time." Taking an entirely new path, they developed a unique characteristic: a brain so sophisticated that it allows us *not* to be animals. Our species repertoire—the behavioral options available to us as humans—is broader. We can recall the past and prepare for the future. We can think, assess, and evaluate our actions. Above all, we can choose and decide in ways unimaginable for the females or males of any other species—which does not make their behavior any less relevant or revealing.

We Are the Egg Makers

Unimaginably long ago, in deepest time, there were no females or males, no eggs or sperm, and no such things as sexual differentiation and reproduction. Simple organisms reproduced by budding (as some plants do) or by splitting into perfect duplicates or clones. Then something happened: Two different cells collided, and, in what some describe as the biological equivalent of original sin, one engulfed the other. For the first time the genes of two organisms merged to form an entirely new hybrid. This random joining occurred again, and again, and again. The new creatures, different from their parent cells, survived—perhaps because combined genes proved hardier or better able to resist parasites or infections. As organisms continued to meld and join their genetic material, the pairing of a larger cell, stuffed with nutrients, with a smaller, faster-moving cell proved most durable. These intrinsically different gametes, or sex cells, came to be known as the egg and the sperm.

Biology, then, provides the answer to the age-old riddle of whether the chicken or the egg comes first: It is always the incredible, evolving egg, with its unique ability to engulf another cell and nourish its genes. Eggs themselves can be as small as a speck or as large as a softball. Some are liquidy, others leathery; some soft and permeable, others encased in protective shells of blue, brown, or speckled white.

As some biologists argue, eggs of every size and hue "cost" more than sperm in terms of the energy and time required to create, protect, and maintain them. Invariably larger, a typical egg dwarfs a tiny sperm. In humans, for instance, the female egg is 250,000 times bigger than a male sperm. This size difference, argues evolutionary biologist Richard

Dawkins, author of *The Selfish Gene*, has given rise to an array of other differences in the relationships of females and males.

In every species, eggs are rarer than sperm, which makes them more valuable. A man produces about as many sperm every half second as the number of eggs a woman ovulates in her entire life. Once the female egg ripens, after decades of dormancy, it remains viable for only about twelve hours, while male sperm may live for several days. Hence, females are the "limiting" sex in terms of the number of eggs and offspring that they can produce. A woman could potentially give birth to a maximum of about twenty babies in her lifetime; a man, at least in theory, can father an unlimited number of children.

Not even scientists can resist anthropomorphizing our big-mama eggs and fast-moving sperm. According to one view, the passive egg, just like a female, sits back and waits for suitors. Sperm, mobile and adventurous, act just like guys, and not very nice ones at that. Sprinting out of the penis, they speed up the vagina. If lucky enough to encounter a ripe egg, the swiftest swimmer invades its boundaries and commandeers its food supply and reproductive machinery. Like a manipulative parasite—or just a selfish cad—the sperm manages to perpetuate its genes with hardly any investment of its own. Thus, says Dawkins, "female exploitation begins." The princess egg becomes hostage of a conniving sperm.

Perhaps. Not all biologists share the same perspective. Some argue that the egg, rather than being a hapless victim, might be the true aggressor. From this view, the female egg seems a mammoth cannibal that castrates and swallows the tiny sperm, harvests his genes, and, having taken him for everything he's worth, proceeds to manufacture a life totally under her control.

Is one or the other of these views true? Recent research suggests that the whole process of fertilization may be more complex than either theory suggests. Sperm themselves may not be as cheap as was traditionally assumed. At least in some species of flies and worms, sperm manufacture consumes so much energy that it shortens the male life span. And not all the 200 to 250 million sperm in a man's ejaculate are created equal. Some are sleek "egg getters," while stockier blockers and multi-headed "monsters" clear their way. But the fastest swimmer in this mob doesn't necessarily win the race. While some sperm rush toward the egg follicle soon after ejaculation, others lie in the uterine lining and patiently wait for ovulation, when the egg becomes ripe for fertilization and makes its way down the fallopian tube. Ultimately one of these sly strategists may be the one most likely to achieve its goal.

The human egg is also not what it was long assumed to be. Rather than a sleeping beauty regally awaiting a sperm's princely kiss to bring it to life, the egg may actually set the entire process of fertilization in motion. By producing pheromones, chemical signals that stimulate scent receptors on sperm (identical to the ones in our noses that detect aromas), the female egg draws sperm to it. Its pull, literally "egging on" the process, may be just as vital to fertilization as the sperm's push.

After sweeping a sperm within its embrace, the egg really sets to work—particularly through the genetic material, or DNA, stored in the microscopic organelles known as mitochondria, which provide energy for all cellular reactions. This "mtDNA" is distinct from the DNA carried by the chromosomes within the egg nucleus. Like the egg and all other cells, sperm also contain mtDNA, but their mitochondria, which power their remarkable journey, are cast off when the egg incorporates the sperm's nucleus. (The transmission of the egg's mitochondrial DNA from mothers to daughters is discussed in Chapter 3.)

In the cellular equivalent of a tune-up, the egg's mtDNA checks for damaged or defective genes in the sperm and produces enzymes to repair some chemically induced mutations—a rehabilitation project not unlike that of the stereotypical bride who finds a good man and immediately devotes her energies to making him better. As a species, we may owe our survival to the egg's unique ability to mend broken genes and to initiate and direct the development of an embryo.

The saga of egg and sperm, the most ancient of specialized cells, has recently taken a new turn. As new treatments for infertility have burgeoned (discussed in Chapter 9), gametes have become commodities, stockpiled and sold at rates set by market demand. Since the advent of artificial insemination, sperm donors have "fathered" tens of thousands of babies. Thanks to technological innovations, eggs "harvested" from female donors have become an increasingly popular option for infertile women. In laboratories around the world, eggs and sperm now form new lives totally independent of their own creators.

We are just beginning to think through the implications of such tinkering with the very cells that create a human being. But this much is clear: The timeless pas de deux of egg and sperm, whatever the new variations, remains central to the ballet of life.

How the Sexes Compete

More than a century ago Charles Darwin destroyed forever the romantic notion of nature as a peaceable kingdom. His radical theory of evolution revealed life as a brutish business in which competition separates weak from strong, fit from frail, "alpha" leaders from also-rans. But as a nineteenth-century English gentleman, Darwin, despite his formidable powers of observation, showed the same blind spot as other scientists of his gender and generation: He missed half of the story—the female half. Convinced that only males compete, he declared that man—like other males—had become "more courageous, pugnacious, and energetic than woman." By failing to compete, he concluded, females of all species had evolved into inferiority.

At first glance, elephant seals, mammoth aquatic mammals whose breeding grounds include northern California, seem to prove Darwin's point. The males—two- to four-ton giants—compete almost from birth. Even as pups, they grab, bite, and slam against each other's necks. By maturity, they have grown natural armor: a thick hide, powerful flippers, formidable tusks. Once a year, when they gather by the thousands in their rookeries, or breeding sites, along the rocky Pacific coast, they immediately begin jousting—literally head to head.

For up to ninety days, the males charge at each other, mauling and mewing. The bellowing winners of their jousts form dominance hierarchies that allow only a few males—just 20 percent of the entire group—to mate with the females that have also propelled themselves onto the rocks. The losers, scarred and battered, become evolutionary duds; the ferocious victors, tirelessly warding off challengers and rounding up stray females, may inseminate several hundred females in the course of a lifetime.

Female elephant seals are much smaller—at most a third the size of the mighty males. Much of the year they spend by themselves, swimming alone in the Pacific. In the winter they migrate to the rookeries to deliver and nurse the pups they conceived the previous year. After about a month, they wean their young, enter estrus (a time of sexual receptivity and peak fertility), copulate, conceive, and swim off to sea.

When marine biologist Joanne Reiter, of the University of California, Santa Cruz, focused on the females, she realized that they too were competing like mad—with each other. They do not fight for food (like the male, the female fasts while at the rookery) or for a mate (all invariably find partners). What they vie for is a prime location on the rocks—large and safe enough to enhance their odds of nursing a pup to ample size and located within screeching distance of the highest-ranking males.

The females who end up in the choicest spots aren't the youngest but, in terms of seal smarts, the savviest. Experienced females arrive earlier in the season and use their greater size and aggressiveness to shove, bite, push, or intimidate younger females. Settling into a good central position in the harem, they are able to nurse longer. As a result, their pups grow to twice the size of those of younger females. When they do wean their pups and are ready to mate, the well-placed behemoths attract the highest-ranking males.

They do so by making the most of the male propensity for knockdown, all-out duels. When a male approaches, a female protests—vigorously and vociferously. Her cries summon larger males who challenge the suitor and force him to back off. The feuding for her favors continues until the fittest—or at least the fiercest—male finally succeeds in mating with her. The younger, less experienced females at the edges of a harem end up mating with low-ranking males because there are no dominant males nearby to push them away. Their smaller pups are only half as likely to survive.

When I describe these his-and-hers competitive styles—brute force versus more subtle jockeying for position—women and men in corporate jungles nod in recognition. "It sounds just like my office," says an executive friend of mine. "If a man wants something—your territory, your responsibilities, even your job—he'll come straight at you with all he's got. The women don't. They go around your back and sabotage you, and that's even harder to deal with."

Of course, not all females and males of other species—nor women and men in more benign work environments—are such tough or wily competitors. More than a few have found a better alternative: cooperation. While some primate females will try anything to keep a rival from mating with a desirable male, others, such as the olive baboons of East Africa, form enduring alliances that serve as the center of group life. These females forage together, groom each other, look after each other's children. When mothers and daughters are in the same group, they maintain an intimate bond for life. The females also form friendships with selected males. These "special friends," as anthropologists describe them, share food, sit or sleep nearby, and protect a female's children in her absence. And when the female enters estrus, she typically copulates first or most often with her special friend, offering him an evolutionary edge without need for brutal confrontation. It's a scenario even a Darwinian could come to love.

The Finickiness of the Female

My husband, an inveterate matchmaker, has given up on my friend Gail. She said that one of the men he'd fixed her up with was too needy; another was too nerdy. One blind date was too immature; another was old beyond his years. Finally my husband threw up his hands and said, "She's just too fussy!" Well, maybe. At any rate, she comes by it honestly. Finicky is indeed something it's just like a female to be—and for good reason.

In most species, females, with their coveted eggs and their greater "investment" in pregnancy, are the courted sex. According to Darwin, their selection of partners allows them to influence the course of evolution. "The power to charm the female," he wrote, "has sometimes been more important than the power to conquer other males in battle."

But such conquests aren't easy. To win a female's favor, some males prance; others pound their chests. Many transform themselves into gaudy self-promoting billboards, festooned with bright colors, hairy tufts, towering antlers, lush manes, curved horns, or cascading feathers. While the males of many species are making such serious fashion statements, females are deciding which most strikes their fancy. But, as anyone who's ever wondered what a particular woman could possibly see in a certain man (or vice versa), there sometimes seems to be no accounting for personal preference. Or is there?

A discerning female of many species, biologists have discovered, may well see more than meets the eye. Consider the female barn swallow, a sucker for a male with a long-feathered tail. So enamored is she with this comely feature that when researchers taped fake tail feathers onto some males and snipped the tails of others, the infatuated female couldn't resist choosing the faux-feathered male. But when the researchers trimmed only half a male's tail feathers, she turned up her beak at this lopsided look.

Length and symmetry, it turns out, are practically irresistible; short and ragged don't merit a second glance. These preferences may not be as superficial as they might seem. A male with long, symmetrical tail feathers has measurably fewer bloodsucking mites (which can stunt his plumage) on his body—and to a bird, resistance to parasites is a definite plus for a potential father of one's offspring.

Males of other species have their own ways of advertising their desirability: The peacock unfurls his rainbow feathers in a dazzling display of reproductive fitness. A rooster shows off his gleaming red comb and wattle—such precise indicators of the presence or absence of infection that professional breeders routinely check them before making their choices. Even the shade of a frog's slimy skin hints of his health status.

In other species, a song says it all. The strength of a bird's courtship ballad, ornithologists speculate, may speak volumes about the size of his territory as well as his own physical stamina. It also may affect the female in other ways. When a male house wren croons to a female, her heart beats faster—and it is thought that this may stimulate the release of hormones that prepare her ovaries for ovulation.

Other suitors woo a female with gifts. A common tern will offer a female a fish; a roadrunner presents a potential mate with a lizard; some chimpanzees proffer morsels of meat. Such courtship feeding—not too different from the classic dinner date—demonstrates to the female that her suitor is a skilled and generous provider. The Donald Trumps of the animal kingdom up the ante: They show off their real estate. In New Guinea, the male bowerbird will build his own equivalent of a Trump Tower—some up to nine feet tall—with sticks, ferns, and leaves, adding decorative flourishes of feathers, flowers, and found objects of every sort. A female, just by surveying his love nest, can assess his strength, stamina, dexterity, hunting and tracking skills, and possibly even his capacity for commitment. If she's impressed, she stays to mate. If not, she flits away.

Yet despite tasty offerings, intricate arias, thoughtful gifts, and posh accommodations, many females will reject what seems to be a perfectly acceptable candidate. This, too, may not be as capricious as it seems. Pheromones, the olfactory chemical signals secreted by both sexes, may be relaying vitally important information about a suitor's true suitability. For instance, a female mouse, given her choice between two seemingly identical and equally fetching partners, will sniff their urine and choose to mate with the male whose major histocompatibility complex (MHC) genes—which produce proteins on the cell surface that help the immune system detect and attack invaders—are least like her own. In this way, she ensures that their offspring benefit from the greatest possible protection from a wide variety of disease organisms.

Women's noses, too, may know things that our rational minds can't grasp. As described in Chapter 7, one woman's pheromones may shorten or lengthen others' menstrual cycles. Pheromones also may influence selection of a potential mate. In intriguing experiments at Switzerland's Bern University, zoologist Claus Wedekind asked forty-nine women at the midpoint of their menstrual cycle (near ovulation), when a woman's sense of smell is keenest, to sniff T-shirts that had been worn to bed for two nights by forty-four men. The shirts were deposited in plastic-lined boxes with holes in the top, and each woman got to sniff seven samples: one brand-new control shirt, three from men with MHC genes similar to their own, and three from men with dissimilar genes.

No one scent appealed to all the women. Some women hated certain odors; some loved others. But the women consistently—though unconsciously—chose shirts worn by men whose MHC genes were most unlike their own. Their scents reminded women of current or ex-lovers; the less-attractive smells of men whose MHC profiles were similar to their own often made them think of a brother or father. In a follow-up study, Wedekind found that no particular combination of MHC genes emerged as more desirable than any other. Difference itself seemed the secret of appeal.

There's plenty of reason, however, to be wary of putting scents before common sense. A rat of the two-legged variety with a favorable immune profile is still a rat. And human noses can be led astray. Birth control pills, for instance, may reverse a woman's natural preferences so she feels attracted to men she might otherwise turn up her nose at—and rejects the most suitable suitors of all. According to the Swiss researchers, women on the pill preferred the smells most like their own. This scrambling of sensory messages may explain why some women complain about a husband's odor—which they'd never even noticed before—after they go off the pill.

Crossed scent signals may also have more serious ramifications. Some couples who suffer repeated miscarriages share more of the same MHC genes than those who successfully conceive and carry a pregnancy to term. At least in theory, a woman's body may have evolved mechanisms to end a pregnancy rather than risk giving birth to a child who, because of a weak immune system, might not have survived to adulthood in the harsh environments of the prehistoric past.

Preliminary evidence suggests that we also may have evolved a mechanism to prevent the choice of an immunologically undesirable mate. In a University of Chicago study, researchers studied the MHC genes in 411 married couples in thirty-one colonies of Hutterites, members of a close-knit religious community who marry among their own. Somehow the most genetically similar individuals, though completely unaware of their MHC profiles, had tended to avoid marrying each other.

In another experiment, biologists at the University of New Mexico added another variable: They measured the male volunteers who provided T-shirts for ear length and width, elbow and wrist width, foot breadth, and lengths of fingers and thumbs and factored in the women's menstrual cycle phases. According to their analysis, the female volunteers preferred the smell of T-shirts worn by the most symmetrical men—but only at the ovulatory stage of their cycles, when they were most likely to become pregnant.

Such research into the biology of mate choice remains new and controversial. Some critics have questioned the methods and possible biases of the scientists. Others have challenged the very notion that scent signals could affect a decision as complex and profound as our choice of a mate. Nonetheless, the questions raised are intriguing—and may yet yield new insights into the age-old question of why opposites attract.

What's Love Got to Do with It?

She is the lover from hell. Elegant in black and red, she exudes an enticing fragrance that suitors cannot resist. The competition among male admirers for her favors is fierce. After killing off all other competitors, one victor approaches. But his is truly a fatal attraction. As soon as he swings into position and penetrates the object of his desire, she releases toxic chemicals that begin to emulsify his body. Yet even as his skeleton dissolves, he clings to her, somersaulting into a position that makes it easier for her to consume his body.

Among species such as the redback spiders of Australia, sex certainly is to die for. Yet from an evolutionary standpoint, the kamikaze lover is a winner: Unlike most males of his species, he manages to find a partner and mate. And because he holds on till death, he fertilizes twice as many eggs as he would have if he'd let go.

Tales of the murderous female redback spider, with her knack for transforming suitors into soup, usually make men wince, but women are intrigued by this turning of the sexual tables. Too often we think of the females of any species as the sexual victims of brutish males. But as reproductive ecologists explain, almost any sexual strategy that a male may try, a female can usually find a way to counter.

A female bird tending to eggs, for instance, will shove a strange male suitor out of the nest. A lemur will attack a male who presumes to approach her sexually without an invitation. Some females have evolved a particularly ingenious way of discouraging unwanted advances. The spider monkey, for instance, disguises her female genitals under what looks like a male phallus. The female hyena has gone even further: She is born with an enlarged clitoris that looks like a penis and swollen labia that resemble testicles. Only the males she chooses as mates ever get close enough to find out the truth.

In the hard-fought battle of the sexes, mothers may actually pass their sexual street smarts on to their daughters. In a series of ingenious experiments, William Rice, an evolutionary geneticist at the University of California, Santa Cruz, observed several generations of fruit flies as they refined complex offensive and defensive sexual strategies. If a female seemed to prefer other suitors, a male would try different ways of attracting or distracting her. If she'd already mated, he'd try to entice her to mate again. But again and again, females countered such seductive moves, even to the extent of producing contraceptive chemicals that blocked fertilization.

Each generation seemed to be born knowing their parents' ploys (scientists have in fact identified a specific gene for sexual strategies in fruit flies) and managed to come up with new tactics. But what would happen, Rice wondered, if only one sex got to put this legacy to use? He allowed forty-one generations of one group of males to mate with certain females and then introduced them to a new, less experienced group of potential partners. The effect was like setting up Casanova and his pals with the virginal students of a convent boarding school.

The insect ingenues fell for every trick of the sons of seasoned Lotharios, who managed to get even females who were already partnered to mate with them. But the males' sexual aggression took an unexpectedly harsh toll on the females: It literally killed them. The increased number of matings and the apparently greater toxicity of the males' seminal fluid shortened the females' life span—an outcome that could have led to the extermination of the entire line of fruit flies. But while such a scenario is chilling, it underscores a brighter reality: In nature, such an extreme imbalance doesn't happen. Fortunately, as Rice observes, "in nonexperimental conditions, females can hold their own."

The same might be said for another form of sexual tit for tat: infidelity. While many have argued that females per se are "naturally" monogamous, this doesn't seem to be the case. By some estimates, only 3 percent of mammals (females and males) are faithful to their mates. Among California mice and titi monkeys—once renowned as models of monogamy—females actually show more interest in other partners than males. Among certain macaques, females "float" from male to male throughout estrus. Female bonobos may have a variety of sexual contacts with several partners in a single day.

Yet according to the egg-and-sperm theory of evolutionary biology, philandering makes sense only for males. With millions of sperm to squander, they can produce more offspring by copulating with as many females as possible. But a female's eggs and pregnancies are limited. Since it takes only one sperm from one male to fertilize a female egg, why should she seek more sex partners?

If love has nothing to do with it, survival of the species just might. According to recent theories that have revised conventional thinking about female sexuality, there may be an evolutionary advantage for those who "diversify" their partners. When females of a species have sex with several males in a short period of time, their sperm, each offering a different genetic legacy, compete, perhaps muscling each other aside, until the hardiest and strongest of all triumphs and penetrates the egg.

In certain species, there may be an additional reason that females lead several males to think a child might be theirs: They may then be less likely to harm or kill it—and more likely to protect and provide for it. At least some primate females may have a more immediate motivation for seeking several partners. Watching estrous chimpanzees strut from male to male for a few seconds of copulation, some women biologists have speculated that perhaps, given the brevity of each encounter, a female seeks out a series of partners not just for long-term benefits to her future children, but for her own sexual satisfaction.

Is Mother Nature Pro-choice?

The father of her unborn child is gone, killed or banished by a challenger. As a powerful strange male approaches—sometimes even at first whiff of his scent—the female unconsciously calculates the advantages and disadvantages of continuing her pregnancy. If its future seems doomed, the fetus, depending on its size or age, is either reabsorbed (resorbed) or expelled. The female soon enters estrus and once again mates and becomes pregnant.

This phenomenon, called the "Bruce effect" for the scientist who first observed it, may occur in mice, rats, and several other species. Although its mechanism is not fully understood, a pheromone secreted by a strange male may trigger resorption or a miscarriage as a means of reproductive expediency. If the chances are slim that an unborn baby will survive after birth or if continuing the pregnancy may jeopardize the mother or her ability to care for her other offspring, nature cuts its losses and moves on. In a study of wild horses in the Great Basin of the American West, when one stallion successfully challenged another for

possession of his harem, 82 percent of the mares that had been impregnated by the deposed stallion in the previous six months aborted their
fetuses.

The Bruce effect occurs most often in younger rather than older
females, often when they are pregnant for the first or second time. Perhaps their still-maturing bodies are more vulnerable to sudden stress. Or
perhaps, in its unique way of "knowing," nature calculates that these inex-
perienced mothers are least equipped to handle the challenge of keeping
a baby alive in times of great peril.

In other circumstances, nature has other options. In marsupials, such
as the kangaroo, a fetus will remain in a state of suspended animation in
its mother's pouch for many months rather than develop and drain
resources from an ill or malnourished mother. During a prolonged period
of stress, the reproductive systems of many females shut down completely, and they do not come into estrus.

Are there parallels in humans? Certainly miscarriage is common. By
some estimates, as many as half of all embryos—most of them blighted by
severe genetic defects—never develop. So many pregnancies end this way
that biologists have described God as "the world's greatest abortionist."
No one ever argues that nature is good or evil, right or wrong, when a
pregnancy ends spontaneously. On the other hand, an induced abortion,
as discussed in Chapter 8, is an act of will, of conscious interference with a
natural process. And so the decision to undergo abortion—never easy or
unthinking—has long been viewed in moral terms.

"Morality" doesn't seem to apply to nature's other ways of controlling population, which include cannibalization and infanticide. Consider
the seemingly guileless guppy, a fish that's taken up residence in millions
of home aquariums. Right before a family's eyes, a female may give birth
one evening; by morning most of the young have disappeared. The
reason: Guppies practice strict population control to retain a ratio of
two females for each male and to ensure that each has at least half a
gallon of water to swim in. In one experiment at the American Museum
of Natural History, a female guppy gave birth four times to a total of 372
young, but the mother ate all but a few shortly after their birth. Six
months after the experiment started, only nine fish remained—six female,
three male.

In the wild, several species regularly engage in the practice of kronism—named for the Greek god Kronos, who devoured his children. When some nesting birds become overcrowded, a mother allows other adults to enter the nest and eat the young. A golden hamster will lick and suckle its pups—but eat the runts of the litter. When food is scarce, the older, stronger eaglet in a nest will kill and eat a weaker sibling.

Hunger isn't the only motive for murder. According to anthropologist Sarah Blaffer Hrdy, author of *The Woman That Never Evolved*, sometimes the circumstances for infanticide—which occurs among lions, hippos, bears, wolves, wild dogs, hyenas, rats, rabbits, chimps, and gorillas—are similar to those that trigger the Bruce effect. After a hostile takeover of a pride of lionesses or a harem of lemurs, the new males kill all nursing pups; this ensures that the females enter estrus and mate with them. Like Mafia "hits," these murders are strictly business—or, rather, evolution. The males have nothing to gain by protecting offspring that are not their own and everything to lose by not impregnating females with their own genes.

Given the sheer biological waste of aborted pregnancies and murdered offspring, one would expect nature to devise its own forms of birth control. But no male of any other species tugs a prophylactic sheath onto his penis, nor does any other female deliberately try to thwart pregnancy. However, there are examples of natural contraception. Among the remarkably productive honeybees—one of the most ancient matriarchies—the queen bee ensures her complete genetic domination by secreting a special chemical that renders the other females in the hive sterile. Among mammals (other than today's well-nourished humans), breastfeeding—the evolutionary invention that transformed the care and feeding of youngsters—shuts down the reproductive system to prevent estrus and limit family size.

Is contraception or induced abortion any more "unnatural"? The answer, argues evolutionary biologist Richard Dawkins, is beside the point. If our species did not control our population by means natural or not, the end result, as he emphasizes, would be "misery even greater than that which obtains in nature."

The Good Mother

Without any possible comprehension of the complex concept of thermoregulation, an Indian python coils her twenty- to thirty-foot body around her eggs and shivers to keep them within one degree of the perfect temperature for incubation. For three months an octopus mother—never taking a break even to eat—guards, oxygenates, and cleans her eggs so they are not smothered by parasitic fungi. A tiny tsetse fly, its nervous system so primitive it consists only of ganglia, zealously guards her young.

None of these creatures, utterly lacking in Bambi-ish appeal, will ever make it onto a Mother's Day card. Yet they undoubtedly qualify as good mothers, at least by evolution's standards: They do whatever they must to keep their offspring alive long enough for them to reach reproductive age.

There are millions of ways different females go about this fundamental challenge. Many, including most insects and fish, follow what's known as an "r" strategy. "R" stands for the rate of increase of the population size, and it is this rate that females try to maximize by producing huge numbers of offspring that sail into the air or swim into the sea.

Although most die, enough survive to keep the species alive. Other females, including primates like us, are "K" strategists, with "K" representing the capacity of the habitat to sustain young. "K" mothers produce fewer children and invest more time and energy in each of them. In mammals, this means that babies drink their mothers' milk, nestle against their warm-blooded bodies, and grow under their nurturing care.

How do "K" mothers know how to do the things they must to provide for their young? In her landmark studies on rat brains thirty years ago, neuroanatomist Marian Diamond, of the University of California, Berkeley, came up with a fascinating insight into the making of a mother. In experiments with male rats, she had shown that providing a novel and challenging environment—in this case, cages filled with mazes and toys—stimulated the growth of new brain cells. Then she studied female rats.

"We found nothing, nothing at all different between those we'd put in enriched environments and those we didn't. We were stunned. We spent a year redoing the study. Only then, when we looked at the data very carefully, did we realize that the female rats that had not been put in an enriched environment had just given birth. And pregnancy alone had changed their brains and actually had caused more growth than enrichment did in the males." Looking back, Diamond, a mother of four herself, feels she shouldn't have been surprised. "It makes perfect sense. Nature is preparing the female rat for the challenge of her lifetime. When her litter is born, she has to be ready for anything. She needs to be operating on all cylinders."

Any new mother would agree. Never in my lifetime have I relied more on instinct than I did in caring for a newborn. Without knowing the reason why, I couldn't keep my hands off my infant daughter. I held her close as she nursed; I strapped her in a Snugli against my chest when I went out; I stroked her downy head as she dozed. "Just like a primate," a biologist friend of mine commented. Primate mothers, in fact, spend the first three or four months of their babies' lives in constant skin-to-skin contact with them. And as scientists have proven, a mother's touch can make the difference between life or death, normal development or permanent lags.

When researchers remove a mother rat from a cage, her pup's metabolism slows down, and its ability to synthesize growth hormones lessens. Regardless of how well it's fed, the pup will not grow normally. Infant squirrel monkeys and macaques separated from their mothers show a dramatic and persistent increase in the stress hormone cortisol—even greater than the spike recorded after an injury or other physical trauma. In the wild, this may be adaptive. Cortisol stimulates the infant to call and search for its mother. But if the mother doesn't return, cortisol depresses the immune system and increases susceptibility to disease. The baby's heart rate and sleep patterns become erratic. If adopted and held by another female, the baby settles down, but its development never catches up.

In the Gombe preserve of Tanzania, Jane Goodall, the famed naturalist who first illuminated the complexity of the lives of chimpanzees, observed signs of severe depression and malaise among six infant chimps whose mothers had died. Four never recovered; the two who did showed dramatic retardation of physical and social development.

Just as mother loss is devastating, mother presence is joy itself. At the University of Wisconsin, scientists found that the opiates in the central nervous system of a rhesus macaque infant soar when its mother holds it near her chest. Perhaps this is why human mothers instinctively hold their babies to the left. The sound of her heart beating—so familiar from the womb—may bring a natural high of happiness.

Not all good "mothering" in nature comes from mothers. Contrary to the contemporary notion that today's "new" men are more involved with their youngsters than any other fathers, many males of other species are devoted parents. In slightly more than half of bird species, males pitch in with nest building, egg tending, and feeding offspring. Some take over certain duties completely or alternate child care. In temperatures that drop to 20 to 60 degrees below zero, the male emperor penguin of the Antarctic keeps his mate's egg warm in the thick fur at the base of his tuxedo shirtfront while she feeds at sea. Alligator fathers spend weeks building a nest with their mates and remain protectively nearby as their offspring grow. The tiny seahorse carries role reversal even further: Impregnated by the female, this aquatic Mr. Mom takes on full responsibility for caring for their brood.

Even the fearsome-looking silverback gorilla is actually what anthropologists call a "big-mama" male—gentle and tolerant of babies scampering up his broad shoulders. If a baby gorilla loses its mother, its father will take it into his nest at night and show special attention to it during the day, shepherding his offspring safely into maturity.

In many species, animal mothers—and fathers—also rely on others to help care for their young. "Alloparents"—caregivers who serve as aunts or baby-sitters—are especially common among primates. Baboon mothers regularly watch out for their friends' and sisters' children, and adolescent females may "practice" mothering skills by caring for infants in the group.

A primate's maternal instincts may even cross species. In August 1996 a toddler tumbled into the great-ape habitat at the Chicago Zoo. While cradling her own infant, a gorilla named Ketsu made her way to the boy's side. The horrified crowd watched apprehensively: Would this hulking beast harm the unconscious child? Would she inadvertently crush or injure him? Not at all. Looking to the zookeeper's door for help, she kept an anxious vigil over the little boy. As Ketsu taught the world, you don't have to be a woman to respond just like a mother.

Sisters Under the Skin?

Sitting together in a sunlit park, I tell an unmarried friend with a new baby about another single mother. Impregnated during a one-night stand, she'd gone through the long months of pregnancy on her own. Completely independent, she provides her baby with everything it needs—a safe place to sleep, nourishment, protection from rain and chill. She takes it everywhere, never leaving it with anyone else. When it howls in fright, she rushes to console it. If it gets into trouble, she rescues it. When its fingernails and toenails grow long, she nibbles them with her own teeth. But some days are so hard and long that she has no energy left to play with her youngster. After the briefest tickle, she takes her baby in her arms and they both settle down to sleep. "It's the story of my life," my friend comments. "Not quite," I say. "I'm talking about an orangutan."

As women, we certainly have a lot in common with other female primates: Our pregnancies are long, our newborns helpless, our children dependent on us for years. We also all tend to be adept tool-users, loyal friends, skillful communicators. And, for the most part (the loner orangutan being a dramatic exception), we like hanging out together.

Yet for all our physical and social similarities to females of other species, women usually assume we must be superior, particularly at a job as formidable as mothering. This isn't necessarily so. Take something every mammal, from wolf to wallaby, does naturally: nursing its young. Early in the twentieth century medical experts, deciding to take a more scientific approach to the nutrition of human infants, advised new mothers to breastfeed their babies no more than every four hours. Children, they insisted, need to learn a schedule.

These mothers soon made a distressing discovery: After nursing, their newborns would rest contentedly for only about an hour. Then they'd start crying—and keep crying until their next feeding. The babies and their weary mothers were miserable, yet the doctors warned that infants would be hopelessly spoiled if their mothers gave in to their demands. Unfortunately, countless sleepless nights and frustrating days passed before the well-educated, well-intentioned "experts" realized that they had ignored a basic biological fact: Human mothers, like other primates, produce very watery breast milk that doesn't provide long-lasting satisfaction. If babies don't nurse frequently, they get hungry and cry—regardless of what the schedule says.

In plenty of other circumstances, of course, intelligence serves us far better than instinct. But we deny or defy our animal heritage at our own peril. We also may miss out on valuable insight—and even inspiration. Certainly, by their very animal natures, females of other species lead lives more restricted than ours. Yet many demonstrate remarkable moxie. As primatologists have discovered, nonhuman female primates may put up with a lot of intimidation from their males, yet they manage to exercise considerable choice in mates and in movements. Males never completely dominate and control their lives, even when they're considerably larger. One reason may be that females cooperate with each other when need be to protect one of their own, for instance, a juvenile female harassed by males. This is something we women, who often have viewed other females as competitors rather than comrades, might do well to emulate.

Jane Goodall once was asked what she'd learned from spending so much time in the jungle amid other species. Her one-word answer: humility. "We used to think that we were unique and that there was an unbridgeable chasm between us and the rest of the animal kingdom," she explained, noting that the realization that we are not so different after all "teaches us a new respect, not only for chimpanzees and the other great apes, but all the amazing non-human beings with whom we share the planet."

Getting to know more about the females of other species also expands our understanding of how we fit into a much bigger biological picture. To me, the impact is not unlike the discovery of long-lost relatives. When you find out that your cousin is double-jointed, you look at your own nimble fingers in a different way. When you study a faded photograph of your great-grandmother, stiff in Victorian lace, you recognize the same dip in the hairline that you see every morning in the mirror. When you hear the staccato echo of your own laughter in an aunt's voice, you smile in recognition. Although you're the same person you always were, one important thing has changed: You now see yourself as part of a family you never knew you had.

CHAPTER 3

Lucy's
Daughters

I am doubly Lucy's daughter—descendant of the three-million-year-old ancestral matriarch whose remains were found in Ethiopia and child of a woman named Lucille born eight decades ago. I can see my mother in me—in the curve of my hips, the jut of my chin, the compact sturdiness of my body. But what of the original Lucy? Does some part of her still live in the billions of great-granddaughters she could claim as her own?

The mirror gives no hints. Lucy—named for "Lucy in the Sky with Diamonds," the Beatles song her euphoric discoverers played endlessly the day they found her skeleton in 1974—did not look like any woman alive today. She was little, only about three and a half feet tall and just sixty to seventy pounds—the size of an eight-year-old girl. By modern standards, she wasn't pretty. Her features were large and coarse, with a low forehead, heavy ridges at her brow, and nostrils that may have flared upward. Her mouth had a prominent jaw with large, bucked front teeth. Thick hair probably covered her sinewy arms and shoulders; her long-boned fingers curved as if she could still swing up into the branches. But Lucy and her kin—*Australopithecus afarensis*, as scientists dubbed them—walked upright. This amazing anatomical feat set them apart from all other creatures.

Lucy, though more than an ape, was not quite a woman. With a small skull and a brain no bigger than an orange—about a third the size of a human's—she probably was about as smart as a modern chimpanzee. While she could neither speak nor reason, her senses were acute. A baby in her arms, she strode—"an accomplished biped," as one anthropology textbook describes her—across the African savanna. She may have used simple tools, like a digging stick, to gather food. Her bones show a still-common female vulnerability to a form of arthritis. Yet at a time when everyday living was perilous, she managed to survive to the fairly ripe age of twenty-five or thirty.

Although the bones of more-ancient two-footed walkers, or hominids, have since been found, the discovery of Lucy remains the most important revelation of modern anthropology. Hers is the oldest, most complete, best-preserved skeleton of any of our early hominid ancestors. And even these millions of years after her death, Lucy, her bones resting in a museum case on regal red velvet, still fascinates everyone who sets eyes on her.

To her daughters and their human descendants, Lucy left a special legacy: She reminded everyone, scientists and nonscientists alike, that the human race owes its existence to the descent not just of man but also of woman—a fact long given short shrift. "The men who dominated scientific discourse in anthropology never saw women," says anthropologist Adrienne Zihlman, of the University of California, Santa Cruz, noting that "there is nothing in the science, nothing in the fossil records" to suggest that female hominids didn't make tools, use fire, create works of art—or provide much of the food that kept the species alive.

In the decades since Lucy's discovery, a new generation of anthropologists (most of them female) has shown that the endlessly fascinating story of man is a woman's story, too. "As a species, we are an unquestioned success; we have grown to be six billion strong," says Zihlman. "Women deserve just as much credit for this as men."

Lucy's line of australopithecines died out, but other hominids—all named "man"—arose to walk the earth: *Homo habilis* (handy man), *Homo erectus* (standing man), archaic *Homo sapiens* (knowing man), and finally modern *Homo sapiens sapiens* (a creature of knowledge and self-awareness). Obviously, hominid women were there at every step on this multimillion-year journey of human evolution. Over these eons, our fore-mothers developed ingenious abilities for adaptation and exquisite survival skills. The savvy, strength, and stamina of these evolutionary champions are part of our human legacy. Understanding these origins helps us see how we got to where we are today and how evolution shaped us in body, brain, and behavior. It also expands our perspective on the possibilities for what we, evolving women in an evolving world, may yet become.

Why Nothing Looks Like a Dame

In the pre-PC days of Rodgers and Hammerstein, the horny sailors of *South Pacific* celebrated the undeniable fact that "there is nothing like a dame." But what intrigues anthropologists is a simple question: Why not? Other female primates have the same hormones, nervous systems, and sexual organs—yet we don't look like them. Only the females of our species have full breasts, fleshy buttocks, and hourglass figures that flare in at the waist and out at the hips. Why did evolution, with a nip here and a tuck there, sculpt women's bodies in these special ways?

The first dramatic changes came when our earliest ancestors, female and male, pulled themselves onto two feet some four or five million years ago. According to studies of fossilized skulls and bones, the first hominids stood tall long before their brains grew substantially bigger than those of other primates. In all probability, the view from their new height helped build a bigger brain. Confronted with so many new challenges, they had to get smarter—fast. But what transformed them into bipeds in the first place?

Theories abound: Perhaps they needed to free their hands to tote food from field or forest. Perhaps as they shed the body hair to which their infants once clung, they had to use their arms to carry their young. Perhaps they had to peer over tall grass or could better traverse longer distances over varied terrains on two feet. Perhaps they stood upright to impress or intimidate, as gorillas do. Regardless of which forces combined to cause this transformation, our ancestors wouldn't have stayed upright for long if this new posture didn't aid and abet what is the primary purpose of every animal on the planet: perpetuation of the species.

This, say the (mostly male) proponents of the sexual-signaling hypothesis, is why womanly figures evolved to look the way they do. Unlike four-legged primates such as common chimpanzees, who thrust upward their bright, swollen bottoms to advertise their sexual availability during estrus, our female ancestors needed other anatomic lures to attract sex partners. Fatty breasts and fleshy buttocks—rounder, whiter, softer, and more prominent than their counterparts in any other species—could catch a male's eye coming and going.

"Some call this the tits-and-ass theory of evolution," observes anthropologist Robin McFarland, of De Anza College. "The basic premise is that women's bodies evolved primarily to please men." She doesn't buy this notion for a minute. In her research, she has focused on something that all female primates have and that modern women have come to hate: fat.

In all cultures and countries, women average twice as much body fat as men—22 to 29 percent, compared to 12 to 15 percent. Even young girls have more body fat than boys the same age. "Females clearly evolved a tendency to accumulate fat for a reason," says McFarland, who believes that our foremothers' survival—and the survival of their children—may have depended on their body fat.

While prehistoric females, with a high-carbohydrate diet and active lifestyle, were undoubtedly thinner than today's women, they still had extra upholstery on their bodies. It not only helped keep them alive during harsh winters, but it may have sustained their ability to conceive, carry, and nourish a child. As modern scientists have demonstrated in contemporary women, if body fat falls below a crucial level, as it can with malnutrition or extremely rigorous physical exertion, ovulation stops, and women become infertile. If this had happened often to prehistoric women—and certainly we have no reason to think they would not have stopped ovulating if their body fat fell too low—it would have been an evolutionary disaster. The dire consequences of too little fat may in fact be the reason that females have more of the lipogenic enzymes that help the body store fat and fewer of the lipolytic enzymes that break it down for fuel.

But for our ancient foremothers, bipedalism posed another challenge: where to store the extra fat. "The possible sites are more limited in humans than in other primates," says McFarland, who notes that the ideal locations are the upper chest and the hip-thigh region—breast-and-buttock territory—because they don't interfere with locomotion.

Women everywhere do indeed store fat in these regions. And at least during and after pregnancy, this fat may serve a vital function. "Body fat is not an undifferentiated gob of goo," explains McFarland. The fat stored in a woman's breasts during pregnancy provides a built-in reserve for the energy demands of breastfeeding. And as a nicety or necessity, the extra cushioning on her buttocks provides a comfy seat.

The anatomical renovations required of a female hominid's body went deeper than fat. Bones had to be rearranged to provide for the multiple demands of upright locomotion, pregnancy, and birth. Evolution's elegant solution was a bowl-shaped pelvis, broader and flatter than a man's, strong enough to support a woman's upper body as she walked and wide enough to accommodate a big-brained, big-shouldered baby. To prevent gravity from tugging at the developing fetus, the uterus and vagina angled forward—unlike the chutelike birth canal of most primates. This design left women with another uniquely female and largely unappreciated characteristic: hips.

Mine, by the way, are too big—or so I've always thought. But I must give them their due: With less generous dimensions, I might not have been able to carry and give birth to a baby that was almost nine pounds. Somewhere in deep time, men must have noticed this correlation between pelvic width, healthy babies, and mothers who survived childbirth. And they liked—or learned to like—what they saw.

How else can one explain an unexpected revelation from contemporary research into sexual attraction? Men today, as always, notice women's figures, and they typically list bosoms (big), bottoms (firm), and legs (long) as their favorite female body parts. But when psychologists have carefully measured the proportions of pinups of yesteryear, as well as of contemporary *Playboy* centerfolds, homecoming queens, and beauty contestants, they found one anatomical feature clearly ranked as most attractive to most men: the ratio of a woman's waist to her hips. Regardless of the actual measurements, women whose hips were about a third larger than their waists ranked as most desirable.

As evolutionary theorists see it, men may have unconsciously learned to assess a woman's waist-hip ratio—or WHR—eons ago. Why? Waist-hip ratio may be a good guarantee of a woman's ability to deliver a healthy infant safely. A slim-hipped woman may be unable to do so; a large-waisted woman may, in fact, already be pregnant with another man's child. As it turns out, WHR also testifies to a woman's health. According to contemporary analyses, women whose hips measure about a third larger than their waists are, not coincidentally, less likely to develop high blood pressure, diabetes, gallbladder problems, and other diseases.

I, who have always had one hell of a desirable waist-hip ratio, find this focus on the functions of women's bodies appealing—if only because it helps us make sense of their reality. Nature designed us to curve, and rather than waging war with flesh and bone, trying to flatten our bodies into the sleek lines of male geometry, we have excellent reasons to appreciate our own.

Designing Females

Just like the finicky females of other species described in Chapter 2, our foremothers learned to be selective about their mates. "Because of our cultural conditioning, we think of men choosing women," says anthropologist Nina Jablonski, of the California Academy of Sciences. "But there's no question that women, just like nonhuman primates, have always had preferences for certain male characteristics." If not for early woman's thumbs-up or thumbs-down reaction to male variations, modern man might well be huge, hairy, and fang-toothed, with a pencil-thin penis and testicles the size of softballs.

The first alteration female hominids made was a matter of scale. In Lucy's day males were about 35 percent larger than females. A size discrepancy this large usually occurs with male dominance over a harem of small and submissive (or seemingly so) females. By the time of *Homo erectus*, about 1.5 million years ago, the hominid size differential began narrowing. Males kept growing, but at a slower rate, and females got much, much bigger. Long before the twentieth-century triumph of the pint-sized nerd, it seems, hominid males learned that they could compete more effectively with brains rather than brawn. And females, who might once have chosen big males to protect them, opted for partners closer to their own size. By size estimates of skeletons from 300,000 years ago, males of that period were about 10 to 15 percent heavier and 5 to 12 percent taller than females—a size difference that has persisted to the present day.

Of course, just like a woman's body, a man's evolved to meet the demands of survival. His arms, like hers, are long—part of our ape ancestry. His skull, like hers, is big enough to accommodate the most sophisticated brain on the planet. His feet, ankles, knees, and legs, like hers, are angled to allow upright walking. But each gender has always had an enormous range of idiosyncratic variations: red hair, pug noses, strong chins, high cheekbones, prominent ears, and countless others.

A man's most appealing physical characteristic, according to recent research, may be symmetry. Just like a female scorpion fly, which somehow manages to mate with the male with the most perfectly matched wings, women tend to choose partners who are literally well balanced—possibly another indication of strong and healthy genes. This evolutionary bonus may explain why the most symmetrical men—in studies involving precise measurements of virtually every body part— report having three times as many sex partners as their more lopsided peers.

As for male sex organs, size does matter—but not in the way a prepubescent boy fears. Consider the penis, a male accoutrement that first appeared when reptiles slithered out of the sea some 350 million years ago. Perhaps dubious of the durability of this precariously placed appendage, nature equipped snakes and lizards with two phalluses. Primate males have only one—but a man's penis is the longest, relative to body size, of all: three times a gorilla's 1.25-inch stub.

Why did man's most vulnerable organ grow larger and more visible over time? Some suggest it was part of male sexual advertising, a way of catching the eye of a potential partner. Male chimps, field biologists note, flick their erect phalluses in the presence of an estrous female. While male hominids may have done the same to impress potential mates, I'm inclined to think that nature was simply being pragmatic. The male penis probably grew longer, as Desmond Morris theorized, "for the same reason as the giraffe's neck—to enable it to reach something otherwise inaccessible." This "something" was the female cervix, gateway to the egg's internal domain.

As female reproductive anatomy evolved, males had to adapt. With bipedalism, the vagina began to tilt forward—a modification that changed the way hominids have sex. Rather than the rear-mounting position most common among animals, women and men, among relatively few species on earth, tend to face each other. In the classic missionary position or its variations, a long penis can extend into the vagina and, most important, deposit sperm as close as possible to the cervix. Given their druthers, human males might well opt for even longer phalluses. In certain New Guinea tribes, men proudly wear decorative penis sheaths that dangle up to two feet between their legs. However, female anatomy set a limit for the human penis: It grew only as long as a vagina and no more.

A man's penis also is thicker than most males'—thicker, in fact, than required for its reproductive mission. "This may have emerged in human evolution simply because Lucy and her girlfriends liked thick penises," speculates anthropologist Helen Fisher, author of *Anatomy of Love*. "A fat phallus distends the muscles of the outer third of the vaginal canal and pulls on the hood of the clitoris, creating exciting friction, making orgasm easier to achieve." And a woman's pleasure also has an evolutionary payoff. According to calculations by British scientists, the contractions of a woman's vagina during orgasm may propel more sperm deeper inside her.

Testicle size itself may reflect female preferences, if only indirectly. On average, men's testicles are exactly that—average, which reveals something about the sex lives of our prehistoric ancestors. Among animals, males who have the most frequent sex with the most partners have the biggest sperm-storing vessels. The bonobo male, for instance, which copulates several times a day with several females, has huge testicles, while the larger but monogamous gibbon, which engages in sex only a few times a year, has tiny ones. The human male is in between.

If women throughout evolution had always been faithful mates (as some have asserted), male testicles would be smaller. If they were sex-crazed sluts (as others have argued), their partners would need sperm factories the size of melons to churn out enough sperm to block other males' contenders. Given this perspective, men might think twice before bragging about big balls: These may be as telltale a sign of female infidelity as a cuckold's horns.

As for actual sperm output, women again have a powerful influence, simply by proximity. The volume of sperm in a man's ejaculate, according to recent research, increases if his partner is away for any period of time. As if to compensate for the possibility that she may have taken another lover, his body produces extra troops to increase the odds that any child she conceives will be his. This automatic adjustment may well have evolved because at least some of Lucy's daughters had multiple lovers in short periods of time. But even a husband's extra output doesn't guarantee he will win what some call the "sperm wars." According to modern techniques for assessing paternity, 10 percent of all babies born in Western nations are not the biological offspring of the men their mothers identify as the father.

The Mating Game

Under the sparkling chandeliers of a hotel ballroom, the year's crop of San Francisco debutantes appear, each on the arm of her beaming father. With a curtsy to the right and a curtsy to the left, they take their place in long lines. Resplendent in virginal white, with flags of gleaming hair and perfect teeth that testify to fortunes in orthodontic enhancement, they sashay back and forth across the dance floor, stopping time and again to bow as they parade their youthful beauty for all to see. The debs giggle self-consciously through the archaic ritual, but year after year, local girls vie to be selected.

Their presentation to society is a sight both comic and touching. It is also one other species might appreciate: an elaborate, socially sanctioned display that sets the stage for courtship, sex, and pair bonding. Of course, it never occurs to these mall-prowling, street-savvy girls or their tuxedoed escorts that they're engaged in a mating dance, but that's exactly what's going on. And as in other species, the females and the males are moving to somewhat different tunes—ones that may well date back to our earliest days in Africa.

Then as now, three things mattered most to males: looks, looks, and looks. In addition to the all-important waist-hip ratio, yesterday's brawny, hairy hominid male—just like his buffed and clean-shaven contemporary counterpart—noticed the sheen of a female's hair, the whiteness of her teeth, the glow of her skin, the fullness of her lips. All of these features testify to youth, health, and fertility—essential for a male wanting to guarantee his genetic future. This gauging of reproductive fitness may be so ingrained that it accounts for the modern male's propensity for automatically checking out any and every female in sight.

For their part, Lucy's daughters noticed that they were being noticed. And long ago in time, they evolved a repertoire of what ethologists call "display behaviors" to draw maximum male attention: the hair toss over the shoulders, the coy smile, the finger twisting around a stray lock, the tongue flicked across the lips, the sidelong glance. Before early woman had mastered the verbal skills to say "Come hither," her body language was blaring the message loud and clear.

Such flirting maneuvers serve another valuable function: They buy a woman the time she needs to determine whether a man might be a suitable mate. While males can assess fertility (accurately or not) with a head-to-toe glance, females, now as always, run the equivalent of a credit check. After studying female preferences in various cultures around the world, evolutionary biologist David Buss concluded that women primarily want good providers of resources for their children. Like the weaverbirds who check out a suitor's real estate before committing, they want to assess what's formally known as "male parental investment," or MPI—a mate's willingness to protect and provide for his offspring. From the perspective of a woman's evolutionary mandate, nothing may matter more than mating well—particularly for the survival of her child.

"The human baby is born more helpless than any other," explains anthropologist Jablonski. "Women must have realized very early on that they would not be able to protect and provide for it all by themselves." They needed partners who would, to use a contemporary term, "commit," providing them and their children with shelter, adequate food, and protection from predators and other dangers.

The female desire for such assets may enhance the appeal of older men (themselves drawn to younger women's fertility). Around the world women tend to choose men a few years older than they are—perhaps because they've had more time to accrue more resources. An added bonus, according to a recent report from the University of Liverpool, is that men five to fifteen years older than their wives are much more likely to sire sons—traditionally the preferred sex among both parents.

Regardless of a potential mate's age, the best test of his potential for commitment may be time. By coyly delaying sexual involvement, a woman can determine which of two categories a suitor falls into: a love-'em-and-leave-'em cad or a dutiful dad. Some women, of course, have always guessed wrong or simply fallen for a charming rogue. But even they may have gotten some evolutionary dividends. According to what anthropologists call the "sexy son" hypothesis, a dashing Don Juan passes on to his children the same genes their mother found so hard to resist.

Women's desire for resources, rather than men's desire for dominance, may even be the underlying basis of polygynous societies, where men take more than one wife. Among the Kipsigis of East Africa, anthropologist Monique Borgerhoff-Mulder, of the University of California, Davis, found that wives would rather share a rich husband than have a poor husband to themselves. "Each of them gets her own house and plot of land, and the wives help each other out and take care of each other's children. They don't understand how Western women can stand being the only wife."

I wonder what these women might make of the complaints I hear from some young women on Wall Street, who regale me with tales of men behaving very badly. Their most egregious offense: They're cheap. Even on formal dates, the men automatically split the tab down the middle and then ask for extra for the tip. Then, more often than not, they hop out of a taxi a few blocks before their date's apartment. "I've had guys who make three times as much as I do stiff me for a taxi," says one thirty-year-old MBA. "I think: If he's cheap now, what would he be like as a husband?"

While I'd like to say that materialistic motives never entered my mind in my dating days, I did marry up—in every sense of the word. My husband, at six foot four, is more than a foot taller. As a short brunette, always the smallest in school classes, I take great delight in having a daughter who is tall and blond (another of my husband's genetic gifts)— and in contemplating a long line of tall, golden-haired grandchildren stretching into the future. But I married up in another way, too. Whatever

I accomplish in life, however successful I've been or ever become, my mother will always take delight in the fact that her daughter married a doctor. For a woman of her time, there was no better guarantee of economic security.

None of this, of course, even crossed my mind when I first laid eyes on my husband-to-be. I didn't shamelessly strut my irresistible waist-hip ratio before him or surreptitiously calculate his lifetime earnings potential. But I am Lucy's—and Lucille's—daughter, and maybe, just maybe, some small unconscious part of me did sit up and take notice. If so, more than twenty years later, for reasons totally unrelated to physical height or financial might, I have to admit I'm glad it did.

The Secret

Not long after her discovery, a funny thing happened to little Lucy: She turned into a babe. Even though her bones gave no hint of her relationships or roles, male anthropologists spun narratives of Lucy's probable life. These theories—dismissed as Kiplingesque *Just So* stories by feminist critics—centered on what they saw as her greatest attraction: continuous sexual receptivity.

Most female mammals engage in sex primarily during their period of peak fertility, or estrus, which may vary from one to forty-five days in length. *Estrus* comes from the Greek word for "gadfly," and that's exactly what a female in heat becomes. It's not so much a question of her wanting sex, but of her insisting on nothing else. And she gets what she wants—a mate, or, in some species, several. Once estrus ends, however, she rebuffs sexual overtures. It may be weeks, months, even years before she engages in sex again. According to anthropologists' calculations, one of our primate cousins, the female baboon, is sexually receptive for only one twenty-fifth of her adult life.

Even after their descent from the trees, our female ancestors probably engaged in sex only for a few intermittent weeks every few years. The rest of the time they were pregnant or nursing. Perhaps, at some unknown time, some females just happened to have sex early in pregnancy or while still breastfeeding—and benefited as a result, perhaps because appreciative lovers provided them with extra food or protection. Extending sexual availability beyond fertile times became our species norm. And so, looking back, anthropologists have pictured ever-ready Lucy, in the words of historian Donna Haraway, as "a reliable, if poorly upholstered, sex doll" whose greatest attraction was her capacity for spending more time "in the position many men have long thought best for women: prone."

The female's nonstop sexual availability had a profound impact on the male of our species. Hominid men no longer had to compete ferociously with other males in order to mate with a female who would be available only for a limited time. This meant they didn't have to bulk up, risk injury, or devote great amounts of energy to warding off competing suitors. Of course, they still had to woo and win females—but their strategies, no longer designed for a day- or week-long battle but part of an extended campaign, switched from might to mind. And as the pressures for all-out competition with each other eased, men may have learned a more adaptive strategy: cooperation, a prerequisite for endeavors such as big-game hunting and transcontinental exploration.

When their reproductive status became invisible, hominid women got a different benefit: a secret. According to the Bible, Eve's great sin was to eat the fruit of the Tree of Knowledge. The forbidden wisdom that she gained—at the price of paradise—was knowledge of good and evil. But the first evolutionary secret that females learned was different: the fundamental link between sex and reproduction.

Our early foremothers—lean, active, living through summer droughts and winter famines—probably had irregular menstrual cycles and, because they were so often pregnant or breastfeeding, relatively few menstrual periods. No one knows when they made the connection between their cycling bodies, sexual intercourse, and pregnancy. Perhaps as they watched the coupling of animals and the birth of their young, women intuited a connection between mating and motherhood. If, as some theorize, the menstrual cycles of fertile women living in small nomadic bands became synchronized—as still occurs among women sharing living space—they may have become pregnant and given birth together in the same seasons of the year. And in the company of other women, they may have come to realize that their bodies carried the seeds of life.

Men eventually shared this understanding, but there were other secrets a man could not know for sure: when a woman was fertile and whether he was the father of any child she bore. This state of confusion may have served women well. Some argue that womanly breasts grew full—unlike those of other primates, which swell only during pregnancy and lactation—to provide additional confusion to the difficulty of figuring out at a glance if a woman is fertile, pregnant, or nursing.

Because only a woman knew if she could have gotten pregnant by a particular man, she could, in effect, strike a bargain with him. In return for protection and provisions—part of the "male parental investment" women still value so deeply—she could reassure him that the child she was carrying or nursing was indeed his. Even though he still could be tricked, early man must have realized it was in his evolutionary best interest to do everything he could to ensure the well-being of the mother of his child. This deal, as anthropologists now see it, may have set the stage for male-female relations throughout time.

Did such hard-nosed negotiating really take place? Almost certainly not in any spoken or even conscious way. But there's no question that hidden ovulation gave women more choice. Rather than being compelled by the spurt of a chemical fire within their very cells, they could choose their lovers more carefully. Whereas an estrous chimp may mate with every male in sight, a hominid female could take time to size up a potential partner. Her brain's decisions came to matter more than her body's urges.

Eventually human pair bonds may have formed as part of the trade-off of paternity assurance for fatherly commitment. No one knows for sure if they endured as long as both partners lived or, as anthropologist Helen Fisher has speculated, only for the three or four years needed to care for an infant and toddler. We also don't know how exclusive such pair bonds were. Even a woman in a stable pair bond may have benefited from an occasional dalliance with another partner, who, if he thought one of her children was his, brought extra food or kept a watchful eye over her young. The women who used their secret knowledge in these ways may have been most likely to survive—and to pass on their sexual strategies (just like the fruit flies described in the preceding chapter) to their daughters.

Nature, in fact, did such a good job at "hiding" ovulation that it wasn't until the 1930s that medical scientists grasped the intricacies of the process and not until 1995 that they realized that fertility peaks before rather than after the surge in temperature that accompanies an egg's release. Even today, with sophisticated ovulation detectors and more reliable contraception options than ever before, a woman's hidden fertility leads to millions of unwanted pregnancies every year. Nonetheless, "this magnificent female trait," as Fisher describes it, has undoubtedly endured for a reason. As in the remote past, it still allows a woman to do something few other females can: to claim the secrets of her fertility as her own.

Puncturing the Paleolithic Glass Ceiling

Like many people, I learned my first lessons in anthropology with my nose pressed against museum glass, staring in awe at dioramas of long-ago life. The scenes were variations on a similar theme: Hunters—spears poised, mouths open in fearsome roars—gathered around a mighty beast. Their bodies were thick-armed and hairy, their teeth large, their features coarse. But there was no mistaking who these bold and wild creatures were—our forefathers. It never occurred to me to ask a question that now seems obvious: Where were the women?

According to one study of eighty-eight dioramas depicting 444 individuals, males appeared in 84 percent of the scenes, usually right smack in the center of the action, running, walking, hunting, carrying game or firewood, engaging in ritual activities. An adult female made an appearance in fewer than half—usually as a faceless "drudge on a hide," head down, nursing a baby or tending a fire.

Is this what it was just like a Stone Age woman to be or do? Not at all. During most of their multimillion-year march from ape to human, female and male hominids were equals in many ways. As nomads, both had the same occupation: foraging. Over many centuries, males came to specialize in tracking, scouting, scavenging, and hunting. But it's highly unlikely that Lucy sat around a cave fire waiting for her mate to bring home dinner. If she had, she probably would have gone hungry many a night, if she survived at all.

Like every other nonhuman female primate, our foremothers had to provide their own food—and according to studies of fossilized teeth and bones, the nuts, berries, roots, fruits, and vegetables they gathered made up the bulk of the hominid diet for millions of years. With the exception of an occasional egg nabbed from a nest or a hand-caught fish, animal protein was rare. And when meat first began to make regular appearances on the equivalent of the dinner table, it was mostly gleaned by scavenging the remains of prey killed by other animals. Even after big-game hunting began, meat probably accounted for only 20 percent of daily calories.

Why, then, do we hear so little about woman the gatherer and so much about man the hunter? Anthropologist Zihlman blames something our prehistoric foremothers could never have imagined—the "Paleolithic glass ceiling." In the eyes of the fathers of anthropology, women's work, however invaluable to their families and the future of the species, didn't seem as significant as men's. The hero of prehistory that captured their imaginations was the hunter: spear-chucker extraordinaire, mighty and brave, towering above the fallen bodies of woolly mammoths and other formidable foes. And hunters were always male—or so everyone assumed.

The Greek historian Herodotus challenged this notion centuries before Christ's birth, when he described a tribe of women warriors who rode on horseback out of the eastern steppes. "We are riders; our business is with the bow and the spear," he quotes them as saying. "We know nothing of women's work."

However, there never was evidence of such a clan's existence—until 1997, when archaeologists from the University of California, Berkeley, reported their findings from a burial ground along the Kazakhstan-Russia border. In it were bones of girls and women, their legs bowed from riding horses, surrounded by weaponry of the hunt, including arrowheads, daggers, and whetstones to sharpen blades.

These women belonged to early nomadic tribes, the Sauromatians and Sarmatians, who date back to the sixth century B.C. The artifacts buried with them indicate that they held high status, performed sacred rituals, and hunted and fought. The body of an adolescent girl had an amulet around her neck in the form of a leather pouch containing a bronze arrowhead; at her side was an iron dagger, at her other side a quiver with more than forty bronze-tipped arrows. A bent arrowhead lay among another woman's bones, suggesting that it had pierced her body in battle.

Did other women of other places and times also ride and hunt? Since hunting requires stealth and strategy rather than strength alone, there is no reason to assume that they didn't—yet anthropologists believe that few, if any, of our foremothers actually did so. The primary reason is that hunting, with its demands for long hours and distant travel, is completely incompatible with child care. Early women opted for gathering— the prehistoric equivalent of a mommy track—so they could forage near home, nurse their babies on demand, and keep toddlers out of danger. As they collected nuts, roots, and berries, they also were able to work in the company of other females—singing, laughing, perhaps weaving vines into baskets and slings.

At some point in time, women also began rubbing together handfuls of plant fibers to create long lengths of thread. With this simple process, they created what may be the most underappreciated invention in prehistory: string, something that Elizabeth Wayland Barber, author of *Women's Work*, describes as "the unseen weapon that allowed the human race to conquer the earth." The String Revolution, as she refers to it, led to inventions of remarkable ingenuity and variety: snares, fishline, nets, packages, tethers, leashes, ropes, cords, tents, covers, blankets—and, not insignificantly, clothing. The quintessentially female arts of needlework, weaving, and sewing date back to between 26,000 and 20,000 B.C.— based on the estimated age of the first large-eyed needles to be discovered. The earliest known fossilized piece of cord has been traced to 15,000 B.C.

Women have been weaving and sewing ever since. Even today, when the most skillful seamstresses may be suturing vital organs in operating rooms, the textile arts haven't gone out of style. Nearly one third of the adult female population of the United States, mostly college-educated women between the ages of twenty-four and fifty-four, sews. And according to a survey by the American Home Sewing and Craft Association, no other leisure activity soothes women more—lowering heart rate, blood pressure, and sweat (three common measures of stress).

Even in the often-frantic bustle of modern times, it's still very much like a woman, her busy days filled with loose ends and unraveling seams, to take up needle and thread to weave order and beauty into her life.

The Grandmothers We Never Knew

My grandmothers died before I was born. I never even knew their names—not until my own daughter, devoted to her grandma Lucille, asked about my mother's mother. Her name, I discovered only then, was Michaelina—far more lyrical than I would ever have guessed. Born in the late nineteenth century in a village in Poland, Michaelina somehow scraped together the means and the moxie to make her way halfway around the world to America. As a young immigrant, she married a miner and settled with him in the anthracite hills of northeastern Pennsylvania. When he died, crushed in a collapsing mine shaft, she brought up four children on her own. Although she spoke little English, she sent her sons to college and her daughters through high school—no small accomplishment for an uneducated immigrant widow of her time and place. She also passed on timeless skills: recipes for the melt-in-the-mouth dumplings called pierogi, a knack for coaxing abundant harvests from spindly tomato plants, and the toughness to make it through tough times. When I finally heard her story, I felt proud to claim her as part of my family history.

Perhaps anthropologists are feeling the same way about the grandmothers whose lives they've recently begun to research. Once they had assumed that prehistoric life was too harsh for women or men to survive to see their children's children. This probably was indeed the norm—but the exceptional women who did live long enough to become grandmothers may have contributed much to their descendants.

Contrary to standard evolutionary thinking, women beyond reproductive age serve—and probably always have served—a valuable purpose. Amid the Hadza foragers of contemporary Tanzania, for instance, field studies have shown that grandmothers are key providers—more efficient and harder-working than younger women. They put in more hours per day (seven, compared to a mere three for girls and four and a half for women of childbearing age) and, thanks to their skill and stamina, they bring in the largest harvests, which they share generously with family and friends.

But a grandmother's contributions go beyond mere provisioning. Rather than producing more children of her own (which is what older men often opt to do, now as always), a postmenopausal woman devotes her energies to her existing children, their children, and her other relatives. And she, who has seen so many seasons, can pass on what genes cannot carry—knowledge earned and learned in the process of living. Throughout time a grandmother who remembered where berries grew even in drought, who knew which herbs to select for healing poultices, who nurtured youngsters when their parents died, helped ensure the survival of her entire tribe.

Grandmothers of the present and the past—working, loving, touching many lives, living on in shared memories—remind us of a basic truth about Lucy's daughters: Without a doubt, the world became a different place and humans became a different species because of their presence. And these remarkable women live on in each of us—quite literally in our very cells.

As discussed in Chapter 2, every female egg contains mitochondrial DNA, or mtDNA, which has the unique ability to repair genetic defects in sperm and launch the development of an embryo. Both females and males receive mitochondrial DNA from their mother's egg, but only daughters can pass it on to their children. Since the egg's mitochondrial DNA reproduces by splitting, rather than combining with a male's genetic material, it changes little over time. Using sophisticated computer analyses to calculate the rate of mutations in mtDNA, scientists at the University of California, Berkeley, have determined that the mitochondrial DNA in today's women is very similar to that of our foremothers. According to their calculations, we are all descendants of a common grandmother, a "mitochondrial Eve," who lived an estimated 100,000 to 200,000 years ago, probably in Africa.

Although the origins of mitochondrial Eve remain the subject of heated debate, there is no dispute over the existence of an unbroken genetic thread linking mothers and daughters through time. Studies of women in 135 different cultures—Europeans, Australian aborigines,

Asians, Native Americans, Africans, New Guinea highlanders—show that all clearly descended from the same foremother, who probably was part of a larger group whose other members' genetic lines simply died out. In 1997, ten years after the identification of mitochondrial Eve, scientists announced the discovery of a male counterpart, a "chromosomal Adam," traced by studies of changes in the Y chromosome, which determines male gender and is transmitted from fathers to sons.

These ties to the past underscore the basic biological fact that we literally all belong to the family of man—and of woman. As women, we are part of a remarkable sisterhood, and also, in one writer's phrase, "walking archives of ancestral wisdom." And as members of the human race, we all—female and male—owe our existence not to Adam's rib, but to Eve's eggs and their life-generating mitochondria, the ultimate gift of the countless grandmothers we never knew.

C H A P T E R 4

The Body of a Woman

Skin the color of fresh rich cream, flower-pink nipples, pillowy breasts, dimpled thighs, moist tendrils of hair. I have walked through the great museums of the world besotted by the sight of women's bodies: goddesses, madonnas, nubile girls, nursing mothers, Botticelli's Venus, Leonardo's Mona Lisa, Degas's ballerinas, Matisse's dancers. Men—Greek gods, martyrs, messiahs, self-portraits of artists as they aged—make an occasional appearance. But the face and figure captured on canvas more often than not belong to a female. And, like millions of others, I cannot take my eyes off her. "Nothing," observes veteran magazine editor T George Harris, "is more fascinating to women and men alike than the female body."

Female and male bodies begin to take their distinctive forms even before birth. Health and height may depend on the sex of the parent who transmits the genes that affect them—and also on whether the embryo itself carries the two X chromosomes that make a female or the X and Y combination that makes a male. In the womb, the mix of estrogens and androgens, different in females and males, sculpts a developing fetus in ways that are similar but not identical. Throughout life, the unique biology of each sex influences strength, stamina, susceptibility, and resilience.

From thick-haired head to high-arched sole, the body of a woman does not look, feel, or function exactly like a man's. It wasn't meant to. As vertebrates, mammals, and primates, the two human sexes have evolved in ways that are exquisitely adapted to the survival of our species. As we have seen, nature equipped the human male with a powerful sex drive (the strongest on the planet), a high rate of sperm production (an astounding 10 million to 50 million per day), and a body large, strong, and fast enough to fend off physical threats. The human female evolved a body equipped for multiple functions, including bearing and caring for children, storing energy, and enduring over the long haul.

On average the body of a woman stands four to five inches shorter than a man's and weighs twenty-five to forty pounds less. Her bones are not only smaller and lighter but, in locations such as the elbow and the base of the thumb, shaped somewhat differently. Her shoulders are narrower, her pelvis wider. A woman takes nine breaths a minute; a man averages twelve. She has fewer sweat glands and fewer red blood cells. A man, for unknown reasons, is more prone to hiccups and, because of greater sensitivity to house dust, more likely to sneeze in a stuffy attic.

Under stress, women unconsciously tend to clench their jaws; men tighten their vocal cords—which may be why they stutter more than women. A woman sleeps more lightly and rouses more easily. "Men forget the world when they sleep," a sleep specialist tells me. "Women stay alert and watchful, almost as if they had one eye open." After surgery, a woman wakens from anesthesia faster—in an average of seven minutes, compared with slightly more than eleven minutes for a man.

These biological differences are not signs of superiority or inferiority, rightness or wrongness, normalcy or deviation. "Nature created two sexes as a grand experiment," says Marianne Legato, of Columbia University. Medical science has just begun to take advantage of this phenomenon by comparing and contrasting the ways in which female and male bodies go about the business of living.

Some women are understandably skeptical about the new field of gender biology. Differences in physiology and anatomy, they worry, somehow imply or may be construed to imply deficiencies—not just in biology but in performance and ability. It has happened many times before. As recently as the nineteenth century, scientists—white and male—devoted themselves to scrutinizing the bodies and brains of women and blacks, measuring every possible parameter to garner proof for their premise that these were lesser beings.

"Women have said to me, 'I'm as good as any man and I can do any task that a man can do as well as he can,' " says Legato. "This may well be so. Nothing in all the data we've accumulated so far implies otherwise." But only by examining the female body and studying the details of how it functions can we expand our appreciation of *all* of human biology. "Learning about gender-specific biology isn't an emotional issue, a feminist issue, or even a politically correct issue," she notes. "It is an intellectual imperative."

Nobody's Rib

According to a literal reading of Genesis, Eve was the original recycling project, assembled from Adam's spare parts. This view, which long dominated perceptions of women, depicts the female as a not-quite-perfect imitation of the male. Yet if there's one thing we now know beyond any doubt, it is this: The body of a woman is no knockoff. With the exception of sperm manufacture, it does everything the male body does—but often in a distinctive way.

Think of what might seem the most asexual of body parts: the liver. It turns out to be anything but. "I consider the liver literally the sexiest organ in the body," says gynecologist Florence Haseltine, president of the Society for the Advancement of Women's Health Research. As she notes, the liver develops differently in female and male fetuses. Although scientists still don't know exactly how or why, "it matters if the liver sees more estrogen or testosterone in the womb—it behaves differently for the rest of its life."

The female liver metabolizes drugs differently, enhancing the effects of some, blunting the impact of others. If a woman of the same weight as a man drinks the same amount of liquor, beer, or wine, she's more likely to get tipsy. Why? The female liver oxidizes alcohol more slowly, so she ends up with a higher blood alcohol level—an effect that's most pronounced premenstrually, when the oxidation of alcohol in the liver is slowest. Even when it outlives its owner, the female liver remains distinctive. For reasons medical experts cannot yet explain, the chance of success for liver transplantation is best when the liver of a woman is grafted into the body of a man.

Like the liver, the heart of a woman is smaller than a man's—about two thirds of its size—and beats to a rhythm all its own. When awake, a woman's heart typically pulses at a rate of 90 beats per minute (bpm), compared with 80 bpm for men. During sleep, her heart rate drops to an average of 66 bpm, his to 56. Her heart also is more likely to skip beats, race suddenly, or "flutter."

"One quarter of women and virtually no men report heart palpitations," notes Legato. The reason may be a uniquely female dip in estrogen that leads to a coronary artery spasm (a sudden constriction of the artery), most likely to occur premenstrually or during perimenopause, when estrogen levels are low. Yet women's hearts stay stronger longer, showing the first signs of heart disease about a decade later than men's and aging at a different rate. However, as discussed in Chapter 5, a woman's heart can "break" in different and potentially deadly ways.

The female immune system, ever vigilant, responds more vigorously to common infections, offering extra protection against viruses, bacteria, and parasites. This may be why Mom is often the last one standing during a family flu siege. Pregnancy turns down the immune response, probably to ensure that a mother's natural protectors don't attack the fetus as a "foreign" invader. This impact is so great that pregnant women with transplanted kidneys typically require lower doses of drugs to prevent organ rejection.

Even the most mundane of bodily functions, such as digestion and elimination, vary in each sex. The chemical makeup of a woman's saliva is different, and foods may taste sweeter or spicier to her. As hormones rise and fall during a woman's menstrual cycle and during pregnancy, her gums swell and become more prone to infection. Food travels more slowly through a woman's digestive tract, so her chances of being chronically constipated are three times greater than a man's.

Universal physiological experiences such as pain and pleasure register somewhat differently in women and men. Based on research on the efficacy of pain medication in both sexes, scientists theorize that the brain circuitry that regulates pain response and relief differs in women and men. Pleasure, too, may travel through the brain via different pathways. In studies of women with spinal cord injuries, researchers at Rutgers University have documented that, despite a cessation in normal nerve function, they remain so responsive to vaginal stimulation that their brains can still register the experience of orgasm.

Women also are more sensual in other ways. Their skin, thinner and estrogen-rich, responds to petal-soft touches. The hairs in the tiny inner channels of the female ear vibrate at a different rate than a man's. A woman's hearing is keener and deteriorates less rapidly than a man's over time. Her nose, smaller and flatter, can detect lower levels of an odor. In one study at the University of Pennsylvania, 1,200 women and men tried to identify forty scratch-and-sniff cards that included scents from soap to skunk; the women consistently scored higher. Even in infancy, baby girls spend more time with scented rattles than unscented ones; boys pay equal attention to both.

Daddy's Girls and Mommy's Boys

"Well, there's no question of who the father is," the waiter says with a glance at my tall, fair husband and daughter and another at short, dark-haired me. "But who's the mother?" We've heard the quip so often that I have a ready answer: "His big genes beat my little ones to the punch."

This explanation may not sound scientific, but it's not terribly off the mark. As scientists have only recently discovered, even genes have gender. According to investigators in the hot research field of genetic imprinting, the sex of the parent whose genes prevail affects the way an embryo develops. "You are different depending on whether you inherit your genes from your mother or your father," says Haseltine, a specialist in genetics.

The human genome, the entire genetic complement of a cell, contains different forms of genes called alleles. As an egg merges with a sperm, usually each parent contributes an allele. However, sometimes something happens that marks or "imprints" a gene in such a way that the allele from one parent is expressed, or fully functional, while the other (the imprinted one) is suppressed and inactive. Of the estimated 80,000 to 100,000 genes that make up a human being, only fifty or sixty are imprinted. Though few in number, they are critical because they regulate key processes such as growth and immunity.

What happens when only a mother's or father's genes hold sway? Experiments—natural and otherwise—give us some answers. In mammals like us, paternal genes are responsible for the development of the placenta, while maternal genes are involved in the differentiation of tissue in the embryo. If only the father's genes are transmitted—as happens in the rare event (an estimated one in a thousand conceptions) when a sperm fertilizes an egg cell lacking a nucleus—only a placenta develops. This "molar" pregnancy grows so rapidly that a woman may require treatment with cancer drugs to halt its spread.

If an abnormal egg cell develops from only maternal genes, it becomes a benign tumor called a dermoid, made up of different types of human tissue, such as bone and nerve, but with no placenta. In laboratory experiments, scientists have manipulated mouse genes so that some mice are born with only their fathers' growth-determining genes and some with just their mothers'. Those with only paternal genes grow to 130 percent of average size; those with only maternal genes are 60 percent smaller.

To evolutionary biologists who view life in terms of the "selfish" gene's drive to survive and reproduce, the bias carried within paternal or maternal genes is another molecular version of the battle between the sexes (discussed in Chapter 2). The father wants his embryonic offspring to grow as large and as strong as possible; from his perspective, bigger is always better. The mother also wants her fetus to grow—but not to the extent that it jeopardizes her well-being or future fertility. If the father gets his genetic way, a huge placenta and a big embryo develop—a reflection of his "selfish" desire to extract as much as possible from the mother of his child, regardless of any harmful consequences to her. If the mother's self-interest prevails, the fetus grows to a more modest size. But it's possible to view this process somewhat differently, as a cooperative venture, with the father—the quintessential provider—supplying the organ of nourishment in utero, the placenta, and the mother—the classic nurturer—overseeing the complexities of development.

The gender of parental genes can also mean the difference between health and disease or alter the course of a disease. For instance, a child can inherit myotonic muscular dystrophy from either parent, but if the gene comes from the mother, the youngster will develop symptoms much earlier and the course of the disease will be more severe. With another neurological illness, Huntington's disease, individuals who inherit the gene from their fathers develop symptoms at an average age of thirty-three, while children of affected mothers typically remain healthy for an additional nine years.

At least one genetic mutation traced to chromosome 15 can result in two different and rare diseases, depending on whether the mother or father passes it on. If the father transmits the defect, a child develops Prader-Willi syndrome, characterized by mental retardation, obesity, and small hands, feet, and genitals. If the child inherits the same defect from its mother, it is afflicted with Angelman syndrome, which causes seizures, unusual movements, a large mouth, red cheeks, and a strange laugh.

The sex of the fetus itself can make a difference in susceptibility to disease. In females, the extra X chromosome acts as a sort of insurance policy. If there is a genetic error on a girl's X, her other X can override it. A boy whose X chromosome carries an abnormal gene lacks a gene on the second X to neutralize the trait. In all, males are prone to more than two hundred X-linked disorders, including hemophilia, color blindness, and Duchenne's muscular dystrophy.

There are other ways that sex makes a difference even before birth. The neural tube—the precursor of the brain, spinal cord, and backbone—develops according to a different timetable in a female and a male fetus. Because of this, each is more vulnerable to a different type of neural tube defect. A male fetus is twice as likely to develop spina bifida, a defect of the lower neural tube. In a female fetus, the upper end of the neural tube is more likely not to close in the first month of pregnancy, and the unborn baby will not develop a normal brain. This condition, called anencephaly, is always fatal.

Both these defects, which often occur before a woman even suspects that she is pregnant, may seem like horrible acts of fate beyond human control. Yet scientists have discovered that they are not inevitable. Women who take folate, a B vitamin, before conception and throughout pregnancy greatly reduce the risk of both types of birth defects and increase the likelihood that a child, whichever its sex, will be born healthy.

What Little Girls (and Boys) Are Made Of

When a biologist's bright young daughter asked how babies were made, she sketched a diagram depicting the X chromosome from the mother and the X or Y the father contributes. "You started like this," she explained, printing XX. "Your brother got an X and a Y." The little girl stared at the block letters and asked, "You mean you and Daddy gave me two kisses, and Mattie got a kiss and a smile?"

This—my all-time favorite explanation of chromosomal sex—adds a grace note of love to the act of conception. It is not entirely whimsical, for the X chromosome does indeed impart the kiss of life. No one—female or male—can take form and grow without it. A girl may have a single X or three or more X's; boys may be born with two X's and a Y, an X and two Y's, or an X with just the tiniest snippet of a Y attached. Some of these unusual combinations have little impact on health and development; others can affect many aspects of an individual's life. Chromosomal sex has turned out to be more complicated than anyone had anticipated, and its lifelong impact more complex and ambiguous. But one fact remains indisputable: An X chromosome is essential for every human life.

The X, a mother's first gift to her child, carries 2,500 to 5,000 genes, including those that regulate muscle development, blood clotting, and immune response. In contrast, the Y, the smallest chromosome, has just twenty or so inhabitants, including highly specialized genes that transform it into what some describe as "a turbocharged fertility factory."

Regardless of their chromosomal makeup, embryos are identical in the first weeks of development. The vital organs—brain, heart, spine—take shape before the genitals. In the beginning, every fetus has a genital tubercle that eventually forms either a female clitoris or a male penis, a mass of tissue called the labioscrotal swelling that turns into female labia or a male scrotum, structures that become gonads (ovaries or testes), and two separate sets of ducts—Müllerian and Wolffian—that develop into female or male reproductive equipment, with the unutilized ducts degenerating.

At about the sixth week of life, genetic signals trigger this process of sexual differentiation. The message to make a male comes from the Y chromosome. But for years after making this discovery in 1959, scientists remained baffled. Some seemingly normal men—an estimated one in twenty thousand—have two X chromosomes instead of an X and a Y, while some women have XY chromosomes instead of two X's. As it turns out, a tiny bit of a Y, containing just 0.2 percent of the genes normally on this chromosome, clings to one of each XX male's X's and is sufficient to trigger normal male sexual development. This exact segment, other studies revealed, is always missing in females with XY chromosomes.

It is not yet clear whether a single gene in this region of the Y is the sole determinant of male gonadal sex, or whether a battery of genes interact to make a male. But we do know that the process is complex—and perilous. Although as many as 130 to 150 males are conceived for every 100 girls (possibly because Y-carrying sperm are lighter, faster swimmers), so many male fetuses perish in the womb that boys outnumber girls by a ratio of just 105 to 100 at birth.

At the Y's signal, undifferentiated sexual tissue in the fetus is molded into testes. As soon as these form, they begin production of androgens, or male hormones, which stimulate a growth spurt in the male reproductive system. One of these hormones, dihydrotestosterone (a precursor of testosterone), stimulates the labioscrotal swelling to become the scrotum. The genital folds fuse around the urethra to form the shaft of the penis; the two sides of the labioscrotal swelling come together to form the scrotum. The Wolffian ducts enlarge and develop into the vas deferens, seminal vesicles, and ejaculatory ducts. Another substance causes the Müllerian ducts, the template for female reproductive anatomy, to shrink and disappear.

Once biologists believed that femaleness was the "default" sex, that is, what an embryo became in the absence of male genes and hormones. This is not the case. As scientists in the United States and Italy have demonstrated, a gene or set of genes for femaleness, located on one arm of the X chromosome, pushes the undifferentiated gonads in a female direction. Under its influence, a woman's lifetime supply of egg follicles—perhaps as many as 400,000—develop, as do the ovaries that store the eggs and produce female hormones, including estrogen. Under hormonal direction, the Müllerian ducts grow into the fallopian tubes, uterus, and the inner third of the vagina; the Wolffian duct system degenerates. The genital tubercle becomes the clitoris; the genital folds become the inner vaginal lips (labia minora), and the two sides of the labioscrotal swelling become the outer vaginal lips (labia majora). By the twelfth week, sexual differentiation is complete. The penis and scrotum are recognizable in males; the clitoris and labia can be identified in females.

The making of a female or male is such an intricate, precisely timed process that it's not surprising that occasional missteps can and do occur. Although relatively rare, they reveal a great deal about how biology shapes our gender identities.

A male fetus with a normal Y chromosome, for example, occasionally lacks receptors—molecular docking sites found throughout the body—for his own sex hormones. As a result of this condition, called androgen insensitivity, "he" is born looking like a "she," with what appear to be normal female genitals, and develops as a girl. However, at puberty, menarche fails to occur. Only then, with medical examination and testing, do a girl and her family discover that she is a chromosomal male in a female body. Most of these individuals think of themselves as females and continue to live their lives as such, although they generally require surgery to create a deep enough vagina to engage in intercourse and, of course, can never have children.

Chromosomal females with another defect, congenital adrenal hyperplasia (CAH), are exposed to very high levels of androgens (produced by their overactive adrenal glands) in the womb. Born with masculinized genitalia—most often an enlarged clitoris and fused labia that may look like a scrotum—they usually undergo corrective surgery and are raised as girls. In childhood many show a greater preference for boys' toys and activities, but as they mature, they look like normal women and tend to be heterosexual. Most marry, and many have children, although their fertility rates are lower than normal. From an early age, they may display the enhanced spatial ability that some see as characteristic of males—possibly a result of prenatal hormones, possibly a consequence of their play with blocks, trucks, and other boyish things—and some researchers have described these girls as more tomboyish and athletic.

These uncommon individuals raise intriguing questions about what it really means, at a fundamental physiological level, to be just like a woman. Is a chromosomal male with androgen insensitivity, who looks and lives as a female, a "real" woman? Is one genetic female, her body and brain shaped by male hormones in the womb, any less womanly than another? What is it, ultimately, that determines whether we come to see ourselves as female or male? The answers may begin before birth, with our genes, chromosomes, and hormonal mix. But they certainly don't end there.

Everyone's Best Friend?

Nature never created "female" and "male" hormones. It simply produced versatile, hardworking compounds with similar but not identical carbon-ring structures. Although both sexes make these steroid hormones, females have higher levels of estrogens, produced mainly by their ovaries, while males have more androgens (including testosterone), produced mainly by their testes. But each sex produces the same hormones. The difference in "his" and "her" hormones is one of quantity, not quality.

The predominant estrogen of a woman's reproductive years is estradiol. As soon as a woman becomes pregnant, estradiol drops—possibly to relax the immune system so it doesn't attack the fetus as an invader—and estriol, the estrogen of pregnancy, takes over. At menopause estradiol production falls, and estrone, a weaker estrogen manufactured in the fat cells, dominates.

As some see it, estrogen in all its forms acts just like a woman—alluring, helpful, protective, nurturing, but with a surprising capacity for mischief. Like the word *estrus*, *estrogen* derives from the Greek for "gadfly" or "frenzy," and it certainly is a molecular mover and shaker. Estrogen, contrary to accusations periodically flung at women, doesn't "rage," but it does range—rising and falling throughout the menstrual cycle and in the form of estriol, surging during pregnancy.

"The Marilyn Monroe of hormones," as some have described estrogen, does more than give a woman curves, soft skin, thick hair, and red lips. As a "sex" hormone, estrogen does indeed endow women with a sumptuous sensuality by maintaining the health of the genitals and promoting vaginal lubrication during intercourse. But as researchers have documented, estrogen does not seem to stimulate aggressive or overt sexual desire; rather, it encourages female receptivity to sexual overtures. In animals, this means assuming a sexually receptive stance—something even a male laboratory rat will do if given high enough doses of estrogen. In women, estrogen's effect is more subtle. As one sex educator puts it, as estrogen rises during the menstrual cycle (as discussed in Chapter 7), it "quietly, gently and unobtrusively" puts out the sexual welcome mat—just in time for ovulation.

Estrogen's impact extends beyond sex and reproduction to virtually every part of a woman's body—strengthening bones, fostering the growth of brain cells, blocking platelets that can clog arteries, altering insulin metabolism, and stimulating production of protective immune cells. By acting on the liver to produce more of the beneficial form of cholesterol known as high-density lipoprotein (HDL), estrogen protects against damaging plaque in a woman's arteries. This favorable effect on blood fats has a practical purpose: It keeps fatty acids circulating in the bloodstream, where they provide a ready supply of glucose during pregnancy. Similarly, by making blood vessels more elastic, estrogen allows a woman's blood volume to expand during pregnancy without causing a dangerous rise in blood pressure.

Although endocrinologists often argue that estrogen is a female's best friend, it can be a fickle one. Estrogen may contribute to a host of medical problems, including autoimmune disorders, asthma, migraine headaches, fibroid tumors, and cancers of the breast, ovary, and uterus. Some of these problems, such as migraines and asthma, flare up as estrogen fluctuates during the menstrual cycle. Others, such as fibroids, diminish when estrogen falls during pregnancy or after menopause.

The length of her exposure to estrogen over the reproductive years—determined by age at menarche and menopause as well as number of pregnancies—may affect a woman's likelihood of developing breast cancer. The longer estrogen's reign, the greater the statistical risk. Long-term estrogen replacement after menopause, an intensely controversial treatment discussed in Chapter 10, adds to this risk—yet epidemiological studies have shown it to be so beneficial to a woman's other systems that, in statistical analyses, it extends life span by an estimated 20 to 37 percent.

At every age, estrogen's influence throughout the body is more pervasive than endocrinologists once guessed. Some tissues, like bone, breast, and blood vessels, not only react to estrogen in the bloodstream but also generate extra supplies locally, using an enzyme called aromatase to convert hormone precursors into estrogen. Two distinctive types of estrogen receptors (alpha and beta) have been located in unexpected places, including the lungs, kidneys, intestines, bladder, and colon—and not just in women.

Estrogen receptors appear in male testes as well as in the very cells that give rise to sperm and regulate fertility in the male. Male mice lacking in estrogen receptors are infertile, with defective sperm and low sperm counts. As experiments with laboratory rats have shown, estrogen actually gives sperm their "reproductive punch" by regulating fluid reabsorption in the efferent ductules, small tubes that produce concentrated semen. Without reabsorption, sperm would remain diluted and incapable of normal maturation.

As men age and their androgen levels decline (though not as precipitously as a woman's sex hormones), their "friendship" with estrogen grows closer. By age seventy-two, according to one study comparing hormonal profiles of the elderly, men have three times the amount of circulating estrogen in their blood as women who do not take replacement hormones.

So vital is estrogen to both sexes throughout life that in all the medical literature there is only one report of an individual described as "deaf to estrogen's call." This man's body produces normal amounts of estrogen but lacks the receptors that allow estrogen to communicate with other cells. At age twenty-eight, when he first sought medical attention because of problems walking, he had reached a height of six feet eight inches and was still growing—and outgrowing his size 19 shoes. Without estrogen, the tips of his long bones had never hardened to halt further growth—a form of closure that happens at about age eighteen in most boys. His bones, deprived of the strengthening that estrogen provides, were as weak and porous as those of a postmenopausal woman of advanced age; his knees were so knocked that his legs splayed outward. Yet in other ways, from beard to body parts, he was completely masculine. His existence proves that life is possible without estrogen (or at least estrogen receptors). However, our bones and bodies are far healthier with it.

So too are our brains. To an extent no one had anticipated, one of estrogen's primary targets is our seemingly asexual organ of thought. This influence begins before birth and extends until death. Estrogen receptors appear throughout the brain, including areas such as the hippocampus and cerebral cortex that have little to do directly with sexual differentiation or reproduction but a lot to do with learning and memory. Estrogen promotes the growth of neurons, including the development of axons, fibers that carry nerve impulses away from the bodies of these cells, and dendrites, the tiny branches that extend outward to receive impulses from other neurons.

In late life, estrogen may preserve the brain's health and help maintain memory and cognition. Neuroscientists now speculate that the male brain's conversion of testosterone into estradiol may account for the much lower rates of Alzheimer's disease (a cognitive disorder marked by impaired memory and thinking) among older men than women. According to several small studies, women taking estrogen replacement therapy are less likely to develop this form of dementia. In some reports of women with mild to moderate cases, estrogen replacement has temporarily improved their ability to concentrate and remember. (See Chapters 10 and 11 for more on this subject.)

Estrogen influences mood as well as mind. "We used to bring transsexual men scheduled for sex-reversal surgery into the hospital for several days of evaluation prior to the operation," recalls psychiatrist Louann Brizendine, who heads the hormone evaluation unit at the University of California, San Francisco. "Every morning they'd line up eagerly for what they called their 'happy pills'—estrogen tablets." Estrogen seems to boost spirits by stimulating the production of receptors that respond to serotonin, a key regulator of mood. In women, low levels of estrogen and serotonin may be linked to depression and other mental disorders (see Chapter 13). In some women who become mildly depressed before or at menopause, when estrogen levels decline, estrogen replacement may restore their sense of well-being or bolster the effects of antidepressant drugs.

At a medical symposium on hormone replacement, a male physician in the audience stood up to make a comment. "If there's one thing about women that I envy, it's estrogen," he said. "If there were a safe way for men to take estrogen supplements, I'd be first in line." He's not the only one. The newest findings about estrogen, Legato notes, "are so exciting that several of my male colleagues are monitoring their own estrogen levels." They expect someday to use an analogue of estrogen that would target only certain organs, such as the heart or brain, without affecting other parts of their bodies. It could be the start of a whole new friendship.

His Hormone, Her Body

In the early twentieth century, scientists went searching for what they called "male essence"—the mysterious substance that made roosters crow and antlers grow. One German research team distilled 25,000 liters of urine from policemen and ground up 2,000 pounds of bull testicles in its quest. Finally, in 1935, Dutch scientists isolated the steroid hormone testosterone from the testes of mice. Although initially heralded as "medical dynamite," this macho molecule lost some of its panache when scientists realized that the "big T," as it's abbreviated, isn't just guy stuff. Women's adrenal glands and ovaries also produce testosterone—although in smaller quantities. The average man has about sixty millionths of an ounce of testosterone circulating in his body at any time. Women have only a tenth as much, an average of six millionths of an ounce. Yet this potent hormone may affect everything from a woman's personality and energy levels to her sex drive, muscle mass, and bone density.

The effects start before birth—in surprising ways. In boys, prenatal testosterone slightly inhibits the growth of the left side of the cerebral cortex, and the right side grows more rapidly. As discussed in Chapter 11, both sides of a girl's brain may develop more equally. But prenatal testosterone may also have more subtle effects on a female fetus.

A girl with a fraternal twin brother, exposed to "his" androgens in the womb, hears just like a boy—no worse than he does, but not as well as other girls. Studies of mixed-sex and same-sex twins have shown that sisters in sister-brother pairs often rank higher in "sensation-seeking" traits, such as taking greater physical risks, than those in sister-sister pairs or girls in general. Some scientists who also happen to be parents of girl-boy twins report, based solely on personal observation, that they see other differences in their daughters that could reflect their exposure to prenatal testosterone—most often an assertiveness (*bossy* is the word they use) that often makes the girl the dominant twin.

Prenatal testosterone also may play a role in the first biological characteristic ever to be linked to sexual orientation in women. Recently researchers at the University of Texas, in a small study, found that the eardrums of lesbian and bisexual women respond to clicking sounds, such as the tapping of a pencil on a desk, with echolike waves that are weaker than those produced by heterosexual women, though stronger than those found in men. This seems to be an effect of prenatal androgen. Could male hormones in the womb also influence female sexual orientation? No one knows, although this controversial finding—which has yet to be confirmed in larger studies—represents the first physiological evidence of a possible connection.

Testosterone flexes its muscles again before puberty, when a girl's adrenal glands churn out testosterone and other androgens that spur the growth of her long bones and strengthen her muscles. From puberty on, the female adrenal glands produce a steady supply of testosterone, while the ovaries, which manufacture roughly the same quantity, vary their output week by week throughout the menstrual cycle. Testosterone spikes at the same time as estrogen—roughly at midcycle or ovulation. In women with high baseline levels of testosterone (20 to 60 nanograms [ng]/deciliter [dl] is considered a normal range), their midcycle peaks may bring them close to those of low-testosterone males.

In the body of a man, testosterone plays many roles, including—as mentioned earlier—the production of estrogen. As noted before, through a simple chemical maneuver called aromatization, the male brain, which contains more receptors for estrogen than testosterone, converts testosterone into estradiol. While male testosterone levels follow both a circadian (daily) and seasonal cycle, they also soar and plummet depending on where a man is and what he's doing. Put a man under the stress of boot camp, parachute training, or prison, and his testosterone will fall. Challenge him to a tennis or chess match, and his testosterone will rise. If he loses, his testosterone will sink. If he wins, it'll climb. Little is known about such short-term blips in testosterone in women—with one exception. A team of Finnish and Japanese researchers has found that a woman's testosterone level rises after alcohol consumption.

In men, researchers have reported that baseline levels of testosterone tend to be higher in actors and football players than in ministers—and in juvenile offenders, substance abusers, rapists, and bullies. Statistics indicate that high-testosterone men are less likely to marry and, if they wed, more apt to divorce. Yet in all these studies, it's not exactly clear which comes first: Does extra testosterone lead to certain careers, to violence and crime, even to bachelorhood, or do these ways of living themselves jack up a man's testosterone?

The few studies (small, controversial, and far from conclusive) that have looked at women's testosterone levels and their career choices are even murkier. In one study of thirty healthy young women followed through the menstrual cycle, the high-testosterone women were the most sexually responsive and career-oriented. Yet, although their lives were filled with interesting pursuits, they (like high-testosterone men) reported more trouble with their personal relationships than those with lower levels.

A particularly intriguing investigation of mothers and daughters followed up a Kaiser-Permanente Medical Foundation research project that had frozen blood samples from pregnant women in the 1960s and then kept track of their children for more than thirty years. Researchers at the University of North Carolina interviewed and obtained blood samples from 350 adult daughters of the women in the original study, asking a range of questions about behavior and lifestyle.

The high-testosterone mothers, it turned out, tended to have high-testosterone daughters, who were less likely to have children and were less enamored of the whole notion of parenthood. The daughters with lower testosterone levels expressed much more interest in family, dressing up, cooking, jewelry, and interior decorating. Yet, as with the men, it's not clear which came first—the hormone level or the personal and professional preferences.

Some historians speculate that Queen Elizabeth I—childless yet amorous, with scanty periods, a spunky spirit, and a receding hairline—may have had unusually high testosterone levels. If so, Elizabeth, who often padded her torso to look larger and lamented that she had "the body of a weak and feeble woman" but "the heart and stomach of a king," probably would have relished the notion.

Although few contemporary women have any idea of their testosterone output, those who discover that these levels are higher than average often take a curious pride in this fact. One women's health advocate conjectures that her high levels of testosterone may account for her feistiness in confronting policy makers. A friend of mine speculates that her high testosterone might explain why everyone in her office says she thinks like a man. A San Francisco newspaper columnist openly yearns for an extra "skosh of testosterone" to help overcome "the second-class citizen habits" of her upbringing, including such seemingly instinctive female responses as shrinking in size and spunk in the presence of a domineering hulk of a man.

Yet while a dollop of extra testosterone may have a certain appeal to women, too much can be hazardous. By some estimates, 15 to 30 percent of women have medical problems caused by overproduction of testosterone or excessive sensitivity to androgens. If testosterone levels rise above 100 to 120 ng/dl, symptoms such as oily skin and facial hair (sometimes heavy enough to require shaving) develop. In time a woman may experience other adverse effects, including balding, infertility, diabetes, high blood pressure, and cancer of the uterus.

Too little testosterone also can be problematic for women, particularly for their libidos. In both sexes testosterone serves as the primary fuel for sexual desire. When a man's testosterone drops to a certain level, he loses interest in sex—though not the capacity for performance. In extensive studies in Canada and Great Britain, women who had their ovaries removed typically reported a loss of libido, as well as a decline in sexual fantasies and intercourse. Estrogen replacement did not restore sexual interest; testosterone supplements, widely prescribed in these countries, did. (This is discussed further in Chapter 10, on menopause.) However, there can be unwanted side effects—acne, facial hair, and potentially harmful changes in blood fats and liver function—as well as beneficial increases in muscle mass and bone density.

With aging, the balance of hormones shifts in both sexes. Just as estrogen takes on new significance for men, "his" hormone may exert more influence as "her" estrogen levels decline. The cells in the ovaries that manufacture testosterone generally outlive the estrogen-making cells, and their output may account for the spurt in energy commonly known as "postmenopausal zest." Even when the ovaries finally shut down production, the adrenals continue to supply testosterone, a hormone that many women are glad to claim as a special friend.

The Weaker Vessel?

They play sports no woman ever participated in a few decades ago. They swim farther faster than any man. Over courses a hundred miles long, they run male challengers into the ground. If Shakespeare had even imagined women like today's female athletes, he might never have borrowed the phrase of the Apostles Paul and Peter and referred to the female sex as "the weaker vessel." In his time, of course, and for centuries thereafter, the very thought that a creature as frail as a woman might attempt a feat as formidable as swimming the channel separating England from France—let alone do it faster than any man—was unthinkable.

At the debut of the modern Olympic Games in Athens in 1896, it still seemed inconceivable that a woman would dare to compete—even though a Greek runner named Melpomene did sneak into the Games and finish the marathon. When women ran in their first official 800-meter race in the 1928 Olympics in Amsterdam, several of the nine competitors collapsed in the heat, prompting newspaper editors to observe that "even this distance makes too great a call on feminine strength" and to pronounce distance running a violation of natural law—not to mention being unladylike in the extreme.

Today both ladies and gentlemen marvel as female athletes achieve levels of performance once thought impossible for women. Their performances not only keep getting better, but they're improving at a rate much more dramatic than men's. Since 1955 women's times in the marathon—an event added to the Olympic roster only in 1984—have dropped by 61 percent, compared to 18 percent for men. In other running events, women, who once ran about 20 percent slower than men, have pared the difference to just 10 percent. In swimming, the time differences are even smaller.

How is it that some women today can swim, run, ski, or skate faster than any man could a few decades ago? The reason is not that men are getting slower or weaker; women are the ones becoming stronger and speedier. In the process they are redefining the potential of the female body.

Will women athletes ever catch up or even surpass men? It depends on the sport they choose. In some endurance events, such as ultramarathon running and long-distance swimming, some women already outperform almost all men. In other sports, it remains unlikely that the gender gap in athletic performance will ever close completely. The reasons lie within the bodies of each sex.

The classic advantage that men bring to athletics remains size. Their bigger hearts pump more blood with each beat. Their larger lungs take in 10 to 20 percent more oxygen. Their longer legs cover more distance with each stride. Their greater proportion of muscle generates more energy. The average adult male, as mentioned in Chapter 2, has roughly twice the percentage of muscle mass and half the percentage of body fat as a woman. If a man jogs along at 50 percent of capacity, a woman has to push to 73 percent of hers to keep up.

Overall, men are about 30 percent stronger, particularly above the waist. A woman's upper-body power is usually only half to two thirds that of an equally well-conditioned man, while her legs have about 70 percent of his strength. With training, a woman's leg strength, compared pound for pound, can equal or surpass a man's. However, the best female sprinters aren't likely to outrun the best males—for anatomic reasons. The angle of the upper leg bone (femur) to the pelvis is greater in a woman, so her legs are less efficient at running. But this doesn't mean she can't run very, very fast.

Differences in body fat and muscle also affect performance. Adult women have ten to fifteen more pounds of fat and forty-five pounds less muscle than men. Even with conditioning, women's bodies remain fatter. Female cadets at the United States Military Academy at West Point, stronger, fitter, and leaner than most women, have roughly twice the percentage of body fat (18 to 19 percent) as their male classmates (9 to 10 percent).

Women's smaller muscle mass also affects their potential strength. With muscle training, women will increase their strength and then plateau after four to six months, when they approach the limits of their genetic potential for improvement. Men continue to make progress for eight to twelve months. There is a similar limitation in aerobic conditioning. Although training improves oxygen capacity for both sexes, a woman's maximum oxygen intake remains less than that of an equally well-conditioned man.

There are advantages as well as disadvantages to female anatomy and physiology. Because they are shorter and smaller, women have a lower sense of gravity and better balance—pluses in sports like gymnastics and diving. Because their tissues and joints are more elastic (another of estrogen's gifts), women are more flexible. And in ways exercise physiologists are just beginning to appreciate, the body of a woman may be superbly designed—physiologically, biochemically, anatomically—to go the distance.

The longer a race—on land, water, or ice—the better women perform. In an analysis of world-record times in running, swimming, and speed skating, researchers at Northeastern University observed that in all three sports the superiority of men's performances diminished with increasing distance. A study of female and male runners, conducted at South Africa's University of the Witwatersrand, found that women were able to maintain a higher rate of exertion for longer periods at distances of ninety kilometers or greater. Another South African study showed that women ultramarathon runners—who run cross-country races of thirty miles or more—have greater resistance to fatigue than equally trained men.

What accounts for women's surprising stamina? The answer may lie in that most maligned form of body tissue: fat. According to studies at Ball State University, women are more efficient than men at using fat as an energy source—and they have a higher percentage of fat available for such use. It may be that by burning fat first, women can put off the depletion of their stores of carbohydrate energy that can cause overwhelming muscle fatigue.

Fat-burning efficiency isn't the only female physiological advantage in endurance events. Several recent studies suggest that women's higher levels of estrogen also may help to delay fatigue, prevent damage to muscles, and increase the delivery of oxygen to hardworking muscles. Another competitive edge, demonstrated in laboratory studies with mice, may come from within the cell itself, where female mitochondria—the cellular structures that serve as power plants for muscles—oxidize fatty acids faster than male mitochondria, making more oxygen available. In research at the Olympic Sports Medicine Center in Barcelona, women competing to become marathon runners for Spain showed no increases in free radicals, tissue-damaging compounds produced by oxygen metabolism, after completing a race. Their male counterparts did.

In the water, female fat has even more advantages. A woman's larger amount of hip fat makes her more buoyant, so her body stays higher in the water. It also insulates her from the cold, so her body temperature doesn't fall as much as a man's. This may explain why no man has managed to break the world record for swimming the English Channel, which was set in 1978 by Penny Dean.

Female performance may improve even more dramatically in coming years. Some coaches calculate that as much as 50 percent of the gap between women and men in athletic performance may be due to early experience and conditioning. In the past, athletic young women often had to break rules and ignore cautionary warnings to train for their sports.

The first woman to win an Olympic gold medal in the marathon, in 1984, American runner Joan Benoit Samuelson, recalls being denied her high school's award as most valuable athlete because she'd violated policy and practiced with boys in order to improve her times. In the past, the majority of girls never got a chance to develop the skills and sports sense that boys did. In the United States, this changed with the passage of federal Title IX legislation in 1972, which literally opened playing fields, gyms, pools, and tracks to all girls. At that time, only one of every twenty-seven girls participated in school sports; today one in three does. Given this equal and early opportunity, tomorrow's female athletes may perform at a level women today can't even conceive of.

Not very long ago no one could have imagined an athlete like Ann Trason, a distance runner who has beaten the world's best ultramarathon runners—female and male. In one twenty-four-hour mixed-sex endurance race, Trason ran 143 miles' worth of circles around a track—four miles more than the male runner-up. To Trason, a biochemist, the challenge of running over extremely long distances consists of three components: physical, mental, and endurance.

"Physical is the only gender-specific area," she says. "Men have more muscle mass, so the strongest man is always going to be stronger than the strongest woman. But I think the physical is only a small percentage of ultrarunning." More important to her is mental preparation, strategizing, problem solving, and dealing with taunts that women aren't up to the challenge. But when she hears that it's just like a woman to give up or slow down, she no longer gets upset. "I just run faster," she says.

Rewriting Destiny

They were students, mothers, lawyers, bartenders. None had been particularly athletic. Several were new mothers who had not gotten back to their prepregnancy weight. The forty-one civilian women who volunteered for a test of female physiological potential at the U.S. Army Research Institute of Environmental Medicine at Natick, Massachusetts, in 1995 were mainly interested in getting into better shape.

Many of the women had never exercised before. Most couldn't do a single push-up, run a quarter mile, or budge a fifty-pound barbell. For six months they worked out under supervision ninety minutes a day, five days a week. By the end of the test period, they could do anything a male recruit in the army might have to do: repeatedly lift forty-pound boxes to a height of fifty-two inches, jog two miles with a seventy-five-pound backpack, perform dozens of deep knee bends with a hundred-pound barbell on their shoulders. Their performance, as one colonel put it, was "awesome."

In its own way, this feat is as impressive as the astounding world records being set by women athletes. Members of the so-called weaker sex not only proved that they could meet or surpass male standards, but that the perfectly ordinary bodies of perfectly ordinary women had capabilities assumed to be beyond any female. The limitations the U.S. Army had once placed on women—like so many others in different places and times—turned out to rest not on actual sex differences but on the cultural interpretation of sex that we call gender.

Depending on the meaning various cultures give to gender, the body of a woman, with its unique and universal female biology, may be weaker or stronger, healthier or sicker, heavier or slimmer. Differences in the care and feeding of girls versus boys or the physical demands and restrictions placed on one sex or another profoundly affect individual growth and development. Feed girls less (as still happens in many poor nations), and they grow up sicker and weaker. Encourage boys to spend hour upon hour throwing a ball or shooting hoops, and they'll hone natural talents into outstanding skills.

Even the nature of work in a society can affect the physiology of gender. When she traveled through Bali, a culture that required little physical exertion of either sex, anthropologist Margaret Mead noted that the arms of the men were as soft as the women's. "If we knew no other people than the Balinese," she wrote, "we would never guess that men were so made that they could develop any muscle."

In centuries past, the same assumption might have been made of women—or at least of those of affluence and privilege who were spared decades of constant work, frequent neglect, and poor nutrition. When women did push the limits imposed by gender and class and tried to become more physical, there was an inevitable outcry. Catherine de Médicis shocked the French court when she took to riding sidesaddle—or, as the French put it, à l'amazone. (She is credited with designing caleçons or calzoni—underpants—to curtail complaints about immodesty and protect "those parts that are not for male eyes" in case of a fall.) In the nineteenth century, when women once again hiked up their skirts—this time to climb aboard the bicycle, then a male form of transportation—medical journals cautioned of potential danger to female physiology. Even in recent decades, whenever women trained for any "male" sports, they were warned of dire consequences—including such far-fetched ones as having their womb fall out or a mustache sprout above their lip.

Perhaps, given a long tradition of such cultural conditioning, it's not surprising that so many women—a third of American females—are sedentary. Yet there's absolutely no reason for women to stay that way, and every good reason for them to get moving. In the last two decades science has shown what good sense always suggested: that the body of a woman—no less than that of a man—is designed for action. While there may always be sex differences in athletic performance, there aren't any in physical fitness. A man may be taller, bigger, or stronger, but a woman can be just as fit and gain as much benefit from regular exercise.

As study after study confirms, no medication, no therapy, no diet, no quick fix can do more for the body of a woman than exercise. Regular workouts, whether they involve walking, jogging, swimming, cycling, or weight training, lower a woman's risk of heart disease, reduce the likelihood of cancer, strengthen her bones, improve circulation, help control weight, and enhance mood. Exercise may also lessen the risk of the disease women fear most—breast cancer. In a study of 25,000 Norwegian women, those who accumulated at least four hours of exercise each week lowered their risk of developing breast cancer by 37 percent.

Ultimately, exercise and healthful habits can do more than prevent illness and enhance women's physical well-being: They can change our sense of our possibilities. Too often gender roles and restrictions have kept women from taking full possession of their female forms. Like short-term renters, we women settle into our bodies tentatively, agreeing to as-is terms and investing little energy in making them stronger and healthier. Yet as owners, we have the prerogative of literally rewriting what once was thought to be part of the biological destiny of our gender.

Consider, for instance, the bones that hold up the female body and put it into motion. Bone tissue is constantly being remodeled, with osteoblasts building up underlying structures and osteoclasts tearing them down in a precisely choreographed cooperative endeavor. At about age thirty in women, the balance between bone construction and bone destruction shifts almost imperceptibly, and bone loss begins to exceed bone formation, although at different rates in different parts of the body. At menopause, this process accelerates, and a woman's risk of fractures and of osteoporosis rises steadily. But this fate is not inevitable.

Although the skeletons of African-American women are more durable than those of Asians and Caucasians, women of all races can build stronger and longer-lasting bones. Scientists have learned that there is a window of opportunity, stretching from childhood into young adulthood, when girls and women have within their power the chance to increase their maximum bone density by as much as 20 percent.

Only two factors are essential: calcium and exercise. Adequate calcium strengthens a woman's bones and lowers her risk of fractures by as much as 60 percent. And exercise, particularly when started early and continued through life, can also improve bone health. According to Purdue University researchers, women in their thirties who played sports in high school have hip bones that are 7 percent denser and have 5 percent more bone mineral overall than those who stayed on the sidelines. But even women beyond age seventy who perform regular strength training may be able to halt bone loss, enhance bone density, and—as an added bonus—revitalize their energy.

Not long ago a fiftyish friend of mine—well past the prime time for bone building—was horrified to discover that she'd lost so much bone mass, she was considered at high risk for fractures. "What am I supposed to do, stay in bed for the rest of my life?" she asked. In fact, doctors recommended the opposite: regular exercise along with some of the new medical therapies that can help rebuild fragile bones. It's never too late, she learned, for women to strengthen both muscles and bones.

This is good news indeed. Since our biology makes us female to the bone, what better place to start building a healthier, fuller range of options for our gender than the skeleton that carries us through our lives? And what better way to start appreciating the body of a woman the way it truly was meant to be—from the inside out?

CHAPTER 5

The Invisible Patient

In an elegant farmhouse overlooking fields of vines, the owners of a Sonoma County winery hosted a dinner party for physicians and their partners. As the men trudged off to tour the grounds, we women gathered on the deck to watch the last rays of the sun turn the coastal hills to gold.

In the fading twilight, the topic turned to our bodies and our health, to the ways we'd been told that it was just like a woman to feel and function and the very different ways we actually do. A competent, confident attorney recalled how doctors had dismissed her complaints of fatigue and depression as all in her head—until tests revealed a thyroid malfunction. A corporate executive told of suffering a seizure after taking a medication she later learned had been tested only in men. A saleswoman in her fifties described her surprise at learning that the strict no-fat diet she'd been following along with her husband was doing her little if any good. Finally a busy obstetrician shook her head: "I never learned about any of these things when I was in medical school fifteen years ago. But what amazes me is that there's still such a huge gap between what's known about women and what we need to know."

"Well, if *you* think there's an information gap, what

about the rest of us?" quipped another woman. "We're talking Grand Canyon."

We are indeed. "What we don't know about women's health is appalling," declares Phyllis Greenberger, executive director of the Society for the Advancement of Women's Health Research. What is still more shocking is that it has taken so long for medical science even to ask. Despite the fact that women make two thirds of all health care decisions, see doctors more often, undergo more tests and procedures, take more medications, fill more hospital beds, and spend two out of three health care dollars, ours is the gender that medicine has long ignored.

The traditional prototype for medical training and research has been the 180-pound white male. His blood pressure, heart rate, and white or red blood cell count defined "normal." Diagnostic tests, laboratory values, prescription medications, and surgical techniques were developed with him in mind. This single-sex focus has proven dangerous, even deadly.

According to the American Medical Association's Council on Ethical and Judicial Affairs, women often have not been evaluated as thoroughly or treated as effectively as men. A woman is less likely to receive clot-dissolving drugs if she has a heart attack or to undergo "aggressive" procedures, such as cardiac catheterization and bypass surgery. If she has kidney disease, she is less likely to receive dialysis or a transplant. Even though lung cancer kills more women than any other malignancy, doctors do not advise diagnostic screening for women as often as they do for men.

This isn't coincidence. Until very recently a discriminatory attitude was "literally taught in medical school," says Nancy Dickey, president of the American Medical Association. "When I went to medical school in the 1970s, women were not valued as much as men. We learned that if a woman had chest pain, she was anxious. If a man did, he had a heart problem."

Even today neither women nor their doctors may be aware of their greatest health threats. In one survey, 40 percent of women identified breast cancer as the number-one killer of American women—as did 22 percent of physicians. In another, 61 percent of women surveyed by the National Council on Aging said they most feared cancer; only 9 percent mentioned heart attack. In fact, heart disease accounts for about 30 percent of women's deaths each year; breast cancer is responsible for just 3 percent. In women over age fifty, heart disease causes 53 percent of deaths.

Women themselves realize they aren't taken as seriously as male patients. In a survey by the Commonwealth Fund, a philanthropic foundation that often focuses on health issues, one in ten women said her doctor would have treated her differently if she were a man; one in four reported feeling patronized or talked down to by physicians; two in five (double the figure among men) have switched physicians because of dissatisfaction with their care. Ever more vocally, women, who've come a long way in so many fields, are demanding that the health care professions catch up.

Why Women Live Longer

Gender, the Women's Research and Education Institute contends, is the single most important factor in predicting a person's life expectancy—more important than race, income, education, or lifestyle. And throughout the industrialized world, the gender that lives longer—by an average of 5 to 10 percent of total life span—is female.

"It's a myth that men mature and women rot," says biologist Estelle Ramey, a pioneer in hormone research, who cites insurance industry statistics indicating that every year, for every 100,000 Americans, 803 men and just 447 women die. The gender difference in mortality rates emerges from the moment of conception. Baby girls are less likely to die in the womb or after delivery than baby boys. Once past age thirty, women consistently outnumber and outlive men. By age eighty-five, there are three women for every man.

This was not always so. Through much of time, the odds favored men—but almost entirely because giving birth so often meant losing life. In ancient Rome, 5 to 10 percent of pregnancies ended in the mother's death. In the Middle Ages, only 39 percent of women, compared with 57 percent of men, lived to the age of forty. Women began to live longer—if they survived childbirth, longer than men—by the end of the eighteenth century. By 1900, the average American woman could expect to live to an age of 50.9 years, compared with 47.9 years for a man. By 1950, women's projected life span had grown to 71.1 years; men's, to 65.6.

According to the National Center for Health Statistics, life expectancy for American women now stands at about eighty, a record high; for men, it's about seventy-three. In other developed nations— Australia, Canada, France, Greece, Italy, Japan, Netherlands, Norway, Spain, Sweden, Switzerland—women live up to two or three years longer than those in the United States, and about seven years longer than men. In the former Soviet Union, life expectancy for females is thirteen years longer than for males. By the year 2020, according to current projections for the United States, the average woman's life may increase by ten years—the average man's, by just six.

Why do men die sooner? "Maleness is a biological risk factor," Ramey contends. "Women have a terrific biological advantage over men. The female of every species of mammals resists stress better than the male, performs better when it comes to chronic physical demands, and outlives the male even when the environment is the same."

As discussed in Chapter 4, the female edge may begin at conception with the extra X chromosome, which provides a backup for defects on the X gene and a double dose of the genetic factors that regulate the immune system. Our other biological ace is estrogen, which, in addition to bolstering immunity, also protects heart, bone, brain, and blood vessels. In contrast, testosterone may blunt immune response—possibly to prevent attacks on sperm cells, which might otherwise be mistaken for foreign invaders. When the testes are removed from mice and guinea pigs, their immune systems become more active.

In men, lessened immunity may lower resistance to cancer as well as infectious disease. Half of all men—compared with a third of women— develop cancer. (Smoking, which for a long time was much more prevalent among men, accounts for some of this difference.) In some cancers, estrogen may somehow protect against distant metastases. This may be why women have a 12 percent lower death rate from cancer of the stomach and lung than do men and a 33 percent greater chance of surviving malignant melanoma.

Testosterone also has been implicated in men's risk of heart disease. Originally designed to equip men with an instantaneous burst of power—essential for survival in Stone Age times—this potent male hormone may surge so intensely that it wreaks havoc throughout the cardiovascular system. Decades ago, in classic laboratory studies of the impact of stress, Ramey forced female and male rats to swim continuously. The males started off strong but sank to the bottom early, while females kept paddling for as long as twelve days. If they were given testosterone injections, the females drowned as quickly as the males. If the males received estrogen, they swam longer.

Men—some men, particularly young ones—also act more self-destructively. Compared to women, they are far more prone to getting into fights, committing crimes, experimenting with illicit drugs, drinking heavily, and driving dangerously. Overall, men are three times more likely than women to die in accidents, mainly in cars and on the job, and four times more likely to die violently. Nine in ten murderers—and eight in ten murder victims—are men. Young men get hooked on drugs and alcohol two times as often as young women. Twice as many men as women die of cirrhosis of the liver; men account for eight in ten deaths from illegal drugs.

Unfortunately, the gender gap in living dangerously is narrowing. About one in four—23 percent—of American women smoke, and lung cancer rates in women have doubled since the early 1970s. Lung cancer now kills more women than any other cancer. Between 1979 and 1993 the death rate for chronic respiratory diseases such as asthma, emphysema, and bronchitis more than doubled for women.

"Women who smoke throw away many of their biological aces," notes Ramey. They have twice the risk of heart attack of other women and two to four times the risk of sudden cardiac death. Their risk of cervical cancer doubles, and they experience menopause as much as two years earlier than other women, thereby increasing the long-term danger of osteoporosis or heart disease. Smokers on birth control pills multiply their risk of a stroke or heart attack by twenty to forty times; women are urged to quit before they begin using oral contraceptives. While women sometimes justify smoking as a means of controlling their weight (on average, cigarettes keep a woman's weight about six pounds below what it might be otherwise), the danger of smoking is as great as being fifty to a hundred pounds overweight.

Drinking like a man also takes a greater toll on a woman's body.

Heavy drinking increases women's risk of heart disease, breast cancer, infertility, menstrual problems, and osteoporosis. Even though men are five times more likely to become alcoholics, women are more sensitive to alcohol's effects and become dependent on alcohol more rapidly. Once dependence develops, they are more likely than men to suffer alcoholic hepatitis, cirrhosis of the liver, and premature death. (Chapter 13 discusses drinking problems in women.)

Is There a Female Advantage?

Not everyone sees women's longer life span as a bonus. It's not that women live longer, some argue, but that they take longer to die. Disease, in fact, spares no one. The sexes differ primarily in their susceptibility to specific illnesses. Before age fifty, men are prone to more lethal diseases, including heart attacks, cancer, and liver failure. Women show greater vulnerability to chronic but non-life-threatening problems such as arthritis, osteoporosis, and autoimmune disorders.

According to the U.S. National Center for Health Statistics, each year women spend 35 percent more days than men in bed because of serious but nonfatal health conditions, such as gallstones, colitis (inflammation of the colon), and anemia. As women age, they're more prone to other chronic problems. In a Commonwealth Fund survey, more than 80 percent of American women age sixty-five to eighty-five suffered at least one persistent illness. However, women and men spend similar proportions of their lifetimes—about 81 percent—free of disability. For men, whose life spans are shorter, this translates into an average of 58.8 years; for women, 63.9 years.

Throughout life, some of the aspects of female biology that confer a certain advantage can also put women at a disadvantage. Our "lustier" immune system, as Ramey describes it, can overreact and turn on our own tissues. This may be why, on average, three of four people with autoimmune disorders, such as rheumatoid arthritis, multiple sclerosis, Hashimoto's thyroiditis, and scleroderma, are women, and why allergic women are twice as likely to experience potentially fatal anaphylactic shock.

Female hormones have negative as well as positive effects. Fluctuations in estrogen may cause flare-ups in asthma, manic-depression (bipolar disorder), and seizure disorders during a woman's menstrual cycle. This hormone also can make a woman's head ache. Migraines are three times more common in women, affecting an estimated 15 to 17 percent of women (compared to 3 to 6 percent of men), and their frequency increases with puberty, pregnancy, and the use of oral contraceptives or postmenopausal hormone replacement. Women also suffer more tension headaches than men in all age groups, races, and educational levels. Those between ages thirty and thirty-nine have the highest rates.

Some unisex diseases, such as diabetes, afflict more women than men. More men develop ulcers and hernias; women are three to four times more likely to get gallbladder disease. Irritable bowel syndrome, the most common disorder of the digestive tract, affects women three times as often as men—and white women five times more than African-Americans.

A woman's urethra, just an inch and a half long—about five times shorter than a man's—allows bacteria easier access to the bladder and increases her risk of urinary tract infections and kidney disease. The impact of kidney disease on women and men also differs. Women whose kidneys fail are likely to suffer ovarian failure, which increases their risk of a particularly virulent form of bone-weakening osteoporosis.

Other diseases also affect a woman's skeleton, but in very different ways. "We've found that women, but not men, with hypertension have higher-than-normal bone densities in their lumbar spines, which is an advantage," says Legato. "Women with late-onset diabetes, but not men, also have less osteoporosis than normal subjects, perhaps because high levels of insulin may promote bone formation or retard bone destruction. We also know that for women, diabetes is a much graver risk for heart disease than it is for men. What do these things tell us? We're still figuring that out."

Yet for all the maladies that single them out, women actually die of the same killers that claim men's lives, though usually at a later age. Heart disease, stroke, and cancer—the same terrible trio that cuts down men in their prime—account for two thirds of women's deaths. Heart disease kills more women overall than any other disease—and, on an annual basis, almost equal numbers of women and men.

Race interacts with gender in complex, little-understood ways that affect any innate female advantage. However, so little is known about the impact of race that, at a recent medical conference, when a speaker displayed a slide summarizing the research findings to date on the course of common diseases in women of color, it was blank.

The life expectancy for a newborn African-American girl is 73.7 years, 5.8 years less than for a white baby girl. Throughout their lives African-American women are more vulnerable than white women to the diseases most often thought of as man-killers, including hypertension, high cholesterol, and heart disease. Twice as many black as white women die of strokes. The death rate for heart disease among middle-aged black women is 150 percent higher than among white women the same age; among those with diabetes, their death rate is 134 percent higher.

Breast cancer rates across all ages are 20 percent lower among African-American women, but of all black women diagnosed with breast cancer, 37 percent are younger than fifty—compared with 22 percent of white women. Mortality is significantly higher among African-American women who develop breast cancer at any age, which is a possible reflection of how social factors, such as economic barriers to diagnosis and treatment, can reduce or remove whatever advantage biology may bestow.

Women of all races are more likely than men to lack health insurance or access to health services. The lower a woman's income and education, the less her likelihood of getting important preventive services, such as an annual Pap smear or prenatal care. Even sexual orientation can have an unexpected impact on women's health. Lesbian women, frequently alienated by physicians who assume all women are heterosexual, tend to seek health care less often—thereby increasing the likelihood that serious illnesses may not be detected early.

One aspect of a woman's life has not proven disadvantageous to her health: her job. Once medical experts predicted that women who worked like men—just like those who smoked or drank like them—would start dying like men. This hasn't happened. As study after study has shown, working women generally are as healthy as—if not healthier than—women who remain at home. The exceptions are "pink-collar" workers in dead-end, low-paying positions, hit hardest by the stress of caring for a family and holding down an unfulfilling job. Their health might well improve if they did indeed work like men.

In an ingenious analysis, sociologists at Ohio State and Harvard Universities calculated the health effects on women of the modern man's work and lifestyle—including having a full-time job, earning a higher income, feeling greater control at work, doing less housework, and exercising more often and strenuously. Their conclusion: In a truly equal environment, women would be just as healthy as men for most of middle age (although less healthy in their twenties and thirties, the peak child-bearing years) and would surpass males in most measures of well-being at age fifty-four. What would happen to men's health if they had to live and work like women—juggling part-time jobs, earning less money, taking lower-ranking positions, doing more housework, caring for children, having little or no time for exercise or personal pleasures? No one's asked.

Unasked Questions

Not long ago, Marianne Legato recalls, a scientist reported his preliminary findings from tests of a new compound on laboratory rats—all male. "What happens in females?" she asked.

"The same," he replied.

"How do you know?" she inquired.

"Because females respond just like males," he answered.

"But how can you be sure if you haven't tested females?" she pressed. Flustered, he insisted that he "just knew."

"I couldn't understand how he could possibly be so sure," Legato says. "Then, finally, it dawned on me: Dolly the sheep wasn't the first clone, Eve was. This man still assumed that women are essentially small men." (No one ever thinks of the converse: men as large women.)

A lack of actual proof for their premises has never gotten in the way of medical experts' assumption that they "just know" the way women are. Aristotle "just knew" that women nursed their babies with blanched menstrual blood stored in their breasts. Medical illustrators in the Middle Ages "just knew" that women were duplicates of men with an inside-out penis for a vagina, an inverted scrotum for a womb, and testicles for ovaries. Voltaire "just knew" that "the delicacy of women's limbs render them ill-suited to any type of labor or occupation that requires strength or endurance." Physicians of the late nineteenth century "just knew" that removal of a woman's ovaries was the best way to "repair" mental disorders—the reason, according to an 1889 report from the U.S. Surgeon General, for 51 percent of such operations.

Even today doctors routinely perform tests, prescribe drugs, and recommend treatments on the assumption that they will be as effective and beneficial for women as for men. How do they know? The truth is they often don't. From 1977 to 1993 the FDA banned women of childbearing potential from participating in the safety tests of new drugs to prevent possible damage to their unborn children and reproductive capacity. To scientists, this offered an advantage: They did not have to take into account such messy variables as women's fluctuating hormones or monthly cycles. As exclusion of women from all sorts of medical testing became common, this ban extended even to women who'd undergone sterilization or were past reproductive age. In a further attempt to keep the science "clean," laboratory researchers experimented only on male animals. As a result, in the landmark studies that shaped many modern medical practices, females were written out—and off.

The landmark Multiple Risk Factor Intervention Trials (known, aptly enough, as Mr. Fit), which studied vulnerability to heart disease, the number-one killer of both sexes, included 12,000 to 15,000 men— and no women. The Physician's Health Study of the potential benefits of taking an aspirin a day to lower the risk of heart attack looked at 22,071 physicians—none of them women. A major evaluation of coffee intake and its impact on stroke and heart attack studied 45,589 men—and no women. Only in 1998 did researchers discover that HIV tests misstate a woman's need for treatment. Even when a woman and a man have the same amount of virus in their blood, the woman is at a more advanced state of infection and at much greater risk of developing AIDS. Incredibly, even a study of the impact of obesity on the risk of breast and endometrial cancer—female diseases—extrapolated from only male subjects.

Aging—something women do better, or at least longer—has been primarily studied in men. In 1958 the federally sponsored researchers who launched what was to become the Baltimore Longitudinal Study of Aging decided not to include women, even though they make up two thirds of the elderly and more than 70 percent of the old old (those over age eighty-five). The reason was what former congresswoman Patricia Schroeder, one of the first champions of women's health research, dubbed "the rest room excuse."

At the time, the investigators had to work out of a single room at the city hospital. The study participants had access to only one rest room, which they had to share with elderly male patients in an adjacent hospital ward. Rather than ask women subjects to use this facility during overnight evaluations, the scientists excluded them altogether. As the budget for this high-profile project grew, the researchers acquired more space—and more rest rooms. However, for twenty years their studies included no women—an omission that did not keep the scientists from entitling their initial four-hundred-page report *Normal Human Aging*.

The very fact that research never took women's menstrual cycling into account has created a black hole in scientific understanding of femaleness. We know that women's bodies work differently at various times of the month, that temperature fluctuates, that fluid volume and weight increase, and that food moves through the digestive system at different rates. But only recently have physicians realized that various diagnostic tests, including cholesterol and blood fat measurements, yield different results at different times of the month and that the timing of medical treatments during a woman's cycle can affect their efficacy—sometimes with life-or-death implications.

According to an intriguing report at an American Society of Clinical Oncology meeting, women who undergo breast cancer surgery during the second half, or luteal phase, of their monthly cycles (days 14 to 28) are twice as likely to suffer a recurrence as those who are operated on earlier in their cycles. Recent research suggests that women with insulin-dependent diabetes may have higher blood sugar levels during the luteal phase of their cycles because fluctuations in sex hormones affect insulin blood levels.

Many medications also have stronger or weaker effects at different times in a woman's cycle and may require adjustments in dosage. However, the doses of most medications—along with their safety and efficacy—have never been tested in women or studied across the menstrual cycle. This may account for the fact that adverse drug reactions, including ones as serious as seizures, are reported twice as often in women.

"More than half of the drugs prescribed today have been tested only in men," says psychiatrist Steven Dubofsky, of the University of Colorado in Boulder, who notes that because of differences in size, absorption, metabolism, and liver function, "there can be tremendous gender differences in both beneficial and adverse effects in women." Yet when Dubofsky tested an experimental medication for Alzheimer's disease, the research review committee banned female participants. "The reason was that women might become pregnant—although the average age in my study was eighty-two."

Even treatments for problems that are more common in women have rarely been tested in them. Research on aspirin's usefulness in preventing migraine headaches, which strike far more women, included only men. Appetite suppressants and diet drugs—used far more often by women—have been tested almost exclusively in men. Men traditionally were the sole subjects of tests of drugs to treat depression, a disorder that affects twice as many women.

The relatively few studies that have been done on pharmacokinetics (how a drug is absorbed) in women have identified potentially significant gender differences. Women metabolize propranolol, a medication used to treat cardiac arrhythmias, more slowly than men. Blood levels of Inderal, used for migraines or high blood pressure, rise higher in women. Other drugs, including acetaminophen and aspirin, several benzodiazepines (antianxiety agents), and lidocaine (a topical anesthetic and a treatment for certain arrhythmias), take longer to clear a woman's body.

Many medications also interact in ways that have a unique impact on women. Oral contraceptives—used by one in five American women between the ages of eighteen and thirty-four—can raise blood levels of some psychiatric drugs so high that a woman on the pill may require only a fraction of the standard dose. Other medications, such as the antiseizure drugs carbamazepine and phenytoin, may decrease the effectiveness of birth control pills and increase the chance of an unwanted pregnancy.

When scientists do study the effects of drugs or other treatments on women, they often learn much that can benefit both sexes. Consider the most significant exception to the no-females-allowed approach to health research, the Harvard Nurses' Health Study, which has followed 121,000 women for more than twenty years. Its participants, who have filled out questionnaires and sent in blood samples and even toenail clippings over all these years, have taught us much about many common health threats—some exclusively female, such as the risk of breast cancer from birth control pills (which seems minimal), and some universal, such as the most effective means of preventing colon cancer.

Yet any research investigation that excludes half the human race—female or male—shortchanges both genders. Learning about human health and longevity by looking only at men, one biologist points out, is like trying to run a successful department store by studying only those that went bankrupt. "More research on women is not a luxury to be indulged in only to pacify feminists, to secure the female vote, or to attract women to a hospital center," says Legato. "Studying women is not so much a service we offer them as an opportunity they offer medical science to improve health care at all levels." Researchers aren't doing women a favor by including them in research protocols. They're doing everyone a service.

The Yentl Syndrome

Felicia, an account manager at a New York advertising agency, worked like a man: Overstressed and underexercised, she put in long hours, smoked a pack and a half of cigarettes a day, and didn't pay much attention to what she ate. At age thirty-four Felicia noticed a burning sensation in her chest when she walked more than a block or two. "I stopped, and it stopped. At first I didn't think it was anything serious. I have a family history of high cholesterol, but I'd never even had a checkup."

Since it was winter, the peak of flu season, Felicia assumed she kept feeling worse because she'd come down with a bug. For ten days she shrugged off chest discomfort, breathlessness, and a throbbing headache. Then one day she walked around a corner in her office and couldn't catch her breath. That's when she got scared. Felicia called her brother-in-law, an intern at a local hospital. At his urging, she went to the emergency room. At first no one suspected a heart attack. "It wasn't like I clutched my chest and fell to the ground," she recalls.

Few women do. And because they don't get the classic symptoms of a heart attack, untold numbers of women complaining of breathlessness or vague pressure in their chest have been sent away from emergency rooms or told to stay home and lie down—advice that may have cost them their lives. Unfortunately, in order to get medical attention, a woman—like Yentl, the girl in Isaac Bashevis Singer's story who had to dress like a boy to study the Torah—has often had to get sick just like a man.

This false and dangerous assumption can occur with many illnesses, but the consequences may be most tragic with heart disease, which many still see as a "guy problem." It is not. Even among women in their forties, heart disease claims more lives each year than breast cancer. Yet a woman's heart, though vulnerable, usually doesn't ache or break like a man's.

Men typically develop the first signs of a heart ailment a decade earlier than women—at thirty-five rather than forty-five. Throughout the reproductive years, estrogen, indeed the best friend a woman's heart could have, prevents the buildup of atherosclerotic plaque in the arteries, boosts levels of the beneficial form of cholesterol, called high-density lipoprotein (HDL), and lowers heart-harming low-density lipoprotein (LDL).

However, estrogen is not a magic potion that guarantees total protection. As Felicia discovered, a woman who has a family history of cardiac disease, high blood pressure, or high cholesterol may develop serious problems even before she reaches menopause. As their estrogen levels fall at midlife, the risk of heart disease rises for all women. After age forty-five, one in nine women has some symptom of heart disease; by sixty-five, one in three does.

"Only in the last eight to ten years have cardiologists realized that heart disease in women has been understudied, underrecognized, underdiagnosed, and undertreated," says Legato. Since then, an explosion of new research has begun to unlock the secrets of a woman's heart. We now know that the same risk factors—high cholesterol, high blood pressure, and obesity—endanger both sexes, but they play out differently in women than men.

A healthy norm for a woman's cholesterol is ten points higher than a man's—210 versus 200 milligrams per deciliter—but this figure matters less than her HDL levels. And even then what's normal for a male may spell trouble for a female. "We don't know why, but women with an HDL under 45 mg/dl are at greater risk, while men don't seem to be at risk unless their HDL dips below 35," says Legato.

In women HDL is such a precise indicator of the heart's current and future health that some describe it as a cardiac crystal ball. Total cholesterol, on the other hand, presents a murkier picture—made more complex by menstrual fluctuations. LDL levels decline in the first half of a woman's monthly cycle. In pregnancy, LDL levels increase and remain high until birth. Oral contraceptives, even those with lower estrogen than the original formulations, raise LDL and lower HDL. Menopause brings a rise in LDL and a small decline in HDL. And after age fifty, other blood fats—the triglycerides—may be a more telling indicator of risk.

Unlike men, healthy women with high total cholesterol may not benefit as much from some cholesterol-lowering drugs, possibly because these medications cause a drop in helpful HDL as well as harmful LDL. In some studies, lowering total cholesterol by drugs, diet, or both, which does reduce the danger of dying in men, provided similar benefits only for women with actual heart disease. In other women, any treatment—dietary or drug—that pushed down a woman's HDL did little good.

Hypertension, or high blood pressure, a unisex risk factor, is more common in older women, but treating it may not be as beneficial as it is in men. "In men, reducing blood pressure by any means reduces the mortality risk by 15 percent," says Legato. "When we use blood pressure medications to lower mild to moderate hypertension in women, their overall risk of dying for any reason actually increases by 26 percent. We don't know why." A better alternative is exercise, which can bring blood pressure down without the adverse effects of medication and can help lessen another serious risk factor: obesity.

For women, extra pounds clearly spell extra danger. Even those who are moderately overweight (10 to 20 percent above their ideal weight) may have twice the risk of leaner women—particularly if they put on weight after age eighteen. In women who add a few pounds with every decade, the risk of heart disease increases—especially if the extra pounds lodge around the waist rather than in the hips and thighs. Apple-shaped women (and men) are at greater risk than pear-shaped ones because midtorso fat seems more likely to move to the bloodstream, where it can build up and clog arteries.

Women also have some unique risk factors, such as age at menopause. In a study of 12,115 Dutch women age fifty to sixty-five, the annual risk of heart disease dropped by 2 percent for every year they continued menstruating. Diabetes is twice as important as a risk factor for heart disease in women as men, and female diabetics have a greater risk of congestive heart failure than males.

Even when women and their doctors recognize that they are at risk, detecting early signs of a problem can be difficult. The first sign of heart disease in a man is usually a heart attack, complete with elephant-on-the-chest, squeezing pain. Women are more prone to "silent" symptoms: shortness of breath, fatigue, discomfort, pressure, nausea, weakness, or pain in seemingly unlikely places, such as the jaw. One woman in her forties had several teeth removed before a cardiologist finally discovered that the sharp twinges of jaw pain had nothing to do with her teeth. The real problem was that her heart was not pumping sufficient blood and oxygen, causing angina that radiated to her jaw.

One form of chest pain, microvascular angina, typically develops in middle-aged, overweight women with high blood pressure and high blood sugar. Notoriously hard to diagnose, women with this condition—sometimes referred to as "Syndrome X"—have no telltale signs of blocked arteries. Nonetheless, this ominous condition increases the risk of cardiac danger sixteen times over that of a healthy woman and six times over a man's.

Testing for this and for other types of heart disease in women remains problematic. Standard diagnostic tests, developed through studies in men only, are less precise in detecting heart disease in women. The traditional treadmill or exercise stress test, which records the heart rate during exertion, is the gold standard for evaluating men. But in women it produces a high rate of false positive (erroneously abnormal) results. A thallium stress test, which uses a radioactive isotope that shows up on an X ray, also is less accurate than in men. Cardiologists knowledgeable about gender differences in diagnostic testing generally recommend evaluation of the female heart with an echo stress test, an echocardiogram that uses sound waves to create a 3-D image of the heart at work.

If tests indicate a problem, the next step is an invasive diagnostic procedure called angiography or cardiac catheterization, in which a thin tube is channeled into the heart via an artery in the thigh or arm. As recently as a decade ago, ten times as many men as women (40 percent versus 4 percent) were referred for this definitive test. Women still remain much less likely to undergo angiography—a critical prerequisite for angioplasty (balloon surgery to unclog arteries) or coronary bypass surgery.

In the past, women undergoing heart surgery tended to be older and sicker, and their death and complication rates were much higher than men's (though they still fared better than women in comparable condition who didn't undergo surgery). More recent studies have found that advanced age and other medical problems, such as diabetes and hypertension, rather than sex itself, are factors that increase the danger. "We're finding that with earlier diagnosis and intervention and with careful surgical technique—crucial because of the smaller size of women's blood vessels—women can do as well as men," says Legato.

Yet women who have heart attacks still are less likely than men to survive over both the short run and the long term. A woman's risk of dying within a month of a heart attack is 75 percent higher than a man's, in part because of a delay in getting help. At the American College of Cardiology meeting in 1998, researchers reported that women typically take an hour longer to get to the hospital than men. And once there, they're often treated less urgently.

According to an analysis of large national databases in the United States, women are 31 percent less likely than men to get clot-dissolving drugs, one of the chief means of limiting the damage of a heart attack, or to receive standard medications like aspirin, the blood thinner heparin, or beta blockers. This gender gap in treatment may be one reason why the death rate for cardiovascular disease has declined faster for men than women in recent years.

However, some advances are offering more hope for women's hearts. Vitamin E intake, according to research in both sexes, can reduce the risk of coronary artery disease in women and men. New medications, such as the blood thinner integrelin, have proved especially effective for women. Women also get as much benefit as men from cardiac rehabilitation—an option that cardiologists often didn't even suggest for them in the past. Given the same opportunity to strengthen their hearts, women continue to show improvements for three years after they start an exercise program; men reach a certain performance plateau within months.

Felicia, whose right main coronary artery was 100 percent blocked, is a latter-day success story. A coronary angioplasty opened her blocked artery—temporarily. It's closed down twice since. "Fortunately, my body has grown its own bypass with new blood vessels. I'm much healthier than ever before: I quit smoking; I lost thirty pounds; I work out five or six times a week; I eat no fat. My cholesterol's gone from 480 to around 200. In a way, I'm lucky. I got a wake-up call that made me realize that women aren't immune to heart problems—and that there's a lot we can do to keep our hearts healthy."

"It's All in Your Head"

In the early 1980s, in her third year of medical school, Vicki Ratner, now an orthopedic surgeon in San Jose, developed unremitting pelvic pain along with extreme urinary frequency and urgency. When treatments for a urinary tract infection didn't work, she was referred from one specialist to another—fourteen in all. "They told me that it was all in my head, that I should find a new boyfriend, that I wasn't cut out to be a doctor, that the only solution was to quit medical school and settle down to a traditional lifestyle." She spent the last two years of medical school in unremitting pain, silently enduring symptoms she'd been convinced were psychosomatic.

Ratner's own search of the medical literature finally led her to an article on a disease she'd never heard of: interstitial cystitis (IC)—a bladder inflammation that typically develops in postmenopausal women. "I found fifty cases exactly like mine. I thought: 'This is it!' " But her urologist was so convinced she was too young for this problem that she had to beg for months to undergo a surgical biopsy, which ultimately confirmed her self-diagnosis. Ratner, who eventually found treatments that relieved her symptoms, went on to start a national organization dedicated to helping others with this condition—an estimated 450,000 Americans, almost all of them women. "The problem is that the symptoms of IC look like a urinary tract infection, but the standard diagnostic tests come back negative," says Ratner. And so women, even with severe pain and an urge to urinate up to sixty times a day, are often told the problem is all in their head.

These words—perhaps the most aggravating uttered by doctors—have echoed in women's ears for years. In a study using videotapes of patient visits, primary-care doctors referred men to medical specialists but suggested that women of the same age with identical symptoms and health histories see a psychotherapist. "There is a reflex in many members of the medical profession to think of women as more emotional," says Legato. "A woman is three times more likely than a man to be told that symptoms are all in her head."

One of her patients, a high-powered corporate attorney in New York City, had developed episodes of very rapid heartbeat at age twenty-five. Her heart would pound so fiercely for hours on end that she felt it would leap out of her chest. Doctor after doctor brushed off her complaints. "I was told that it was because I was working too hard, that I was drinking too much or drinking too little, that I was too anxious," the woman recalls. Finally she decided to attend a talk on women's hearts given by Legato.

"My heart started beating fast during the session, and Dr. Legato looked at me, listened to my symptoms, and said, 'You have a real problem, and you need treatment. I want you in my office tomorrow morning.'" Around-the-clock testing with a portable cardiac monitor revealed a textbook case of a disorder called Wolff-Parkinson-White syndrome, in which a tiny bundle of extraneous muscle cells in the heart causes potentially deadly disturbances in the heart's rhythm. Within two weeks of surgery to correct the defect, the attorney was back at work—and she's been feeling "absolutely sensational" ever since.

In twenty years of medical reporting, I've heard variations on this story dozens of times. It took seven years for one woman I interviewed, sandbagged by pain and fatigue, to discover the underlying problem was lupus erythematosus, an autoimmune disorder. Another woman, told that her bouts with diarrhea and stomach pain were wholly psychological, was eventually diagnosed with irritable bowel syndrome, a digestive malady that is three to five times more common in women. Other women, who'd developed genital burning, itching, and excruciating pain during intercourse, were told they were sexually repressed. Several years passed before they learned they had vulvodynia, a little-understood but treatable inflammation of the tissue that surrounds the opening to a woman's vagina and urethra.

Why are women's health complaints so often missed or dissed? "Rather than admitting they just don't know or don't have a test to document and quantify the problem, physicians deny that a problem exists," says Ratner. "They blame the patient by suggesting that the problem is stress-related or all in her head. And it can be hard for a woman to convince a physician that she's in excruciating pain if she looks healthy."

Pain, perhaps the most subjective of symptoms, has long been viewed as a troublesome female complaint. In studies in which women and men have been subjected to the same provocation, women generally give it a higher pain rating. Women also routinely report more pains in more places than men do and experience more pain following injuries such as fractures. The reason may lie in brain chemistry, which fluctuates with the menstrual cycle. Some pain problems, such as migraine headaches, often strike when estrogen, the neurotransmitter serotonin, and the soothing brain chemicals called beta endorphins are low. Many of the pain-that-has-no-name syndromes that doctors once dismissed as psychological have turned out to be real and specific—and to have actual names, including endometriosis, dysmenorrhea (menstrual cramps), fibromyalgia (a neuromuscular disorder), mitral valve prolapse, microvascular angina, vulvodynia, irritable bowel syndrome, and interstitial cystitis.

Yet even though these and other painful problems single out women, until 1996 no one had ever studied sex differences in response to pain medications. In a study of forty-eight women and men undergoing removal of their wisdom teeth, researchers at the University of California, San Francisco, discovered that a class of pain relievers called kappa opioids provided much greater and longer-lasting pain relief to the women. "Biologically men and women do not obtain pain relief in the same way," concluded chief researcher Jon Levine, who speculates that the reason may be sex differences in the number of receptors for this type of drug or in basic brain circuitry.

The female-friendly kappa opioids, which do not cause side effects such as sleepiness, nausea, confusion, and addiction (as codeine and morphine, both mu opioids, do), had all but been discarded prior to Levine's research. The reason: They'd been tested only in men—whose continuing complaints of pain after taking kappa opioids were never dismissed as all in their heads.

Is there any proof to back up the premise that it's just like a woman to seek care for phantom pains or trivial or nonexistent health problems? None at all. Researchers from the University of Amsterdam, in a five-year study of more than nine thousand female and male patients seeking primary care, found that fewer than 20 percent of women's "excess" visits involved vague physical symptoms with no known medical cause. The vast majority of the women who sought help had serious, legitimate problems that fully warranted medical attention.

The more frequent problem, says Ratner, is that physicians discount what women are saying so thoroughly that women come to doubt their own judgment. "There's something drastically wrong when male physicians are so ready to trivialize and negate women's experience," she says. "Women have to remember that they are the best judges of their own symptoms. Their lives may depend on it."

Becoming Visible

In 1970 some of America's most distinguished gynecologists—all male—testified before the U.S. Senate on a matter that would touch the lives of millions of women: a patient information insert for birth control pills. These learned experts contended that the insert should not include information on possible side effects and complications. If you caution of possible headache, several argued, it would be just like a woman to say the pill had given her one. If you discuss possible heart disease risk, it would be just like a woman not to use the pill at all. A noisy group of women marching outside disrupted the hearings to demand the full information women needed to make responsible, intelligent decisions about their fertility and their health.

The women won this political battle, one that many look back on as the opening salvo in a revolution that has since transformed women's health care. By making themselves visible and vocal, women have challenged and changed the American way of giving birth, the standard medical approach to breast cancer (which used to mean that a woman

anesthetized for a surgical biopsy might wake up with a radical mastec-
tomy), the once-soaring rates of cesarean deliveries and hysterectomies,
the use of potentially dangerous IUDs like the Dalkon shield, and the
medical profession's pervasive view of women as second-class citizens
deserving of only second-class treatment.

Times are changing indeed. "Never before have women meant so
much to so many," observed one report on the booming business of
women's health centers, which are sprouting up across the country. There
are journals, seminars, and associations for physicians interested in women's
health and for women interested in their own well-being. Women are
finally being recognized and treated with respect—partly because they
are the health care industry's biggest consumers, partly because they have
become too visible throughout society for anyone to ignore, particularly
politicians.

"Throughout life people are taught that if you're sick, you go to
the doctor for treatment," says Ratner. "The reality for women's health
is that it has taken a political act, sometimes an act of Congress, for the
medical community to sit up and listen." This is exactly what happened in
1989, when an investigation by Congress's General Accounting Office
documented the huge gender gap in medical research. At the time, only
14 percent of National Institutes of Health funds were earmarked for
women's research (it's since risen—but only to 16 percent), and NIH
employed more veterinarians than gynecologists (who numbered just
three).

Outrage over the GAO's findings eventually led to unprecedented
women's health legislation, a mandate for inclusion of female participants
in research studies, and the establishment of an Office of Research on
Women's Health. Other federal agencies—the Public Health Service,
the Centers for Disease Control and Prevention, the Food and Drug
Administration—have since created women's health offices, and federal
spending on women's health issues has increased more than sixfold.

But the agenda for women's research has come not just from the top
but also from the grassroots, particularly from women who decided to
make visible a disease their mothers and grandmothers would never have
discussed in public: breast cancer. In 1990 the United States spent about
ten times more on AIDS research than on breast cancer, even though
breast cancer claimed roughly six times as many lives. Through persistent

and highly public lobbying, breast cancer advocates won more and more funding for research—now more than $550 million a year.

Today no single women's health research project is more visible than the Women's Health Initiative, a fifteen-year, $625 million study that is following 164,500 postmenopausal women to assess methods of preventing heart disease, breast and colorectal cancer, and osteoporosis. Although criticized by many—for reasons such as excluding premenopausal women and not adequately integrating women of color into the study population—this project has already made an important statement. "Before it was hard for me to question the doctor, but I am getting much bolder now," says one seventy-two-year-old participant. "I've learned that women's ailments deserve attention." She's not the only one.

Not coincidentally, the increased visibility of women in research studies has paralleled their increased visibility in medical science. Rather than just complaining about doctors, women have *become* doctors. The number of women physicians has quadrupled in the last twenty years. Today, in more than twenty medical schools in the United States, women make up at least half of the student body. Overall, they represent 43 percent of all medical students. In other nations, the percentage is even higher—up to 75 percent in Argentina, for example.

Today's female medical students have come a long way from the 1870s, when the first women at the University of Edinburgh school of medicine were greeted with obscenities and mud flung by male students. Inside the lecture hall they found a sheep, another "inferior animal" seeking medical education. In France the first female doctor to demand to be allowed to serve an internship was burned in effigy by her classmates. The University of Michigan constructed walls so its first women students would not hear certain lecture material in the presence of men. In time, curtains replaced the walls and then gave way to a simple red line on the floor that served the purpose of keeping women in their place.

Although many medical schools have banned once-widespread pranks, such as tying pink bows around the penis of a female student's cadaver, sexism hasn't disappeared. In a 1998 analysis of surveys from 4,502 female doctors, nearly half reported some form of gender harassment, including unwanted sexual advances. And the subject of women's unique health needs still doesn't get the attention it deserves in medical school curricula.

"I sat in medical lectures, considering myself a feminist, and listened to professors explain that they couldn't study women because their cycles would ruin the science," recalls a physician who graduated from medical school in the 1980s. "I used to nod and think, 'They're right. We can't have women screwing up research.'" In a 1995 survey of graduating medical school seniors, 44 percent of the women—and 22 percent of the men—rated coverage of gender differences in medical conditions as inadequate.

Because of this lack, some physicians and policy makers are advocating creation of a primary-care specialty devoted to women's health that, like pediatrics, would offer comprehensive care tailored to the unique needs of female patients. Others argue that, rather than teaching some doctors a great deal about women, medical schools should make sure that all physicians know at least some fundamentally important things about them. The still-better option, says Legato, is integration of gender-specific information in physiology, anatomy, pharmacology, pathology, psychiatry, and other specialized fields into every aspect of medical teaching and training.

Whichever approach prevails, the focus on women isn't going to go away. One guarantee is what some call the "feminization" of the profession as more women enter clinical practice. As a medical reporter, I've interviewed hundreds of doctors of both sexes—more than enough to realize that gender alone doesn't guarantee empathy or competence. Some of the most caring and dedicated physicians I've met are men; a few of the most arrogant are women.

Yet on the whole, women "doctor" differently. For one thing, as demonstrated in videotaped sessions with patients, they listen more, smile more, and make more eye contact than their male colleagues. In one study, women doctors also spent more time with patients than men—23.5 minutes versus 18 minutes—and gave more positive feedback, offered more medical information, and tried harder to build partnerships with patients than male doctors did. According to other research, they perform Pap smears and breast exams twice as often as male physicians. And some women (I among them) feel that female doctors give gentler pelvic exams.

Female physicians also practice what they preach. In studies comparing their health-related behaviors with women in the general population, female doctors were less likely to smoke or drink heavily, more likely to undergo regular screening tests such as mammograms, and much more likely both to prescribe and to use hormone replacement therapy.

Do women patients want women doctors? In a *New York Times* poll, the majority of women said they'd prefer a female gynecologist (even though their own was more likely to be male), and younger women said they would trust a female doctor more. But what women want even more are physicians who know and appreciate women's health and medical needs.

In a survey by the Partnership for Women's Health at Columbia University, 87 percent of respondents said it's important for their doctors to know the differences in female bodies. And women want doctors—regardless of sex or specialty—to listen to them and to speak with them clearly and without condescension. There's something else we'd like as well: to be seen, really seen, as people as well as problems, as serious individuals whose concerns merit serious consideration.

After years of getting all my health care from a gynecologist, I developed a condition clearly beyond her expertise—aching wrists (a writer's occupational hazard). I gathered names of physicians and chose a well-respected internist, who happens to be a woman. After evaluating my wrist problem, she scheduled a complete physical for the following month. "Unless there's something else you're worried about that can't wait," she added. When I mentioned an odd growth I'd noticed on my back, she made a note to check it during my upcoming exam.

Almost out the door of the examining room, she turned around and said, "I can tell you're worried about it. Let's look right now." In a matter of minutes she'd checked out the mole, pronounced it benign, and moved on to her next patient. Would another doctor—a male one—have picked up on my unspoken anxiety? Would he have taken the time, there and then, to deal with it? I'm dubious. As I left my new doctor's office, feeling greatly relieved, I smiled and thought, "Now *that's* just like a woman."

PART TWO

The Dance of Life

There were seeds
within her
that burst at intervals
and for a little while
she would come back
to heaviness,
and then before a surging miracle
of blood,
relax,
and reidentify herself,
each time more closely
with the heart of life.
"I am the beginning,
the never-ending,
the perfect tree."

May Sarton,
" 'She Shall Be Called Woman' Part 10"

CHAPTER 6

Girls in Bloom

They cuddle koalas and pandas as they sleep, paint their fingernails midnight blue, forget to brush their teeth, and adore double fudge marshmallow ice cream cones with extra sprinkles. At home they sing in the kitchen; at school they giggle in the hallways; on their way across a courtyard, they burst into coltish leaps. Sigmund Freud described school-age girls as "little men," and they are indeed good fellows: cheerful, companionable, hardy, loyal—and feisty.

When I ask my daughter, Julia, and her "tween-age" friends whether they would choose to be girls or boys, they immediately answer, "Girls!" Who gets the better deal in life? Once again they chorus, "Girls." Why? Julia gives me an eye-rolling, how-could-anything-be-more-obvious look and replies, "Girls kick butt!" I resist the temptation to answer in retro-sixties speak and say, "Right on!" Yet at the same time I wonder: What will these spirited girls have to say a few years from now?

As our daughters—so lovely and loving—emerge from the protective cocoon we've spun around them, we parents worry. On the way to womanhood, a lamenting chorus tells us, girls become an endangered gender. They "hit the wall," as some researchers put it, and lose their sense of self. They silence their voices, take to the sidelines, drop out of science, lose ground in math. Their bodies become a battleground. They starve and binge, obsess over being too fat or too flat, tumble into the temptations of drugs, alcohol, and sexual experimentation.

This, we're warned, is what it's just like a girl to do these days. And so whenever parents of girls on the cusp of adolescence get together, we worry: Is the news all bad? Must girls shatter like mouth-blown glass in the seismic jolt of puberty? Will our daughters inevitably be short-changed at sports, passed over in the classroom, poisoned by a society that sets them up for sexual exploitation?

The truth about girls, just like the truth about women, is never that simple. But it may be even harder to get at because of popular untruths about adolescents of both sexes. "Teenagers have gotten a bad rap," says adolescent psychiatrist Lynn Ponton, of the University of California, San Francisco, who notes that the teen years usually are not a season in hell for girls, boys, or parents. As large-scale epidemiological studies have consistently shown, about 80 percent of teens successfully negotiate this life passage without significant trauma.

Adolescence itself may be as misunderstood as the young people passing through it. For our prehistoric ancestors, what we think of as a transition was a lifetime. Although no one knows for sure, some anthropologists speculate that our earliest ancestors may rarely have outlived their teens. For them, living fast, risking big, and never thinking about tomorrow—behaviors that seem immature these days—were survival strategies that may in fact underlie the typically adolescent urge to pack a lot into a short time.

Through most of recorded history, childhood was brief and ended abruptly. Young people often left their family homes before or soon after reaching sexual maturity. In the Middle Ages and Renaissance, a girl of noble blood might be betrothed and trundled off to her fiancé's household at seven or eight, married at twelve, and a mother by fifteen. Even before reaching their teens, her poorer peers might be sent away from home to work as servants, farmhands, or factory laborers. According to records from the eighteenth century, about 80 percent of European country girls left home at about age twelve—two years before their brothers—to earn money for their families and, if they were lucky, to scrimp together enough for a modest dowry.

The concept of "adolescence" as a distinct life stage didn't win scientific recognition until 1904, when an American psychologist, G. Stanley Hall, published a monumental book on the subject. Its very title—*Adolescence and Its Relation to Psychology, Anthropology, Sociology, Sex, Crime, Religion, and Education*—testifies to the scope and significance Hall accorded this transition. This newfangled notion expanded the years of childhood dependence, deferred the onset of adult obligations, and transformed families, schools, and other institutions.

Hall—an exponent of the nineteenth-century Romantic tradition—not only carved out new territory for this life stage but established that the terrain could be treacherous. Reflecting the Sturm und Drang perspective of his times, he conceptualized teens as tempest-tossed, impulsive individuals with "a peculiar proneness to be either very good or very bad."

Decades later we still think of teens as going to extremes, in ways that seem (and sometimes are) more perilous than ever. And we blame their behavior on almost everything: the raging hormones of puberty, the psychological forces that sabotage self-esteem, the social values that glorify danger. Yet what's often lost is the big picture, the view of adolescence as a normal biopsychosocial experience of astounding complexity, one that follows no one set pattern, that does not typically lurch between extremes, and that varies with the uniqueness of every adolescent—and with her or his gender.

Adolescence isn't inherently easier or harder on either sex; girls and boys each get their set of knocks. In terms of physical danger, boys are at greater risk—in large part because they put themselves there. Of the various "risk behaviors" that teens engage in, Ponton notes, boys "excel" at all but two: disordered eating and pregnancy (although, of course, they play an undeniable role in conception). Boys are more likely to drink and drive, to experiment with illegal drugs, and to engage in daredevil exploits. And perhaps because such showy behaviors have always drawn a lot of attention, boys—bad boys, especially—long personified the troubles of teendom.

Except for those who wound up pregnant and unwed—never an uncommon occurrence—teenage girls were unseen and unheard. This, as we've learned in the last two decades, is part of the problem. Many of the risks teen girls face are silent ones: higher-than-ever expectations (to be smart, skinny, or both), devastating loss of self-confidence, soul-crushing depression. Yet it doesn't have to be just like a girl—and it is, in fact, *not* like most girls—to be pulled down and under by these forces. To assume otherwise does girls a disservice. If we come to think of teenage girls as "alien sociopaths" (a term used in a recent British medical journal) or lost souls, what else can we do but throw up our hands and abandon our hope—and our daughters?

Most parents don't, and this in itself gives today's girls a great advantage. Through much of history, being a girl meant being dispensable, without value except as property to be transferred or as a bride to be bartered. "Outside my father's house, I am nothing," a girl of ancient Greece wrote in one of the few fragments of female writing preserved since classical times. Her future, as she well knew, would involve only two journeys: one to the house of the husband her father chose for her and one to her grave.

For girls today, poised on the brink of many journeys, adolescence is neither the first nor the last stop. But before they can get a good fix on where they are and map out directions in which they might head, they have to understand where they've been. Freud, it turns out, was wrong about young girls: They are not "little men." From their first day of life they are uniquely female. And they blossom, inside and out, in ways that only a girl can.

Girls Rule!

They scrawl it on their hands, the ink squishing into the soft folds of their palms. They print it in block letters across their notebooks. They scratch it into the sand of beaches and the bark of trees. In primary schools, "Girls rule; boys drool" has become a modern mantra, one that, at the very least, captures a fundamental truth about childhood: Girls and boys experience it differently.

Some say parents are the reason. New mothers and fathers, describing their one-day-old infants, use words like *soft, sweet,* and *delicate* for girls and *strong, active,* and *robust* for boys. In one experiment, women playing with six-month-olds were more likely to encourage the diaper-clad babies they thought were boys to crawl or to try to walk while cuddling and comforting the infants they thought were girls.

Others contend that sex differences begin even before birth. Because of "hard-wiring" of female and male brains in the womb, they argue, girls just weeks old pay more attention to faces; boys are just as likely to smile at blinking lights. Baby girls respond more to language, are more sensitive to touch, gaze into others' eyes longer, and vocalize earlier. Girls sit up on their own sooner, boys crawl more quickly—yet both walk at about the same age.

Which influence ultimately proves stronger: nurture or nature? Neuropsychologist Marc Breedlove, of the University of California, Berkeley, who is a leading expert in the study of sex differences, used to favor nurture. Then his third child—and first daughter—was born. "Before she could talk, the thing she most wanted to do was go into her mother's closet and put on shoes. She was born into a house filled with boys and their toys, but they never interested her. At six, we'd argue with her every day because she'd only wear dresses, never pants. This is a girl whose mother wears a dress around three times a year. And here I am, a psychology professor at Berkeley who must know what I'm talking about because I have several pieces of paper that prove how smart I am. But she doesn't care. She just likes dresses."

If there is a frilly-frock gene, my daughter, who lived in nothing else for years, also inherited it. As a toddler, Julia so adored baubles and beads—the gaudier the better—that she piled them onto her arms and around her neck. For her first preschool Christmas party, she appeared in a tiara. I, whose workday wardrobe consists of sweatshirts and cutoffs, was dumbfounded. We gave her a toy truck; she used it as a doll bed. When I took her and a friend's son—both around four—to play with a collection of oversized stuffed dinosaurs, she immediately formed a cluster of mommy, daddy, and babies. He assembled the tyrannosaurus troops into battle lines.

As Breedlove now sees it, there's a word for people who believe society alone molds children into sex roles: *childless*. Parents quickly learn otherwise. "I'm now convinced that boys and girls start out a little bit different at birth," he says, "but they get more different as they grow up." Because of innate differences in their brains, girls and boys may seek out different experiences, even as infants, and respond to them in ways that change their brains still more, causing even greater divergence. At least in theory, if girls and boys grew up with truly equal environments and experiences, they might be more similar in aptitudes and attitudes as adults. But they would never, ever be the same.

Don't try telling this to a toddler. Reveling in what psychoanalysts call the "omnipotentiality of the young," very young children assume anything is possible. Girls think they can do whatever their dads can, and boys believe they can do anything their moms do—including giving birth. When a young psychiatrist's son declared that he was going to have a baby—just like his mommy, pregnant with her second child—she did a study of other mothers of sons and discovered that nearly half of the young boys had fantasized about being pregnant. One therapist recalls meeting with a new mother who was nursing her baby during their session; her young son sat by her side, a teddy bear pressed to his own chest.

"Until around six or seven," a psychologist explains, "children think, 'I'm a boy today but I could become a girl tomorrow'—and vice versa." Somewhere in the preschool years, this prospect starts to seem unsettling. Girls bedecked in tutus and boys in Batman capes become fiercely feminine or masculine—much to the horror of parents trying to foster androgyny. During this period, Barbie and her male superhero counterparts reign supreme. The fact that these icons bear little resemblance to real women and men doesn't matter; their over-the-top embodiment of femaleness or maleness (including big hair and big weapons) is the secret of their appeal. Eventually, as youngsters realize they are and will forever be girls or boys, they relax their gender expectations—and their standards for acceptable apparel. By second grade, even my bejeweled daughter had switched to jeans.

By the age of six, Freud theorized, youngsters have also struggled with Oedipal conflicts: a young boy's desire for his mother, a young girl's passion for her father. But girls, as Freud saw it, also longed for something else—a penis (or, as some interpret it, the power and privilege it represents). "There truly is such a thing as penis envy in girls," says psychiatrist Lois Flaherty, of the University of Pennsylvania, noting that this concept "went from being universally endorsed to being universally dismissed. However, now we know that there also is a male counterpart that is equally influential."

Certainly parental response to children's preoccupation with their genitals has changed. "When my son was about three, he started saying, 'I have something you don't have: I have a peepee,'" a no-nonsense friend of mine recalls. "I told him I have something better. It's called a vagina, and it makes babies. That totally shut him up." One wonders what turn psychoanalysis might have taken if Freud's mother had ever said the same.

Differences between little girls and little boys extend beyond anatomy, showing up even in the games they play. Contrary to common misconception, girls' play can be, in its own way, as competitive as boys'—and even more complicated. "It's amazing to watch," says Robin Hayden, a multimedia executive in Silicon Valley who volunteers at her sons' preschool. "The boys say, 'Give me that,' and whoever can hold on longest wins. The girls' play is incredibly convoluted; there's so much negotiation going on: 'First, I'll play with the toy for ten minutes, then I'll let you borrow it, then we'll share for a while.' When there's a dispute, the boys will say, 'You took it, and it's mine!' The girls let loose a whole arsenal: 'I don't like the dress you're wearing. Your mother wasn't here yesterday, and mine was. The snack you brought last week tasted terrible. I'm not inviting you to my birthday party, and I'm not getting you a birthday present, either.'"

Contrary to other false assumptions, girls don't always stick to the rules or stop playing when conflict erupts ("Imagine how many Goody Two-shoes there would be if they did!" comments an expert in girls' development), nor are they confined to girlish roles. All in a day's play, they can switch from Barbie to baseball, from dress-up to digging in the dirt, from fairy princess to king of the hill. And they're more likely to join the guys in a game than boys are to "cross the border," as one psychologist puts it, and play with girls.

"Girls have much more freedom to engage in atypical gender behavior than boys," Flaherty observes. "It's not considered a big deal if a girl refuses to wear dresses, but there's great anxiety if a boy wants to put on a dress." Parents may boast about the fearless tree climbing of a tomboy daughter; they keep mum about a son's fascination with his mother's makeup or jewelry.

Even sports-loving, fence-climbing, all-guy boys are more likely than girls to run into rough patches in early childhood. In the cozy, maternal classrooms of the primary grades, girls sit still longer, concentrate better, tend to be more cooperative and compliant, and become the teachers' pets. Although young boys receive more attention at school, most of it is negative, a barrage of reminders and reprimands. Much more prone to learning disabilities, they often lag behind on reading and handwriting. As discussed in Chapter 11, the reason may lie, at least partly, in their brains. In general, girls and boys may use different clusters of neurons in learning to read and different skills in solving math problems.

The problems young boys encounter aren't confined to the classroom. "I see a major gender difference in children every time I look into my waiting room," says a child psychiatrist. "There usually are nine or ten boys for every girl." A long list of childhood disorders—bed-wetting, hyperactivity, attention deficits, conduct disorders, learning disabilities, dyslexia, stuttering, depression—strike boys more often than girls. To my daughter and her friends, this lopsided demographic only confirms what they so heartily believe in: the essential excellence of girlness.

It also testifies to the stultifying socialization of boys. Psychologist Carol Gilligan, of Harvard University, a pioneer in studying the silencing of girls, has turned her professional attention to boys. (Her personal attention was always there: She is the mother of three sons.) "I think boys are at risk in early childhood because their initiation comes sooner," she says. "Girls are ignored until the edge of adolescence."

The problems for boys, she notes, start when they feel forced to separate from their mothers, usually before age six, in order to become "real" guys. "What we are discovering is how vulnerable boys are, how under the surface, behind that psychic shield, is a tender creature who's hiding his humanity. I often say about my own boys, who are now grown, that I feel that the world muffles the very best qualities in them, meaning their sensitivity."

The emotional and social sensitivity that girls display from early childhood (also discussed in Chapter 12) becomes more intense through the years—and may become at least a temporary liability as they hurtle toward maturity. For boys, adolescence represents a kind of second chance. For girls, it is something else entirely.

The Last Hurrah

From a distance, their bodies outlined in a glow of sunlight, it's hard to tell if the middle-schoolers on the field are girls or boys. Cloaked in oversized sweatshirts and baggy jeans, the sixth-graders chase each other in an elaborate game of capture the flag. What they do not realize—what we parents sense with a wistfulness that feels like wisdom—is that they are at the end of a personal era.

"Twenty years ago we thought that girls went from childhood to adolescence to adulthood," says Flaherty. "Now the idea of a phase prior to adolescence is very important." Some analysts thought of the preteen years as the "last fling of phallic fantasies," when girls were able to pretend for a little longer that they were boys. Such sexist assumptions have faded. It's not so much that girls want to be boys—a thought any self-respecting preteen of the female persuasion would reject as outrageous—but that they feel free to do or be anything: wear lipstick and shoot hoops, bake cookies and earn black belts, grow up to be actresses, astronauts, or both.

Yet beneath the surface of their no-frills bodies, starting much earlier than anyone once guessed, great changes are under way. Standard charts on sexual development, based on British white girls of the 1960s, no longer apply. In a 1997 analysis of growth charts from 17,077 girls age three to twelve, researchers at the University of North Carolina at Chapel Hill found that by age eight, 15 percent of white girls and 48 percent of African-American girls show signs of sexual development (the reasons for this racial discrepancy are not known). The mean ages for breast development are 8.87 years for African-American girls and 9.96 years for white girls; for pubic hair, they are 8.78 years and 10.51 years, respectively. African-American girls begin menstruating at a mean age of 12.16 years; white girls, at 12.88 years.

The hormones that propel a girl toward her physiological future are the "male" androgens. At age seven or eight, a girl's adrenal glands begin to release weak androgens (plasma dehydroepiandrosterone and dehydroepiandrosterone sulfate) and then more potent ones (including testosterone). Under their influence, the long bones of a girl's legs, thighs, and arms grow, and her body proportions change. Her hips widen; her waist becomes fuller; her weight climbs. There is a 120 percent increase in body fat in girls before menarche—a normal and necessary change essential for reproductive maturity. Yet this normal weight gain may cause girls, or their figure-conscious parents, to assume that they're getting fat—and may account for the alarming finding, in a 1996 survey in the United States, that 40 percent of nine- and ten-year-old girls are trying to lose weight.

"Adrenarche"—the maturing of the adrenal glands—brings other changes: higher energy, athletic ability, muscular prowess. Roughly two years before boys her age, a girl stretches upward and sprouts hair under her arms and around her genitals. Sweat glands become more active, and girls develop a body odor. Their skin becomes oilier and more prone to pimples. Testosterone and its brother androgens also may have an impact on girls' behavior. Long associated with belligerence in males, androgens may contribute to the surprising mean streak that emerges in middle girlhood, a time of cliques, clubs, and verbal cruelty. "Boys duke it out in the playground," a fifth-grade teacher observes. "Girls do just as much bullying—but they don't use their fists."

Adrenal ripening also fosters a sexual awareness that adds a new intensity to girlish crushes. After years of being oblivious to physical charms, girls suddenly look across a crowded playground and, as biologist Martha McClintock, of the University of Chicago, puts it, start to "notice—with a capital N" that someone, whether of the same or the other sex, looks particularly good to them. They feel a zing that may not be sexual in the adult sense but definitely carries a charge. A year and a half to two years later, as the reproductive glands churn out much greater amounts of sex hormones, sexual desire kicks in.

The early adrenal activity is simply the overture for reproductive development. The tiny pineal gland, buried deep within the brain, sends a message to the hypothalamus, the conductor of the endocrine system, and the pituitary, the concertmaster, to start the reproductive symphony. Literally as girls lie sleeping, the pituitary sends pulses of two key hormones—luteinizing hormone (LH) and follicle-stimulating hormone (FSH)—through their bloodstreams. These messengers signal the ovaries to manufacture more of the main female sex hormone, estradiol, which increases at about age eight or nine and stimulates the growth of the breasts, uterus, vagina, and pelvis.

The metamorphosis of puberty follows an orderly sequence through five developmental phases, called Tanner stages for the researcher who meticulously chronicled girls' growth. In Stage I, girls, hairless and streamlined, show no signs of sexual development. In Stage II, breasts begin to bud, mainly just in the areola (the region around the nipples); a few hairs sprout under the arms and on the labia; and a girl's growth spurt begins, propelling her upward by as much as three inches in a single year. In Stage III, her breasts become fuller; the nipple and areola begin to project. More hair grows in the genitals and armpits; her vagina enlarges, and her clitoris grows. About 30 percent of girls first menstruate at this time. In Stage IV, the breasts and external genitals are well developed; menarche (first menstruation) occurs, and pubic hair becomes moderate to abundant. In Stage V, female sexual development is complete. Estrogen seals the ends of the long bones of the arms and legs, and growth slows. Girls generally add only two more inches in height after menarche.

The complete process of reproductive maturing takes about four years—although some girls develop in just a year and a half, others in five. As dramatic as the visible transformations can be, the invisible changes are often more disconcerting. Giddy in the morning and glum in the afternoon, young girls—and their families—may feel buffeted by unsettling mood swings.

"Emotionally, young girls are going along on a two-lane street, then puberty hits, and all of a sudden they're speeding along on a super-highway," observes psychiatrist Louann Brizendine. "The pulses of the reproductive hormones greatly expand a girl's emotional range. She becomes incredibly sensitive and empathic—which, from an evolutionary perspective, makes sense, since these are wonderful traits for a mother to have. But her awareness that what she says can hurt people and her vulnerability to being hurt may affect how she sees herself, so she turns inward and becomes more introspective."

This is, in fact, what psychological research on girls has shown. Prior to puberty, young girls comment freely on what they observe, protest violations of trust, and tell the truth—even if it gets them in trouble. "Look at Uncle Joe's nose!" a nine-year-old girl sings out at a formal dinner. "It turns red when he drinks." "Say something in French," urges a proud mother who's just returned from Paris with her ten-year-old. The girl delivers a brief but beautifully accented sentence; the translation (accompanied by a mischievous grin on her face and a burning blush on her mother's) is "Who cut the cheese?"

"There's a certain smugness among ten-year-olds, which I really love—but that's supposed to break down," says psychologist Barbara Sommer, of the University of California, Davis. "In normal cognitive development, around age twelve you're supposed to lose childish egocentrism and recognize you're not the center of the universe or the smartest person in the world. And it shakes your confidence." She speculates that girls may reach this stage earlier, while boys remain "locked for a longer time in a self-centered world where they don't even see reality."

The exuberance of a girl's preteen years reminds me of another transition: at about age one, when babies just learn to walk. Their pride in this astonishing feat fills them with joyous energy. "Today I'm walking," the newly vertical baby, glowing with self-satisfaction, seems to think. "Imagine what I'll do next!" A few months later, reality crashes in: The toddler still can't go as fast and as far as she'd hoped. And as she lurches into dangerous territories, her parents constantly say no. The thrill of reveling in her new skills gives way to the frustrations that make the "terrible twos" so trying for both child and parent.

So too with this transition. A taste of independence thrills "tween-agers." The first time my daughter prowled through a mall with her friends, she called to tell me she'd found heaven. These neophyte shoppers, carefully counting out allowance money for lip gloss and barrettes, are new to the world's wares and ways. They have yet to crash into the limits of personal finances or parental patience, to discover the boundaries of realms where they dare not go. And if they do tiptoe into dangerous territories, they soon scurry back under the protective safety nets of home and family, willing to remain, for just a bit longer, little girls.

Early Bloomers

At her annual girls-only lecture on menstruation, the school counselor passes around samples of tampons and sanitary napkins. Soon some of the fifth-graders are shooting tampons from their plastic applicators like skyrockets into the air. Others strip off the adhesive and stick maxipads onto their foreheads. One girl is stuffing slender "junior" tampons up her nose; another sticks them in her ears. At first glance, it might seem that these girls don't know tampons from toys. But their hijinks betray both the natural playfulness of their age and unspoken uneasiness about a subject they know is not a childish one. While most of the girls dissolve in giggles, a few sit silently, as if trying to will themselves into invisibility. They are the ones who've gotten their periods and know full well that menstruation is no game, but a basic part of the business of being female.

It is a lesson more girls are learning at earlier ages. Ever since 1900 the average age for menarche, or first menstruation, which had been 14.8 years, has slowly and steadily been dropping at the rate of about 0.3 years per decade. In surveys in seven Western countries in the 1960s, menarche occurred between the ages of 13 and 13.5. As noted above, many American girls start menstruating before their thirteenth birthdays—some much earlier. Pediatricians once defined precocious menarche as occurring at age eight; now this is considered within normal range.

Why are so many girls developing womanly bodies so quickly? The primary reasons are salutary: improved nutrition and good health. Girls today are bigger, taller, and better-fed, and they have a higher percentage of body fat (one of the triggers of sexual maturation). At menarche, girls' bodies weigh an average of 101 to 103 pounds, with about 24 percent fat.

The littler and leaner a girl—as a result of malnutrition, illness, extreme dieting, or rigorous exercise—the later she reaches menarche. Genetics also play a role. Early- or late-developing parents have children who tend to follow their timetable. Identical twins, who generally grow and mature more slowly than singleton girls, reach menarche about two months apart; fraternal twins, no more genetically similar than other siblings, tend to differ by about twelve months.

Early menarche per se isn't new. In the Roman Empire, some counselors advised marriage and intercourse before a girl's teens in order to prompt menstruation—and prevent the seduction of innocent virgins. In Shakespeare's depiction of Verona, Juliet probably was no older than thirteen—and presumably sexually mature when she fell passionately in love with Romeo. Medieval records make note of marriages of girls of twelve and births to mothers as young as fourteen or fifteen.

Poorer girls have traditionally matured later than more affluent ones—a possible consequence of malnutrition, hard physical work, and greater susceptibility to infectious diseases. In the eighteenth and nineteenth centuries, when girls of all classes were prone to tuberculosis and other "wasting" illnesses, the average age at menarche increased to seventeen or eighteen. In poorer nations today, it remains high—in Bangladesh, for instance, it is just under sixteen; among certain New Guinea tribes, it is about eighteen.

Other environmental factors also play a role. The endless light made possible by the harnessing of electricity may have accelerated girls' development. According to some theorists, chemical additives or growth hormones, fed to dairy cows and beef cattle, may be tampering with female physiology. Certain illnesses, such as hypothyroidism, accelerate menarche; others, such as diabetes mellitus and ulcerative colitis, delay it. One study found that left-handed girls reached menarche sooner; another, of girls in Peruvian mountain villages, found that those living at higher altitudes matured later. Even the seasons may play a role. A prepubertal girl's height increases twice as fast in the spring, with peak growth reported between March and June. The greatest weight gains occur in the autumn, and girls are most likely to have their first period in the late fall or early winter.

Although menarche is a physiological event, some of its triggers may be psychological. According to studies in the United States and New Zealand, certain types of stress at about age seven—frequent parental conflict or a father's leaving the family—accelerate development, so that a girl begins menstruating four or five months sooner, sometimes even earlier, than her age peers. This may be an evolutionary adaptation—nature's rush to ensure that a female lacking a protective male will have the opportunity to reproduce. In the wild, as noted in Chapter 2, new males who take over a harem of females often slaughter their young. In these dire circumstances, juvenile females may imitate the sexual overtures of a mature female in estrus—almost as if they realize that sham maturity is safer than childish vulnerability.

Whatever its complex causes, early menarche can be potentially hazardous both physiologically and psychologically. As discussed later in this chapter, an early-developing girl often faces a harder emotional struggle as she adjusts to life in a womanly body. "For girls who go through sexual maturation early," one child psychologist comments, "the experience can feel like the ground slipping under their feet in an earthquake."

First Blood

At any age, menarche, the first of the female "blood mysteries," can trigger ambivalent feelings. "I was at school when my period started," a Japanese woman in her fifties tells me. "I didn't know what was happening, so I said I was sick and went home. My mother explained that I had a special box, like a drawer, inside me, and that was where the blood came from. I said, 'I don't want it. Can I give it back?'"

This is not an unusual reaction. Preteen girls, "itchy with the work of sprouting," as one writer put it, usually look forward to getting their periods as testimony to the fact that they are growing up. They expect to call their friends and share the big announcement with at least four or five other girls. But what is exciting in theory is complicated in reality. When menstruation turns out to be much more messy and mundane than they'd imagined, girls would just as soon go back to the way they were—and they no longer feel much desire to talk about it.

Although most of the taboos that long shrouded menstruation (discussed in Chapter 7) have finally been dispelled, today's girls—though better-informed, thanks to sex education classes, informational videos, and Internet sites (including a Tampax-sponsored "cyberzine")—still have a visceral response to the sight and smell of their menstrual blood. In teen magazines, young readers recount mortifying stories of blood-soaked skirts or tampons spilling out of purses. In studies of college students, even those who said they had plenty of technical information often felt unprepared for the normal feelings of fright, embarrassment, and discomfort.

Advertisements and educational materials tell girls only partial truths. They depict radiant women who never have menstrual accidents, never complain of cramps, never even take a break from their biking and hiking and swimming. Girls who can't cope as well may assume there's something wrong with them. And even those who feign nonchalance may be unclear on certain concepts. One friend recalls that her well-prepared daughter was stunned when she brought up the subject of overnight protection. "You mean it doesn't stop when I sleep?" the girl asked.

Curious or baffled, girls are most likely to turn to their mothers for answers. In one study, 75 percent of the girls told no one but their mothers that they'd gotten their first period. The fact that they share something uniquely female offers a special opportunity to mothers and daughters. "A girl's first period is a distinct event, usually marking an inevitable turning point in the communication about sexuality between mother and daughter," psychologist Bruna Zani noted in a study of teens in Bologna, Italy. "A boy's first ejaculations never form the background for an exchange of information between parents and sons." The "talk" that never happens, the silence about the workings of a male body, she theorizes, may be one reason why "boys attribute less importance than girls to information provided by their parents."

In some cultures, a girl's coming of age is celebrated with rituals that give thanks for what some tribal nations call "the blessing of blood." In an annual feast, Navajo girls who'd begun menstruating would run footraces to show their strength and would perform skits to honor the goddess Changing Woman. Among the Mbuti of Zaire, menarchal girls would live in a menstrual hut for a year. There older women would teach them about their bodies and bring food to fatten them up and make them more beautiful. Before returning to the village, the girls would run through the forest singing to proclaim their womanhood.

In my trendy home state of California, mothers sometimes host celebratory "circles" to welcome newly menstruating girls into the sisterhood of women. Girls themselves, self-conscious and private, say that what they want most is reassurance that their experience is normal and love and support from their mothers. In one study mothers liked the idea of responding to menarche with the statement, "Our little girl is growing up." Psychologists preferred a different statement: "Something special has happened," which allows room for a girl's mixed emotions.

As for symbolic gestures, mothers liked the idea of a toast to the girl or a meal in her honor. But the girls said they'd prefer a hug and a token, such as a locket or flowers. They also want—like women of all ages—to hear the truth, not just about the mechanics of menstruation, but also about the meaning it has had in their mothers' lives and the potential meaning it may have in theirs.

The Psychobiology of Change

Blood and bodily transformation are the stuff fairy tales are made of. At the brink of womanhood, Sleeping Beauty pricks her finger and falls into deep sleep. Snow White, she of the bloodred lips, bites the poisoned apple and collapses. Cinderella experiences the ultimate makeover; Rapunzel extends a life-saving braid. And in the end, girls no longer, these young women find love and lifelong happiness.

These stories, told and retold for centuries, capture the essence of female adolescence, a time when a young girl's body and world change completely. Physically, girls undergo the most profound transformations since infancy. Seemingly as they sleep, flesh they lived in their whole life slides up, down, around, about. Breasts bud. Hips curve. Hair sprouts in unexpected places.

The transformation of a boy into a man, although not without its awkward and embarrassing phases, is far less dramatic—and less potentially traumatic. After some initial misgivings, as psychologists have documented, boys come to like their bigger, stronger, hairier bodies (although those who remain short or scrawny or become painfully pudgy or pimply do not). Most boys, like most girls, experience an initial drop in self-esteem around puberty, but as their body image steadily improves, their self-esteem rebounds more quickly.

Girls too may feel an initial delight in their new figures—and the attention they draw. With brand-new breasts and rounded hips, they take to wearing tight sweaters and short-short skirts—much to their mothers' horror. (The fashions may vary from era to era, but the look—"baby tart," as one friend puts it—and the responses of parents remain the same.)

"I remember dressing in tank tops in eighth grade and liking it when guys honked their horns at me," a college senior recalls. "When I got to be fifteen, I suddenly realized that I didn't want that kind of attention. It made me feel cheap." Perhaps the early surge in testosterone—a hormone that fuels sexual desire and display—encourages such preening by preteens; the quieter female sex hormones, along with growing awareness of undesired reactions, may eventually modulate this urge.

As hormones shift and body parts morph, girls have to come to terms with a completely new figure. When researchers ask girls of different ages to draw female figures, the premenarcheal girls show little, if any, sexualization: They sketch sticklike silhouettes with happy faces. The postmenarcheal girls draw womanly figures with full breasts and hips, often dressed in sexy clothes. But when girls look in the mirror, they may not know quite what to make of their own unfamiliar figures, ones that rarely bear much resemblance to the fleshless females they see in the media.

This too may explain why girls start looking toward others for feed-back, sending out their exquisitely sensitive psychological antennae to pick up signals of approval or approbation. In his research, psychologist James Pennebaker, of the University of Texas, has found that at puberty a gender difference appears in emotional experience. Boys tune in to their own body signals and become more adept at "reading" their inter-nal states. Girls turn outward, ignoring their own responses and react-ing to what they sense others want or feel. (This research is discussed in Chapter 12.)

Unfortunately, many of the messages the outside world transmits to girls are at best mixed and at worst downright toxic. To succeed in a world run by male-made rules, a girl realizes she's going to have to achieve just like a boy. Yet all of her conditioning, all of evolution's cues and society's pressures, underscore the importance of acting just like a female—of flaunting her fertile body, of attracting male attention, of being sweet as well as smart, sensitive as well as successful, sexy and yet not sexual. It's an impossible agenda, and girls who buy into it—few can resist its omnipresent drumbeat—set themselves up to fall short.

Because girls get a physiological head start at puberty, maturing an average of two years before boys, they also are more likely to tumble into a developmental warp. While they no longer look like little kids, they still think like children, with cognitive skills lagging behind physical maturity. The fullness of their new figures may look like fatness to them. Their monthly bleeding may feel like a betrayal by their body—or at least a burden. They may misread sexual overtures and find themselves in situations they aren't sure how to handle.

Early maturers typically encounter the greatest difficulty. Intrigued by the adult world that suddenly opens before them, girls who look older find that they are treated as if they were indeed older—by strangers, schoolmates, teachers, even parents. Compared with their younger-looking peers, they're more likely to stay home alone, to take on baby-sitting and other jobs, to wear makeup, to hang out with older kids, and to start dating. In his research, Stanford University psychiatrist Chris Hayward found that they are more likely to develop "internalizing symp-toms," such as depression and poor self-esteem.

Faux maturity presents other dangers to young girls, particularly those who begin to date. These early maturers are more likely to engage in sex at younger ages (often under pressure, if not outright coercion, from the older boys they date) and are at higher risk of sexually transmitted diseases and pregnancy, as well as depression, panic attacks, and eating disorders. Yet such dire consequences are by no means inevitable. "Early puberty isn't a major risk factor for emotional problems," says Hayward, "but if it occurs along with other risks—such as a family history of depression, chronic illness, or abuse of any kind—it adds to a girl's vulnerability."

So does upheaval—or what a girl perceives as upheaval. If she changes schools just as she starts menstruating—a common occurrence for those who move into middle school at age twelve—she may feel overwhelmed by the need to adapt in every way and every place in her life. Family changes also can be traumatic. Statistically, parents of teen girls are much more likely to divorce than those of teen boys, possibly because families may feel a greater need for the father to remain present for his sons. This can be difficult for girls, who are at a stage where they are trying to sort out how relationships work—and who may feel resentful or rejected if their parents' marriage fails.

Boys, meanwhile, are going through changes of their own—ones that researchers are just beginning to explore. Rather than focusing on their bodies, as girls do, pubescent boys get serious about achievement. In seventh or eighth grade, realizing that they need to get good grades to get into a good college to get a good job to earn a good salary for a good life, many hit the books. Others get intensely involved in sports. Their lives revolve around accomplishment, both in the classroom and on the athletic field. If they do well at least in one important arena (which these days might include cyberspace savvy), their self-esteem rebounds. Girls, preoccupied by appearance and more internally focused, may lag behind in self-confidence well into their late teens and beyond.

In a survey of a thousand fifteen-year-olds, New Zealand researchers asked the teens to check off the positive attributes they felt described themselves. "Both boys and girls checked off a lot," Flaherty reports. "But they were different." A third of the boys—but fewer than 20 percent of the girls—saw themselves as attractive. The boys saw themselves as good athletes, confident and skilled, while the girls were more likely to describe social characteristics, such as being reliable and good friends. "The boys defined themselves through activity," says Flaherty. "The girls saw themselves in the context of their relationships."

While it is just like a woman at any age to value relationships, adolescent girls become so eager to please that, as one therapist puts it, "they bend themselves into pretzels." Tuning in to others' voices, they pay no heed to their own. This can lead to a crisis in confidence. In a 1997 Commonwealth Fund study of 3,586 girls and 3,162 boys in grades five through twelve, the girls were consistently more likely than the boys to be self-critical and self-doubting. More than a quarter of the girls said they did not like themselves, reported suicidal thoughts, said they were sad many times or all the time, or felt like crying most days or every day.

Yet some groups of girls, such as African-Americans, show remarkable emotional resiliency. According to the American Association of University Women's landmark report *Shortchanging Girls / Shortchanging America*, black girls have a greater sense of self-esteem than girls of any other ethnic group. In high school, 58 percent say they are happy with "the way I am"—compared with 30 percent of white girls and even lower percentages of girls in other ethnic groups.

No one suggests that African-American girls have it easy. Statistically, they are more likely to come from single-parent families, lack economic security, and have few incentives for academic achievement. Yet at the very least they are more comfortable in their own skin. In a 1995 survey University of Arizona researchers found that 70 percent of African-American teens—compared to just 10 percent of white girls—were happy with their weight; even overweight black girls rated themselves as happy and saw beauty as an attitude, not an external characteristic.

African-American girls also tend to stand up for themselves—perhaps because they are given what psychologists describe as "greater permission to argufy" than white girls. And most important, they have an often overlooked advantage. "Look at their mothers," says psychiatrist Kathleen Pajer, of Allegheny Medical Center in Pittsburgh, who is studying teen girls who get in trouble with the law. "Black girls come from a matriarchal culture in which strong women are the ones who keep the family together." And, as discussed later in this chapter, strong mothers, to a remarkable extent, help keep girls strong.

Girls at Risk

In one nerve-fraying week, I talk with two women on opposite sides of the American continent about their teenagers. At fifteen, the daughter of an East Coast friend—shining in my memory as a golden-curled cherub of two—has swallowed an overdose of aspirin and admitted a propensity for slashing her skin. On the West Coast, another friend's thirteen-year-old daughter lost twenty pounds, almost a fifth of her body weight, in three months.

I hold my breath as I listen. If any girls were to sail smoothly through their teens, these two should have led the fleet. They had grown up in loving homes in quiet, big-treed suburbs. Their parents had Ivy League educations, distinguished careers, and long-running marriages. When the girls were little, their mothers had cut back their work hours to provide hands-on care. They had festooned their houses for birthday parties, cheered at soccer games, chauffeured the girls to ceramics and music classes, and fretted over every nuance of their academic and emotional needs. I'd watched with admiration from the sidelines, hoping that someday I would do as good a job. Now I wondered: What could possibly have gone wrong?

Nothing surprising, says Ponton, who explains that these girls were doing what all teens try: taking risks. Some take small risks, like staying out past curfew. Others find healthy ways of testing their limits through adventurous sports like rock climbing. A not-insignificant minority, like these two girls, risk their own well-being. In general, teen boys, perhaps fueled by testosterone's high-octane kick, take risks that are more physical and obvious, including drinking and experimenting with drugs (although more girls today smoke—slightly more than boys, in fact, and white girls more than African-American girls; a dubious interpretation of liberation). However, the most dangerous risks that girls tend to take involve food and sex.

"Disordered eating"—a term applied to a variety of abnormal and potentially unhealthy eating patterns—is the most common risk behavior among preteen girls. "The only group that has experienced a demonstrable increase in eating disorders in the last forty years has been girls eleven to fifteen," Ponton reports. Also at high risk are teens with chronic medical conditions, such as asthma or diabetes, and competitive athletes in sports, like gymnastics, that prize petiteness.

Alarmed by what they see as bodily bulges, girls may swear off sweets, then meat, then pasta, then bread, then almost any food containing significant calories—or nutrients. Some start on a temporary diet and can't seem to stop restricting their eating even after they reach their target weight. Fewer girls today induce vomiting after eating, Ponton notes, but laxative abuse is growing, with girls sometimes taking ten to twenty doses of laxative a day. And, wanting to be trim as well as thin, many "binge" on exercise, working out for hours at a time.

The triggers of such behaviors vary. A father's offhand comment about love handles at her waist or a coach's unthinking remark about moving her "big butt" gets terribly distorted in a young girl's mind. One therapist describes confused girls as "creating a little world of control around what they eat as a substitute for dealing with change." If their weight falls low enough, they actually can stop some physiological changes, such as regular periods and breast development. And, as they realize, this is no mean feat.

"The only thing I thought I could succeed at was being thin," says a girl in therapy for anorexia nervosa. "It was the one thing I could do right." But weight loss, once it reaches a certain point, takes on a life of its own. Starvation itself or the chemical imbalance it causes in the brain wreaks havoc with perceptions and critical judgment. Weight becomes an obsession, and even as they become thin to the point of gauntness, girls cannot recognize that they are in grave danger of long-term physical complications (such as osteoporosis) and even of death.

Other girls subject their bodies to different risks, such as self-mutilation with razors, scissors, cigarettes, or other objects. "The first time I took a paper clip and gouged it into my skin, harder and harder, I just sort of thought about how it felt, analyzed it, focused on it," one girl recalls. "It was like I was an observer, and afterward I felt like I'd proved something to myself—that I could control my pain." Most often "cutting" is a symptom of a larger problem, such as depression. And it too, if unrecognized, can become increasingly dangerous.

Until puberty, boys are more likely than girls to become depressed. By the end of adolescence, rates of depression, as noted previously, are two to three times higher in women than men. The hormonal upheaval of menarche itself may make some girls vulnerable. Some researchers now believe that certain girls may be hypersensitive either to their own sex hormones or to cyclic changes in hormone levels. In surveys of young people in the United States, New Zealand, Canada, and Puerto Rico, the likelihood of severe depression doubled in girls in the year after the onset of menstruation. Those who become depressed at menarche are at risk of subsequent depressions after childbirth or at menopause—and possibly premenstrually as well.

In adolescence, as at other times of life, other factors can increase susceptibility to depression. One of the most significant is abuse—verbal, physical, or sexual. A barrage of critical or belittling comments, whether directed at a teen's looks, intelligence, or behavior, can hit like body blows, leaving painful though invisible scars. The other types of abuse are shockingly common. According to recent studies of American teens, as many as one in four girls has been sexually or physically abused, sometimes by a parent or another adult, sometimes by a date who forced her to have sex against her will. In addition to becoming depressed, these girls are more likely to engage in dangerous risk behaviors, including smoking, drinking, drug use, and unsafe sex. Stressful life events—parental divorce, serious illness, a beloved grandparent's death, a move, a change in schools—also make girls more susceptible.

Signs of a girl's vulnerability may show up before adolescence. Studies of eleven-year-olds suggest that those who subsequently become depressed are self-conscious and dissatisfied with their appearance, worry about potential losses (such as their parents dying), show emotional "overcontrol," and express great concern about popularity as well as about moral issues. Often depression in young girls goes unrecognized until it leads to destructive behaviors, such as disordered eating, substance abuse, or self-mutilation. This delay can have a long-lasting impact. An episode of depression, if unrecognized and untreated, can alter the brain in such a way as to increase the risk of other episodes throughout life.

In some instances, a girl's emotional distress can be so profound that it affects her body as well as her mind. In a nine-year study of 716 boys and girls, followed from preadolescence to adulthood, Columbia University researchers discovered a surprising correlation between emotional problems and stature—but only in girls. Intense anxiety (one of the few childhood mental disorders more common in girls than boys) stunted the growth of preteen and teenage girls, sometimes by as much as one to two inches. It may be, the researchers speculated, that girls experience anxiety more intensely, causing a fall in levels of growth hormone, which stimulates bone and muscle development. Yet although the girls' mental distress was severe enough to slow or stop growth, neither their parents nor their family doctors had noticed anything wrong.

Even when parents do sense something amiss, they may assume it's something their child will grow out of. This is often a false hope. If parents don't confront teenagers who are repeatedly engaging in dangerous risk taking, their youngsters are likely to take bigger risks, says Ponton, who advises parents to state calmly what they've observed and why they're worried. "It's never easy," she concedes. "When you confront kids and say you think they are abusing laxatives, vomiting, cutting themselves, whatever, they will lie and tell you they are not doing whatever you suspect. That's the first reaction. But in therapy kids tell me that they are glad their parents picked up on what they were doing. They get angry, but underneath they're scared, and they want help."

After a few hellish months of slammed doors, hateful words, and sleepless nights, my friends' daughters—thanks in no small part to their parents' persistence and some professional counseling—stepped back from the brink of self-destructive behavior. "Sometimes I think every little thing we did mattered and sometimes I think nothing did, that we were just lucky," says one of the mothers. "But I think what was most important was that we didn't stop trying."

Why Smart Girls Don't Have Sex (or Kiss Much, Either)

In my day, bad girls teased their hair, slathered on makeup, and "did it" with their boyfriends. Of course, that was in the dark ages before the sexual revolution reverberated into the Catholic neighborhoods of northeastern Pennsylvania. Today the definitions may have changed, but the double standard, which long condoned and even encouraged sexual experimentation by young men, still sets different rules for girls. Today a "good" girl may have sex—but only with a boyfriend she loves. "Bad" girls earn their reputation by having sex just like boys—without serious commitment to a relationship.

Various studies, while they measure different behaviors in different groups, do suggest that not all teens are rushing into sexual involvements. Federal statistics based on a major national survey conducted in 1995 and released in 1997 suggest that the age of first intercourse, which had decreased steadily for two decades, is rising. Among girls age fifteen to nineteen, 50 percent reported that they'd had intercourse—down from 55 percent in 1990. (As might be expected, the percentage of girls who'd lost their virginity rose steadily from 21.4 percent of fifteen-year-olds to 38 percent of sixteen-year-olds, 49.6 percent of seventeen-year-olds, 62.7 percent of eighteen-year-olds, and 72.4 percent of nineteen-year-olds.) Among boys from fifteen to nineteen years of age, 55 percent said they'd had intercourse—down from 60 percent in 1988.

Statistics apart, we know little about why teens do or do not become sexually active. With boys, explanations focus on the physical—the assumption (unproven and quite possibly untrue) is that testosterone, which surges in their teens, heats up their sex drive. For girls, most of the theories emphasize psychological and sociological factors, such as a girl's desire to please, while her hormonal changes or sexual desires are dismissed—if even mentioned at all.

In one 1996 survey of 720 American teenage girls, most said girls engage in sex because they think they will lose their boyfriends if they don't or because boys pressure them into sex. "Girls trade sex for love, and boys say they love them to get sex," says Deborah Tolman, of the Wellesley Center for Research on Girls and Women. "Girls don't realize they are entitled to have their own feelings and desires and to expect others to take them into account."

Other less-expected factors also influence girls' sexual choices. According to the National Survey of Family Growth, 42 percent of girls who grow up with both biological parents have sex before age twenty, compared with 60 percent of those from single-parent homes. What does the presence of two parents have to do with teenage sex? No one knows exactly, but their influence may reverberate in everything from age of menarche (which may occur later than in single-parent homes) to closer monitoring of where girls are and what they're doing. Parental education also makes a difference. According to Child Trends, a research group in Washington, D.C., 10 percent of girls with college-educated parents lose their virginity before age fifteen, compared with 26 percent of girls whose parents had a high-school education or less.

However, the strongest predictor of sexual abstinence may be a girl's own intelligence. According to researchers at the University of North Carolina at Chapel Hill (whose study gave this section its title), there is an inverse correlation between a girl's intellect and a range of sexual activities, from light petting (known as necking in my day) to heavy petting to sexual intercourse. The brighter a girl is, the longer she delays each step of the progression from kissing to petting to intercourse, even when she's dating or going steady.

Are smart girls less interested in sex, less attractive to boys, more aware of the potential negative consequences of sexual involvement? Do they avoid sex to safeguard their lofty educational aspirations? Are their sexual attitudes more conservative? Are they busier with school activities or more closely monitored by their parents? After two years of studying two hundred African-American and white girls (mean age 13.8 years and all past menarche when the study began), the conclusion that the North Carolina researchers reached was: none of the above.

The bright girls were as attractive as others, even more intrigued by the subject of sex, and no more or less conservative or cognizant of pregnancy risks. Their reasons for abstaining from sex defied obvious adult explanations. They were not trying to safeguard their educational goals; they weren't too busy; their parents weren't more restrictive.

However, the "smart girls" in the North Carolina study did know, if in ways adults cannot quite fathom, something that other girls too often learn the hard way: that sex at an early age is a perilous experience, physically and psychologically. Looking back, most fifteen-year-old girls who've already lost their virginity tell interviewers they wish they hadn't. As one girl put it, "I gave away part of me I can never get back before I even knew what it meant."

Why Girls End Up in Trouble

At a Christmas service, the ministers of our church—a woman and a man—acted out a mini-drama, with one playing Ann, mother of Mary, and the other portraying her father, Joachim. Both wrestled with a timeless dilemma: the pregnancy of their teenage daughter. Outraged, Joachim wanted to get his hands on the male who had taken advantage of Mary's innocence. Ann, though also dubious of Mary's story about an angel's visit, nevertheless argued that their daughter, their cherished only child, still needed their love. Yet neither of them could get past a troubling question: Why? Why did Mary—always such a good, loving, obedient girl—end up in trouble?

Two millennia later, parents—along with teachers, politicians, policy analysts, and a host of others—are asking similar questions. Teenage pregnancy remains the most unimpeachable gender difference of adolescence, the only exclusively female kind of trouble. And today it's not just a personal crisis; it's a political hot button, with some accusing teenagers of becoming pregnant solely to qualify for government support.

Because of the growth in population, more teens in the United States—about a million a year—become pregnant today than half a century ago. However, the *rate* of teen pregnancy is actually far lower than in the Ozzie-and-Harriet fifties, when the birth rate for teens age fifteen to nineteen reached an all-time high of 90 births per 1,000 girls. Since 1991 the teen birth rate has declined by 12 percent; in 1996 (the most recent year for which statistics are available) there were 54.7 births per 1,000 girls. Of these teen mothers, the highest percentage—approximately 45 percent—were Caucasian; less than 30 percent were African-American; the rest belonged to other racial groups. And the overwhelming majority were eighteen or nineteen, old enough to qualify as legal adults.

Few of these girls consciously tried to conceive. By most estimates, 85 to 95 percent of teens who become pregnant did not intend or plan to do so—whether or not they loved their partners, hoped to get married, or used contraception. Obviously they engaged in sex, but this fact alone explains little beyond the basic biology of conception.

"By and large, the reasons girls have sex are different from why they get pregnant," says psychologist Nancy Adler, of the University of California, San Francisco, an expert in decision making in adolescence.

"Having a baby is, unfortunately, a side effect of having sex." Girls who do not engage in intercourse—whether the reason has to do with intelligence, environment, or religious or personal conviction—eliminate the risk.

Yet most girls who engage in sex don't become pregnant. Knowledge and the use of contraception are crucial reasons why. In Scandinavian nations, where teenagers are just as sexually active as in the United States, teen pregnancy rates are three to ten times lower. Young people in these countries learn at an early age that birth control is an essential part of sexual responsibility and have ready access to contraceptives and to counseling in their use. In this country, efforts to offer contraceptive counseling or to distribute condoms in schools often run into opposition, despite studies showing that neither increases the likelihood of teen sex.

American girls also find themselves caught up in old-fashioned good girl–bad girl stereotypes. "A simple way of showing that one is a 'nice girl' is to be unprepared for sex," Adler explains. Even bringing up the subject of birth control may indicate a girl is interested in sex (whether or not she is), knowledgeable (which she often isn't), and experienced (something no "nice girl" should be). Not knowing what to say to a boy, not daring to do anything to protect herself, a girl may let herself be "carried away" into unprotected sex. Not surprisingly, about 20 percent of teenage girls become pregnant within a month of first intercourse with a partner; half do so within six months. (This may be changing, however, since recent reports suggest an increase in condom use by teenagers during their first sexual experience.)

Another common misconception is that older men pressure girls into unprotected sex. According to a recent government analysis, only about 20 percent of the children of teenagers are fathered by men much older than the mothers. Most fathers of children born to girls of fifteen or sixteen are teenagers themselves; older girls have older partners, often in their twenties. Regardless of their age, fathers aren't likely to do what men in previous decades considered the "right thing" and marry the young woman carrying their child. Most teen mothers—60 percent of white girls and 90 percent of black girls—remain single. (This is not limited to adolescents: Teenagers account for only a third of all births to unmarried mothers in the United States.)

Every girl who finds herself pregnant has a unique story to tell about the whys and hows (although none can match the tale Mary told Ann and Joachim). However, two common threads consistently emerge from the often confusing and contradictory analyses that have been done of teen mothers and their motivations: They are often both poor and poor students. While poverty and lack of educational achievement do not directly cause adolescent pregnancy, their influence is too great to dismiss or ignore.

In comparisons between the United States and Scandinavian nations, poverty rates in the United States tend to be higher by about the same proportion as birth rates among adolescents. According to government data, American teenage girls who live near or below poverty income levels account for six of seven births to adolescent mothers. Girls living in more prosperous regions or states are statistically no more likely to give birth than their Scandinavian age peers.

Compounding poverty's impact is a lack of scholastic ability and opportunity. In one study of sixty-four teen mothers, most had been academic underachievers prior to getting pregnant; many had serious but undiagnosed learning disabilities. More than half lagged a grade level or more behind in reading, yet only two had undergone any educational evaluation and counseling.

With all the doors that education can open closing before them, academic underachievers like these girls may, consciously or not, view pregnancy as a misguided chance for success—even if they don't set out to get pregnant. In a recent analysis, National Center for Health Statistics researchers documented a direct relationship between fertility and educational achievement. Girls with less than a high-school education are more likely to become pregnant as teenagers and to have more children than those who complete secondary school.

What does this suggest about preventing pregnancy? Certainly it's not enough to exhort girls to just say no, to threaten them with loss of government support, to harangue them to believe in the promise of a future that they don't see as particularly bright. We need to lift girls out of poverty and to offer them education and opportunities that provide alternative paths to personal fulfillment. Only then can girls who might otherwise bear children in their teens learn what the "smart girls" in the University of North Carolina study already know: that in making sexual decisions about her body, a girl's best asset is her mind.

The Girl Who Cut Off Her Nose

In eleventh-century France, as was the custom at the time, the parents of a young girl named Ode arranged her engagement to a suitable member of the nobility. Ode protested, but her parents dismissed her desire to enter a convent and pursue a celibate religious life. At her wedding ceremony, Ode absolutely refused to give her required consent. Her parents and the groom's family were aghast. The members of the wedding procession didn't know where to turn or what to do. Ode, with fierce single-mindedness, disregarded the uproar. Brushing everyone aside, she returned home. To prevent any further attempts to marry her off, the determined girl cut off her nose.

It was a quintessentially adolescent act—horrific but dramatic, irrational yet undeniably effective. Ode's parents, who in all probability were acting in what they saw as their daughter's best interest, had no choice but to allow her to enter a convent. There she lived a life of such virtue that she became a saint of the Roman Catholic Church.

Almost a thousand years after Ode's defiance, teenage girls still use their noses to outrage their parents—by piercing them. At a certain level, they are sending the same message as Ode: "You can't tell me what to do. I'm no longer a child. If necessary, I would indeed cut off my nose to spite my face."

Although at times it may seem that parents and teenagers have made little progress over the last millennium, we have learned important lessons. The most important—yet most often overlooked—may be how much we need each other. In 1997 the National Longitudinal Study of Adolescent Health, the largest-ever study of American adolescents, published the initial findings of its survey of ninety thousand students in grades seven through twelve. Its most unexpected finding was this: Parents matter.

Girls and boys with strong emotional attachments to their parents are less likely to use alcohol or drugs, attempt suicide, engage in violence, or become sexually active at an early age. Although no teen is immune from internal demons or external pressures, those who feel loved and understood, and who feel they are paid attention to, are more likely to avoid dangerous risk behaviors. More than the actual amount of time parents spend with them, what matters most to teens is a strong personal bond, a sense of "connectedness." Although the researchers also recorded problems—in girls, greater emotional distress and more suicide attempts—this study marked an important difference from others. Rather than asking once again, "What's wrong with teens?" it raised a more important question: "What do teens need?"

This in turn leads to two different questions, each equally valid: What do boys need (the subject of another book) and what do girls need? The answers, despite considerable overlap, are different. Tinkering with girls so they fit better into man-made worlds—"remedial masculinization," as some call it—doesn't work. Girls need recognition that they are unique and worthy of attention. They also need more than reassurance to bolster their flagging self-esteem. Telling girls they're capable means little; they have to learn to believe in themselves by doing, by challenging themselves to become all that they might be.

The key to a girl's self-esteem may be the very same thing that makes adult women feel good about themselves (as discussed in Chapter 12): a rich variety of experiences and interests. As recent studies have shown, involvement in all types of activities boosts girls' self-esteem and body image. Sports in particular offer girls the chance to value themselves for the ways their bodies function—for how fast they cross the soccer field or how well they guard on the basketball court—rather than just the way they look. Girls who are physically active, whether in a team sport like volleyball or a solitary pursuit like swimming, also are more likely to challenge other limits, to tackle difficult classes in math and science, and to retain a healthy sense of their own worth and ability. Once again the psychobiology of being female comes into play: Learning the limits and possibilities of their bodies seems to open girls up to the potential of their minds.

Girls also need to see real-life role models—if only to counter the images of brain-dead bimbos that still monopolize the media. A recent survey of images aimed at teenagers found that women in movies or on television are far less likely than men to be seen working, using their intelligence, or focusing on issues other than romance, hair, and personal appearance. But with just a little parental nudging, girls can see women of more substance, literally and figuratively. I talk often with my daughter about the women I interview for magazine pieces: an Olympic gold medalist studying to be an orthopedic surgeon, a nurse blinded in an accident who now trains guide dogs, an African-American attorney who heads an FBI white-collar-crime unit. We also talk about women we both know: her friend's mother who's chronicled the exploration of the *Titanic*'s wreck, my friend who raises funds for innovative museums, a neighbor who fought to save an open-space preserve for horses to run free.

Of course, girls need real men in their lives, too—men who take them seriously and treat them with respect. And no man matters more to a girl than her father. Yet of all kinship ties, father-daughter relationships have been studied least. The assumption long has been that there is nothing to say other than the observation that fathers, unnerved by the sexual ripening of their little girls, often pull away, physically and psychologically, when adolescence looms. Such distancing is neither desirable nor destined, however. Girls who get attention from their fathers may be less desperate to do anything to find it elsewhere. And the father's role in the household also has a more subtle impact. Girls who grow up in egalitarian families in which both parents have careers and share household responsibilities are less likely to go into an academic slump in sixth and seventh grades than girls whose parents adhere to more traditional roles.

Nonetheless, more than anything else—by their own admission— girls need their mothers. In an American Psychological Association symposium on adolescence, one consistent finding emerged: What matters most to a teenage girl, troubled or not, is her mother. Warm, empathic mothers who show affection, listen carefully, and make a real effort to talk and socialize help ease the strain of their daughters' journey through these years. Girls who see their mothers as strong and supportive experience fewer symptoms of depression and feel better about themselves. According to adolescent specialist Flaherty, "A mother's self-esteem has more influence on a girl's self-confidence than any other factor."

Still, while mothers can offer a great deal, daughters need to discover their own truths. One is the realization that they too are strong. Their bodies, which may seem like alien space forms during puberty, are built to endure over the long haul. Their intense feelings, which now sweep over them like summer storms, will enrich their life with an emotional richness they cannot yet appreciate. Their mental abilities, when finally given the chance to flower, are demonstrably astounding. Educators may bicker over which sex scores higher on aptitude tests, but girls aren't waiting for the resolution of the debate. Around the world, more girls than ever before in history are attending colleges and universities, earning advanced degrees, and pursuing almost any career imaginable.

But this is not how the world looks from a girl's perspective. A twenty-year-old whom I've known and loved since her birth sends me a college paper entitled "Surviving Adolescence." In it she eloquently describes "what girls need to make adolescence more 'do-able' and less scary." Her wish list includes positive role models, media portrayals of girls "who look like them, not like cocaine addicts," positive ideals, and realistic goals. What she pleads for, on behalf of all girls, is "a society in which adolescence for girls is a journey of self-discovery and pride, rather than one of pain and loss."

This is not an unreasonable or impossible request. But if it is to happen, we have our work cut out for us. To make such a journey, girls need grown-ups to fight for opportunities, to open closed doors, to ensure their safety. They need protection from sexual predators, any form of abuse, all aspects of discrimination. Above all, they need us to believe in them and their strength as they dream big, try hard, fail where they may, and pick themselves up to face another day.

This isn't easy for them—or for us mothers, with our protective lioness instincts. On a blustery summer day I stand on a pier overlooking San Francisco Bay and watch my daughter's sailing class as twenty-five-knot winds buffet their tiny crafts. Again and again the wind overturns Julia's little boat. Almost trembling with trepidation, I wait for her yellow-haired head to bob above the surface of the water. If I could, I would take on Neptune himself, calm the winds, warm the frigid water, pluck my daughter from the sea, and set her safe on shore. Instead, I telepathically send her a message: *"Forza!"*—a word the Italians use to cheer on their athletes. With all the might she can muster, Julia rights her boat, grasps the helm, and steers once more into the wind.

Most girls do. By the end of adolescence, they emerge from the long metamorphosis into womanhood as bigger, stronger, smarter versions of their former selves. What we—mothers, fathers, loved and loving ones—can offer as they make their way through this sometimes daunting passage is our faith, even at the darkest moments, in the strong, resilient, and wiser women they are in the process of becoming.

CHAPTER 7

Riding the
Moon

The first assignment in an introductory college art course was to make something shocking. The students came up with an array of grotesque creations: sculptures of bizarre beasts, exotic erotica, scenes of violent massacres. But nothing proved more unsettling than a plain white box a quiet young woman brought to class. Unlatching the door revealed a tampon, suspended by its string and saturated in dripping red paint.

Of all bodily fluids, none has the visceral impact of blood, the sign of injury, illness, death—and also life. The Romans thought of menstrual blood as *sacra*, both sacred and accursed, with the power to heal and the potential to destroy. And every month a woman's menstrual cycle does indeed lift her up toward the timeless and bring her down to touch the tangible realities of the female body.

No other biological process may be at once so mundane, mysterious, and misunderstood. Contrary to common misconception, the shedding of blood is not itself the main event, but an anticlimax. The menstrual cycle is fundamentally an act of creation, of ripening, release, and renewal, a defining female rhythm that affects far more than our reproductive capacity: As they ebb and flow, these hormonal tides may enhance our creativity, sharpen our senses, improve our coordination, heighten our sensuality, speed the flow of ideas through our minds and of words from our lips. And the cycle's significance extends beyond women.

"It's not just a woman's cycle; men respond to it, too," says psychologist Diane Schechter, of Columbia University. "The menstrual cycle controls the sex lives of both genders, men as well as women. It is the chemical dance that drives the species."

This duet, as old as time yet eternally new, occurs among only a few mammals—humans and apes among them. Rather than menstruating, most females of other mammalian species experience estrus, a time of sexual receptivity and fertility, and engage in sex only then. The evolution of a more or less monthly menstrual cycle (the root of the word *menstrual* comes from the Greek for "month") allowed human females to have sex even when they weren't fertile, a biological bonus that became part of our genetic legacy (as discussed in Chapter 3).

Menstrual cycling has no counterpart in the male. Only women, and all women, do it—teens, matrons, virgins, mothers, regardless of class, culture, race, or sexual orientation. In prehistoric times, when light came only from the sky, menstrual cycles may have become synchronized with the phases of the moon and fertile women may have entered their "moon time" together. Even amid artificial constellations of electric lights, today's women still "ride the moon." It remains a truly remarkable journey.

Modern women menstruate far more often than our foremothers, who were almost continuously pregnant or nursing. In their entire lifetimes they may have had only fifty to one hundred periods (some anthropologists place this estimate even lower). Over the centuries, as women bore fewer children, breastfed less (if at all), and lived longer, their lifetime number of periods multiplied. These days a woman can expect to menstruate for almost four decades, cycling some four to five hundred times.

Any process that occurs so regularly over so many years in so many people certainly qualifies as a legitimate subject for scientific investigation. Yet research into the menstrual cycle has lagged—partly because of male scientists' lack of interest and partly because of women's reluctance to explore this aspect of their biology.

"I get letters from women asking me to stop studying the menstrual cycle," says psychiatrist Donna Stewart, chair of women's health at The Toronto Hospital. "On the one hand, there is tremendous fear that even talking about hormonal variations somehow stigmatizes women and will be used against them. On the other, women with severe menstrual disorders feel that research on the positive aspects of menstruation could keep them from getting the help they need. Menstrual research is a terribly politically incorrect arena to be working in, and scientists enter it at their own peril."

Yet ignorance about the menstrual cycle has proved decidedly perilous to women. Those who sought help for menstrual symptoms were routinely told that their problems were simply part of being female, that their bodies were programmed for monthly pain and discomfort. Only in the last quarter century, as great numbers of women have entered the public domain, bringing their biology in all its complexity with them, have scientists begun to take menstruation, its complications, and its clinical implications for many medical conditions seriously.

In 1977, when the Society for Menstrual Research convened its first assembly, only a hundred researchers attended, and their findings were not considered suitable for coverage in family newspapers. In 1997 its twentieth-anniversary session drew participants from around the world. These researchers—mostly women—had amassed more data on the menstrual cycle than ever before in history.

There is even a Museum of Menstruation, tucked into a nondescript suburban street outside Washington, D.C. It is an Alice in Wonderland kind of place filled with objects almost never seen—in public, that is. The exhibits—curiouser and curiouser—feature "sanitary bloomers" and rubberized "aprons" from Victorian times, early magazine ads for Kotex and tampons, and artworks with menstrual themes. The museum's very existence is a testimonial to a subject that has inspired shame, apprehension, and confusion, but little public recognition.

Women and scientists alike are still struggling to find ways to think and talk about a process that is both a harbinger of health and a source of symptoms, one that is perfectly natural, altogether normal, yet also, as one British wit put it, "the original bloody nuisance." Some individuals of both genders insist that we place far too much emphasis on a function that is as unremarkable as digestion. Others contend that ignoring or dismissing monthly fluctuations can set women up for a no-win battle with their own biology.

To me, the menstrual cycle seems not just female but strikingly feminine, one of those cooperative, turn-taking, constantly communicative ventures that women so often undertake. Only in its case, our brains, hormones, and reproductive systems join together in a month-long conversation. The more we learn about what they're saying, the better we can understand the rhythms of our lives and appreciate an essential part of our womanly natures, the "surging miracle of blood," in the words of poet May Sarton, that makes a woman

> as distinctively part
> of the universe as a star—
> as unresistant,
> as completely rhythmical.

Changing Woman

In a shady grove, a storyteller recounts tales of Changing Woman and her child. Journeying around the world, they come upon a river too wide to cross. Changing Woman turns into a giant turtle and carries her child across on her back. When they come to sky-high mountains, Changing Woman becomes an eagle and flies her baby to the other side. When they are attacked by bloodthirsty beasts, Changing Woman transforms herself into a lion and chases them away. When winter winds rage around them, she grows a pelt like a polar bear and snuggles her baby in its warmth. Changing Woman can become a wolf that runs through the forest, a falcon that soars above the clouds, a dolphin that dives deep into the sea. And yet one thing about this remarkable female never changes: the love in her heart.

Although our powers may seem less dazzling than those of the heroine in this mythic tale, we all are changing women. "Men, poor old things, seem to just stay on in the same groove for their whole lives," Germaine Greer once observed. That's not a woman's style. A woman will change anything and everything—her mind, her style, her hair, her politics, her opinion. In Verdi's *Rigoletto*, the Duke of Mantua's irresistibly hummable refrain, *"La donna è mobile,"* is usually translated as "Woman is fickle," but *mobile* also means "changeable." Although this trait drives some men crazy, it may help keep women sane and strong. In nature, change is a sign of health.

While male hormones, vital signs, and mood states also fluctuate, female biology is more responsive to changes around us as well as within us. When winter melts into spring and autumn fades to winter, melatonin, a brain chemical that influences migration and mating in many animals, rises or falls only in the female of our species. "When it comes to seasonal change," one expert in biological rhythms observes, "men just don't get it."

Why does "the music of the spheres," the unspoken dance of planets, sun, moon, and stars, resonate only in a woman's body? Perhaps in deepest time the survival of a woman and her children depended on her recognizing the best seasons to conceive, to give birth, to find food for her family. Perhaps from the dawn of human existence, women looked to the sky, to the sun's light and the moon's glow, for comfort and inspiration. We still do. Without light, our moods slump, our energy flags, our menstrual cycles become erratic.

"We don't know exactly how or why," observes psychiatrist Barbara Parry, of the University of California, San Diego, "but a woman's sensitivity to light affects her sleep-wake rhythm, her release of various hormones, and her menstrual cycle." In one study of nearly two thousand women with irregular cycles, she found that a low-intensity night-light placed near their beds during the three days around ovulation helped establish regular menstruation. In other studies, she has demonstrated that exposure to bright light can ease premenstrual mood symptoms.

The menstrual cycle also changes in response to other cues. Physical or emotional stress can cause it to shorten, lengthen, or stop altogether. Pheromones, the silent chemical messengers discussed in Chapter 2, also affect it. Sigmund Freud, who meticulously charted the cycles of the women in his household, noted a tendency among women "affectively linked" (emotionally connected in some way) to menstruate in harmony. In experiments with female lifeguards and other women sharing close quarters, University of Chicago biologist Martha McClintock confirmed this same synchronization and speculated that pheromones were the reason. In 1998, thirty years after her original work, she offered proof for this premise. When compounds taken from the underarms of one group of women were dabbed under the noses of others, the recipients' cycles either shortened or lengthened, depending on whether the first group of women were at the beginning or middle of their cycles.

Why should pheromones have such an effect? No one yet knows, although evolutionary theorists suggest that this strategy may somehow have helped in attracting males or in damping competition from other females. It also could have served a more supportive purpose. Regular cyclers may have boosted the fertility of those with irregular periods and enhanced their chances of conception.

The menstrual cycle may also respond to other influences. Women who engage in frequent sex with a man (or those dabbed regularly with male pheromones) tend to have a greater number of regular cycles, whereas the cycles of women who are celibate or have only sporadic intercourse are more irregular. And sexual orientation may have an effect. When she charted the cycles of twenty-nine cohabiting lesbian couples, anthropologist Wenda Trevathan, of New Mexico State University, found no evidence of menstrual harmony.

The Scarlet Letter

When she overheard her older sister giggling with friends about periods and pads, a ten-year-old asked her mother what they were talking about. "It doesn't concern you now," her mom said. "When you're older, I have a book that you can read." The curious girl scoured the family bookshelves until she zeroed in on the title she thought her mother had been talking about: *The Scarlet Letter*.

We women, gathered around a kitchen table, howled at this story, but all of us identified—not just with its teller but with the infamously adulterous Hester Prynne. We'd had our share of acutely embarrassing menstrual moments when we might as well have had a bright red *M* for *menstruating* emblazoned on our chests. And we'd all sensed an unspoken shame in our body's betrayal by blood.

"I was fifteen and the last of my friends to get my period, so I was happy when it happened," a vibrant executive in her thirties recalls. "My parents had just gotten divorced, and my dad had shacked up with a woman who didn't seem much older than I was. My mother gave me some Kotex and dropped me off at my dad's house. Obviously she had told him. He said—in front of his current babe—'So my little girl is a woman now.' I wanted the earth to open up and swallow me. I can still re-create the experience of feeling so abysmal, so dirty."

Certainly boys' bodies also do embarrassing things: Their voices break, their penises pop up at inopportune times, their dreams leave stains on the sheets. Yet these are mainly temporary trials; boys outgrow most and learn to control the rest. Girls encounter a different reality: As discussed in Chapter 6, they have to learn to anticipate and manage a complicated physiological process—preferably without calling attention to it.

Shameful feelings about this process date back through time. Al-though legends of ancient matriarchies suggest that menstruation once inspired awe, most often it triggered loathing. Menstrual blood was feared as a potent toxin that could spoil milk, destroy crops, sour beer, drive dogs mad, shatter glass, dull swords, and sicken even the most virile males. Its shedding was deemed so disgusting that women felt they had to keep a normal, fundamentally female process secret.

An ancient Persian myth portrayed menstruation as a consequence of the serpent's seduction of the first woman. Jewish rabbis, who saw menstruation as God's curse for Eve's original sin, wrote canonical law banning menstruating women from the presence of untainted men and requiring them to undergo a ritual bath when their periods ended. Other ancient societies feared the touch, breath, even the gaze of a men-struating woman. "What power!" observes one researcher, noting that if women had indeed possessed such abilities, they'd have gotten a lot more respect.

Early scholars tried to explain the biology of menstruation—but got it hopelessly wrong. Hippocrates described it as a form of detoxifica-tion, analogous to perspiration in men. Aristotle believed that menstrual blood contained a substance that a man's sperm "concocted" to create a fetus—a belief that persisted, with variations, into the eighteenth cen-tury. One theorist believed menstrual blood had three components: one for nourishing a fetus in utero, another for transformation into breast milk, and the third a venomous element eliminated during delivery. Others postulated that the menstrual flow served to "irrigate" male ejaculate so that it would adhere "to female parts." It wasn't until the nineteenth century that London physician John Power connected ovulation and menstruation, although he wrongly asserted that women were most fertile when menstruating.

History, which paid little attention to women's public lives, all but ignored their private cycles—except for those of women as famous as men. The daughters of England's son-hungry Henry VIII, Mary and Elizabeth, were plagued by menstrual problems. Mary, dubbed "Bloody" for her persecution of Protestants, suffered from amenorrhea. Her half sister Elizabeth—the Virgin Queen—also had infrequent periods (or so said gossipy laundresses). Joan of Arc, burned at the stake at age twenty, supposedly never menstruated—perhaps because of her rigorous lifestyle and lean frame. Marie Antoinette bled so heavily on the night before her execution that she stained the white chemise she had planned to wear and hid the soiled garment in a crevice in her rock-walled cell. Elizabeth Barrett Browning reportedly became addicted to the opium she took for her disabling cramps.

Even in the early twentieth century, medical experts postulated that mental activity during menstruation could interfere with ovulation and destroy feminine "capability." The president of the American Gynecological Society cautioned schools for women to recognize their students' instability during menstruation and to allow for adequate rest. The Philadelphia County Medical Society contended that women should be barred from medical training because their cycles rendered them constitutionally unfit to deal with crises in the practice of medicine.

When she learned the facts of menstrual gynecology as they were understood at the turn of the twentieth century, Martha Carey Thomas, who grew up to become president of Bryn Mawr College, recalled being "terrorstruck lest I, and every woman with me, were doomed to live as pathological invalids in a universe merciless to woman as a sex." One of her contemporaries, the physician Clelia Mosher, showed that it wasn't biology that was causing much menstrual suffering. In a study of college women between 1890 and 1920, Mosher noted a much higher incidence of menstrual cramps in the "Gibson girl" era, when some fifteen pounds of heavy clothing were draped from a girlish waist squeezed to an eighteen-inch circumference. As skirts grew shorter and skimpier and waistlines eased outward, the incidence of crippling cramps dropped.

Pseudoscience countered common sense in the 1920s with the reported identification of "menotoxins"—substances in a menstruating woman's saliva, urine, perspiration, milk, tears, even the air she breathed—that could cause a bouquet of roses to fade within a day. These alleged poisons turned out to be atypical globulins, which exist in even higher levels in nonmenstruating women and have no pernicious effect on flowers or anything else.

Why have so many myths—often too absurd to merit a moment's belief—surrounded women's menstrual cycles? Freud believed they sprang from a blood phobia, an ancient human terror that may have served "aesthetic and hygienic purposes." Theodor Reik argued that the origin of menstrual taboos went deeper—to men's ambivalent views toward women. On the one hand, a man may be irresistibly drawn to a woman; on the other, he struggles to restrain powerful sexual urges. Thus, men come to see women, with their tempting flesh and repugnant blood, as sources of both desire and disgust.

Male ambivalence about, if not antipathy to, female bleeding may have influenced men's interpretation of menstrual rituals in other cultures. When male anthropologists wrote the first descriptions of menstrual huts in various foraging societies, they depicted them as places of banishment, where women, shunned by the group, stayed in shameful exile. Yet when female anthropologists eventually interviewed women in these societies, they got a very different impression: that the women looked forward to their days off from the hard work of their daily lives and enjoyed the opportunity to laugh and relax in the company of other women.

Molimina: The Ways We Change

A classic British advertisement for what is discreetly called "feminine protection" features a photograph of a tampon in a cardboard applicator and an unforgettable headline: "If men were shaped like most tampons, the human race would have died out by now." An overstatement, perhaps. But if women didn't menstruate, we truly might have become extinct. Yet although our species owes its survival to the menstrual cycle, many people know little about *molimina*, the medical term for the normal changes a woman experiences each month.

The average menstrual cycle is twenty-eight days long, although a range from twenty-one to thirty-five days is considered normal. The first day of bleeding marks the beginning of the cycle, which is divided into two halves: the follicular stage, which culminates in ovulation (the release of an ovum, or egg cell), and the luteal stage, which begins after ovulation and ends in the shedding of the uterine lining.

As the follicular stage, the time of ripening of an egg follicle in the ovary, begins, a woman is most like a man—hormonally, that is. Her levels of estrogen and progesterone may overlap with typical male readings. Throughout the follicular stage, the pituitary gland increases production of follicle-stimulating hormone (FSH), which signals the ovaries to waken several immature egg cells, or oocytes, nestled in their follicles, from their long sleep. Usually only one oocyte reaches full maturity; the others disintegrate. The ovaries also secrete estrogen, pushing blood levels higher. The pituitary gland then cuts back on FSH and stimulates production of luteinizing hormone (LH), which triggers ovulation—the release of a mature ovum from the follicle. Messages travel back and forth along the hypothalamus-pituitary-ovarian axis to ensure that just the right amounts of the various hormones are released at exactly the right times.

After emerging from its follicle, the ovum makes the journey of its lifetime to the fallopian tube for a possible rendezvous with a partner's sperm. Following ovulation, body temperature climbs and remains elevated. Potassium, at its highest at ovulation, falls afterward, while the sodium in a woman's blood—lowest at ovulation—rises.

The corpus luteum, the remnant of the ruptured egg follicle, orchestrates the changes of the second half—the luteal stage—of the menstrual cycle by secreting progesterone, which, together with estrogen, causes the uterine lining, or endometrium, to thicken in preparation for implantation by a fertilized egg. In effect, a woman's body sumptuously furnishes an internal nursery for occupancy by a fast-growing, energy-draining human fetus.

Usually without realizing it, women consume more food (a smart move to nourish a beginning pregnancy) in the early luteal stage—the ten days following ovulation. About one third of women report a weight gain of one to five pounds during the luteal stage—a consequence of water, sodium, and chloride retention as well as increased food intake.

If fertilization and implantation do not occur, the pituitary gland shuts down production of LH and FSH. In the late luteal or premenstrual phase—the six days before menstrual bleeding begins—the corpus luteum disintegrates, and estrogen and progesterone levels fall. As discussed later in this chapter, most women experience some symptoms—physical, psychological, or both—during this time. Many common disorders, including allergies, asthma, depression, migraine headaches, epilepsy, and autoimmune diseases, tend to flare up; this phenomenon, dubbed "premenstrual exacerbation," may require adjustments in the medications women take for these conditions.

Each month's cycle ends with the shedding of menstrual blood, which is actually a combination of blood, endometrial cells, and mucus from the cervix and vagina. Darker in color than the blood that flows through our arteries and veins, it also has a distinctive odor and texture—similar, as one researcher puts it, to "an oil-based paint, with small particles suspended in a thick fluid."

Women typically bleed for five or six days, most heavily on the first three days, with the most profuse flow on day two. An estimated 90 percent experience at least occasional pain during their periods, particularly those in their teens and early twenties. Like other menstrual problems, dysmenorrhea, pain during menses, was long thought to be in a woman's head, an indication of her psychological conflicts about being female. However, we've learned that cramps have a specific biological cause: high levels of prostaglandins, hormonelike substances that cause muscle contractions and control the dilation and constriction of blood vessels. Painkillers that block prostaglandin synthesis, such as ibuprofen, provide relief.

Perhaps the most remarkable aspect of molimina is not how many changes occur during the menstrual cycle but how well women take them in stride. Although long viewed as a sign of feminine frailty, the menstrual cycle is in fact a testimony to female fortitude. "There's been so much emphasis on pathology related to the menstrual cycle that we tend to forget its normalcy," says psychiatrist Judith Gold, who chaired the American Psychiatric Association's task force on premenstrual disorders. "The vast majority of women may experience some symptoms before or during their periods, but they function, and function well, throughout."

The Inner Flow

You wake up, and the world seems new. Ideas flood into your mind. Filled with energy, you make plans, set goals, tackle projects. As days pass, you're drawn into the world, intrigued by new people and ideas, open to suggestions and possibilities. You're extroverted and friendly. You delight in everything from a favorite tune on the radio to a flower's sweet smell and satiny sheen.

What's going on? Nothing extraordinary, just the perfectly normal emotional changes—psychological molimina, one could say—that occur during the follicular stage of the menstrual cycle. As levels of estrogen, an up-and-at-'em hormone, and testosterone, the hormone that sparks sexual desire as well as energy, rise, women typically feel eager for challenge, interested in new ideas, and willing to take risks.

Just prior to ovulation at the end of the follicular stage, FSH and LH surge, and women open up even more. Vision becomes more acute; the senses of touch and smell sharpen. Women are less aware of pain; feelings of aggression and anxiety are low. This is the time of the month when they are most likely to feel not just happy but elated, to fantasize about sex, and to seek out sexual encounters. Without consciously deciding to do so, a woman may return a flirtatious wink or respond with unexpected passion to a partner's embrace. Even though there is little scientific evidence, some experts think we may be at our most engaging at this time. Waitresses, for instance, have reported that they get higher tips at midcycle, right around the time of ovulation.

As the luteal phase, the second half of the menstrual cycle, begins, progesterone dominates, and some internal barometer shifts. Women tend to stay closer to home. They want to think through their ideas, mull over the possibilities that had seemed so irresistible a little while before. Their senses are somewhat muted; their euphoria diminishes. Rather than drinking in every sensation, women tend to block out what is happening around them.

The luteal phase is a time for evaluation and reflection, a psychological ebb tide. Thoughts take on a negative slant; a woman sees the glass as half empty rather than half full; she worries more. In one intriguing experiment, when different emotionally charged words were spoken through headphones into women's right and left ears, those in the luteal phase of their cycles heard fewer of the positive words.

As discussed in the following section, the late luteal phase—the six premenstrual days before bleeding begins—is often emotionally intense. But attention has mainly focused on the negative aspects of this time. "Hardly anyone ever asked women what they liked about being premenstrual," comments psychiatrist Stewart. When she posed this question in a survey of a hundred women, two thirds reported at least one positive change: increased energy, greater sexual interest and enjoyment, an urge to tidy up or get things done, more attractive breasts, and more creative ideas. More than 20 percent of the women cited five or more positive changes.

"The one thing women mention most is feeling more energetic," says Stewart. "But they use this energy in very different ways—some have sex, and some straighten up the office or vacuum the living room." The premenstrual surge in sexual arousal, pleasure, and orgasm, documented in other studies, may be a consequence of engorged blood vessels or of a woman's realization that this is one of the "safest" times of the month for sex. The tidiness urge is harder to explain, but it may be similar to the nesting tendencies many pregnant women report in the final weeks before delivery.

In Stewart's study, 95 percent of women also mentioned at least one negative premenstrual change, most often feeling more emotional, tearful, irritable, moody, or unable to keep a lid on their feelings. Yet even these changes may serve a purpose. A premenstrual outburst, the emotional equivalent of house cleaning, may clear away tensions that have been building for weeks. And many women feel that the issues that surface at this time often are important but neglected concerns deserving of their attention.

The nature and intensity of psychological changes over the course of the menstrual cycle vary greatly among women, yet are most often benign. In her studies at Columbia, psychologist Schechter has found that, contrary to common assumption, "women cycle much more in positive emotions than negative ones. They feel varying degrees of well-being rather than going back and forth between positive and negative mood states." Those who slump into the lowest lows at one time of the month often report higher highs at other times in their cycle. "These women don't see it as a bad thing to move up and down in their cycles," she says. "To them, it's worth it."

Do intellectual abilities also fluctuate with a woman's cycle? Many have claimed they do, even arguing that women should avoid taking crucial examinations, such as qualifying tests for college or graduate school, at times when they might not perform at their best. Such concerns don't seem at all justifiable. In a review of the highly controversial studies—few in number and erratic in quality—that have been done, psychologist Barbara Sommer, of the University of California, Davis, found scant scientific evidence for significant menstrual variability. In general, regardless of whether they are ripening an egg, ovulating, dismantling their internal nursery, or shedding their endometrial lining, women can think abstractly, add, subtract, multiply, divide, remember, speak, define, and coordinate their movements equally well.

However, there are some measures—most of dubious relevance to daily life—that may vary through a cycle. Some women do better at "disembedding," that is, finding hidden patterns or words, when estrogen levels are low, as they are before and during a woman's period. Some do poorly on backward subtraction (a skill even accountants leave to calculators) prior to ovulation. And in one especially curious (and irrelevant) study, hand steadiness in holding a revolver declined in the premenstrual phase.

The Premenstrual Puzzle

My husband, Bob, and I are discussing one of those topics that long-married partners rehash as often as Thanksgiving turkey: I want him to carve more family time out of his crowded schedule, or one of us needs to bail the other out of some sticky social situation, or we're debating once more the pros and cons of a bigger house. The discussion is perfectly calm and rational. I present my arguments logically; he responds or rebuts. Then, without warning, some lever beyond my conscious control flips, and tears flood into my eyes. A certain look comes over Bob's face, and he says, "Ah, you're getting your period!" And I know that he's just discounted everything I've been saying.

As any woman who's been in this situation knows—and every one I know has—nothing can be more infuriating than the double whammy of a premenstrual meltdown coupled with an intellectual put-down. Yet as it's always been just like a woman to menstruate, it's always been just like men to doubt us—in either ability or stability—because we do. This is never more true than in the infamous premenstrual period—"hell week," as a friend refers to it.

In most women, emotions do intensify at this time. Something that may have been nagging at them all month long becomes more insistent, and rather than denying irritation or frustration, they let it out. Does this mean that there is something wrong with every woman who bursts into tears or snaps at her spouse the week before her period? Not at all. Most women report one or more premenstrual symptoms, but symptoms alone do not a syndrome make.

As defined by a National Institute of Mental Health consensus conference, a diagnosis of premenstrual syndrome, or PMS, must be based on daily ratings of symptoms, physical and psychological, that indicate a change in intensity of at least 30 percent (some contend this threshold should be higher) in the six days before menses compared with days five to ten of a woman's cycle following menstruation. While other countries prefer the term "premenstrual tension," or PMT, studies in North America, Great Britain, Australia, Italy, Switzerland, Nigeria, China, and India have documented a similar constellation of symptoms in women. These include physical changes, such as fatigue, headaches, bloating, food cravings, appetite changes, aches, breast tenderness, and dizziness, and psychological symptoms, such as mood swings, tearfulness, irritability, nervous tension, sadness, anxiety, persistent anger, sleep problems, and poor concentration.

Because few studies have defined PMS consistently, estimates of how many women actually have this problem vary greatly. On the basis of its review of four hundred articles and more than six hundred clinical cases, the American Psychiatric Association task force on premenstrual disorders estimated that 20 to 30 percent of women have complaints, ranging from mild to severe, that could be categorized as PMS—far fewer than the percentage of women who think they have it.

"PMS may be the only psychiatric problem that more people are willing to say they have than actually do," says Stewart. "We see a lot of overattributing to PMS, because it's more acceptable to say you're premenstrual than that you're depressed or having a problem at home or work. Study after study shows that PMS is not a serious problem for most women, yet the myth persists that women as a whole are incapacitated. Even women believe it and expect to feel unwell."

The best way for an individual woman to sort out puzzling premenstrual symptoms from true PMS is to keep a daily record of mood, energy level, and overall sense of well-being over two monthly cycles. In studies in which women did so, as many as 40 percent were able to rule out PMS. Often charts reveal that symptoms believed to be premenstrual actually wax and wane along with job or family stress or that mood swings occur throughout the cycle, rather than just premenstrually. Or the variation in symptoms over the course of a cycle may be slight.

A diagnosis of PMS depends on a woman's subjective evaluation of cyclic changes as well as their timing and severity. Symptoms must occur or intensify only before her period and must interfere with her ability to function normally—that is, to take care of her family, do her job, and cope with daily responsibilities.

A significant percentage of women evaluated for PMS actually suffer from depression that intensifies premenstrually. The symptoms are similar to those of PMS (fatigue, appetite changes, sleep difficulties, low mood, and decreased concentration), but they never go away completely. During most of the month these women manage to get by, but as their periods approach, they feel much worse. Proper treatment for such depression—with medication, psychotherapy, or both—is important, since even moderate premenstrual depression increases a woman's risk of a major depressive episode at some time in her life (see Chapter 13).

What actually causes PMS? Standard laboratory tests have revealed no abnormalities in reproductive hormones, ovarian physiology, or the neuroendocrine network linking the brain and the ovaries. However, recent studies suggest that PMS is, as scientists at the National Institute of Mental Health put it, "an abnormal response to normal hormonal changes." For unknown reasons, some women seem especially sensitive to cyclic fluctuations in estrogen and progesterone, possibly because of their effects on neurotransmitters, such as mood-regulating serotonin.

Medications that boost serotonin—primarily the antidepressant selective serotonin receptor inhibitors (SSRIs) such as Prozac (fluoxetine) and Zoloft (sertraline)—have proven effective for PMS, whether women take them only during the second half of their cycles, use low doses (half the amount given for depression), or take a daily half dose for two or three weeks, with a full dose in the premenstrual period. In clinical trials, these medications offered significant relief to about 60 to 70 percent of women with PMS or a more severe problem called premenstrual dysphoric disorder (discussed later in this chapter).

If the SSRIs don't work, physicians may prescribe the antianxiety drug Xanax (alprazolam) for use throughout the luteal phase or the days before menstruation, with the dosages tapered off after a woman's period begins. Another alternative is the antianxiety agent BuSpar (buspirone), taken at a low dose throughout the menstrual cycle.

No single treatment is effective for all women with PMS, but careful diagnosis and a systematic approach to potential therapies help most feel better. Some benefit from increased light. About 70 percent of women with PMS experience fewer symptoms during the summer. In her clinical research, psychiatrist Parry has found that both sleep deprivation (for half a night, either from 9:00 P.M. to 1:00 A.M. or from 3:00 to 7:00 A.M.) and phototherapy (exposure to bright lights for one to two hours every morning for a week or to dim red evening light) relieve symptoms.

Many women report improvement with other nondrug alternatives, including stress reduction (through relaxation exercises, yoga, and meditation), a healthy diet (made up of carbohydrate-rich, low-protein foods, which may boost serotonin production), regular exercise (particularly aerobic activities like walking and jogging), vitamin supplements (a daily multivitamin together with no more than 50 mg of vitamin B_6), and increased calcium. Others have tried evening primrose oil, herbal supplements and teas, and other natural therapies, but their efficacy and safety have not been demonstrated by scientific studies.

Just as with other aspects of the menstrual cycle, the most impressive fact about premenstrual symptoms and PMS is not how many women experience them, but how well they manage despite them. According to research in Australia and the United States, few women diagnosed with PMS ever take time off from work because of this condition, nor do colleagues notice any change in their job performance. "Women have probably always had premenstrual symptoms, yet they've always done what they had to," comments Gold. "Isn't that just like a woman?"

Women on the Verge

As a psychiatry resident at UCLA, Barbara Parry had never seen a psychotic patient like this woman before, and she never forgot her. The woman clearly had lost her grip on reality. She saw skeletons in the closet. She heard voices telling her to kill herself. Then one morning, several days after the woman's admission to the psychiatric ward, the patient looked up as Parry entered the room, greeted her by name, and calmly wished her a good morning.

"I was sure that someone had given her antipsychotic medication, but when I checked her chart, I saw that she hadn't gotten any drugs. But there was a note that the woman's period had started." As Parry discovered, this woman suffered from a potentially life-threatening mental disorder that occurred only in the week before her menstrual period. This condition, now known as premenstrual dysphoric disorder (abbreviated as PDD or PMDD), is rare, affecting an estimated 3 to 5 percent of women. But it is real and can be extremely serious.

Some people describe PDD as "PMS on steroids," and the border between severe PMS and PDD is not clear. Researchers do not yet know whether PMS and PDD are two points on a spectrum of premenstrual disorders or two biologically distinct conditions. To be diagnosed with PDD, women must have at least five symptoms (confirmed by daily charts), including depressed mood, feelings of hopelessness or self-deprecating thoughts, marked anxiety or tension, significant mood swings, or persistent anger or irritability; their symptoms must markedly interfere with their daily responsibilities, whether in working, caring for a family, or interacting with others. Psychotic symptoms, like those of the UCLA patient, are unusual but can develop. All symptoms must improve within a few days of the onset of menstrual bleeding and must not occur in the week after menstruation ends.

PDD sufferers often show clear biological differences from other women. Their sleep tends to be more fragmented throughout their cycles, and they respond differently to phototherapy. "If you expose normal women to bright lights, they will advance their sleep rhythms by two hours; women with PDD don't," says Parry. "It may be that women who develop PDD aren't as physiologically flexible as others; they may not be able to make the small modulations that are necessary to maintain stability over the long haul." The same treatments used for PMS—serotonin-boosting medications, antianxiety drugs, and phototherapy—are often effective in women with PDD. In extreme cases, physicians may use powerful drugs called GnRH agonists that shut down the menstrual cycle completely, but because of their side effects (which include menopausal symptoms and increased risk of osteoporosis), they are rarely used for more than six months.

PDD is the only menstrual problem that is considered a psychiatric disorder. In the 1980s, when researchers first proposed such a designation, the very notion set off a furor. Protesters marched on psychiatric convocations. Labeling any menstruating women as mentally ill, they argued, might mean that all women would fall under suspicion: Ancient menstrual taboos would take on new life, working women would be shut out of high-level jobs, and mothers in divorce cases would lose custody of their children.

A panel of the nation's most distinguished female psychiatrists and psychologists—"the cream and evaporated milk" of the distaff side of the profession, as one observer put it—convened to consider the matter. They spent four years reading the scientific literature, analyzing and reanalyzing data, writing, talking, faxing, meeting, telephoning, discussing, debating. Some believed that a serious but treatable premenstrual mental disorder did exist and, however politically unpopular, had to be acknowledged as such. Others remained convinced that any categorization of a menstrual problem as a mental disorder would do women more harm than good.

Ultimately, PDD—but not PMS—was included in the appendix of

the newest version of the standard psychiatric diagnostic manual; this placement acknowledged that it is a real problem but indicates the need for further research. Despite the dire predictions, the "raging hormones" debate has not reignited—nor have the courts been crammed with cases involving PDD either as a justification for discrimination or as a defense for illegal behavior.

"I'm not surprised," says Parry. "It is very hard to be diagnosed with PDD. You must have symptoms only premenstrually, they must be severe, and there can be no other cause, including life stress or depression. But there are women I see who are suffering with this disorder. And because we've finally acknowledged that something is seriously wrong, they're able to get treatment and feel better."

Blood Secrets

If necessity is the mother of invention, menstruation has been midwife to some of women's cleverest concoctions. Using sponges, moss, cotton bolls, coconut fibers, and papyrus, our foremothers fashioned all types of sanitary protection. In the fifth century B.C., Hippocrates described tampons made of lint wrapped around lightweight wood. In Rome, women reportedly used wool; in Africa, they rolled grasses into absorbent bundles. Eventually Western women came to rely on washable pads of soft cotton or flannel, held in place by various diaperlike devices and belts—and, in Victorian times, covered with layers of bloomers, slips, and skirts.

Modern disposable sanitary protection dates back to World War I. French nurses, working long shifts tending the wounded, improvised by using cellulose bandages for napkins. The material, they noticed, provided much longer-lasting protection than cotton. After the war, Kimberly-Clark, the giant paper manufacturer, oversupplied with bandages, used the absorbent material it called "cellu-cotton" to create Kotex. Although not the first disposable, its name, as advertisements noted, served as a code word, so women could ask for sanitary napkins without having to mention menstruation. The first German disposable pads contained a slip of paper that a woman could give to a clerk to request additional boxes without saying anything at all. As more stores stocked and displayed disposable napkins—usually in the no-man's zone next to sewing patterns in the notions department—sales soared.

In 1931, after years of experimentation, an American physician, Earle Cleveland Haas, filed a patent application for an intravaginal "catamenial device" (from a physiological term for menses). He later coined the name Tampax from a combination of *tampon* and *vaginal pack*. Despite initial worries about possible harm to virginal young women and concern about toxic shock syndrome in the 1980s, tampons have become the most popular form of protection among European and American women (in developing nations more women use external protection). *Consumer Reports* included tampons on its list of fifty "small wonders" that changed modern culture. Along with other menstrual products such as anti-inflammatory medications to relieve cramps and hormonal contraceptives that regulate cycles, they have certainly revolutionized the ways women "manage" menstruation.

In an era when girls begin menstruating earlier and women (who spend far less time pregnant or nursing than in the past) menstruate more often, the menstrual cycle has become all but invisible. No one knows which woman in the lecture hall, at the starting block, around the conference table, or in the operating room is menstruating. And no one need know. With birth control pills, women can manipulate the timing of their periods. In the future, with the refinement of drugs that can suppress menstruation entirely or techniques like menstrual extraction (the aspiration of the endometrial lining), they may be able to stop doing what it's always been just like a woman to do.

Will they choose to? In the feminist heyday of the 1970s, Germaine Greer declared that no woman would menstruate if she didn't have to. On jagged-nerve, bad-cramps, stained-skirt days, most women have felt the same way. Yet in a World Health Organization survey of attitudes toward menstruation among women of all socioeconomic classes in ten countries, 71 percent said that, despite the very real inconveniences and occasional discomforts, they would not choose to stop their menstrual cycles—even for the sake of complete contraceptive protection.

A woman's age and life stage may well affect her opinion. Teenage girls fumbling with pads might well opt to be spared the monthly visits of what we used to call "my friend." But in time, many women come to appreciate the secret knowledge carried by their blood. In my twenties I'd greet the first telltale signs of menstruation with a certain relief, thankful not to be pregnant. Years later, yearning for a baby, I prayed not to bleed, not to face yet another round of disappointment.

The menstrual cycle, as women learn as they move to its rhythm, is nature's exercise in hope. Month after month, year after year, it signals change and rebirth, wakens us to new possibilities, entices us with prospects of what might be, expands our own notions of who we are and what we might do in our lives. Time and again it tells us a secret: that we are in for some changes.

When their menstrual cycles finally end, women are often surprised by their own ambivalence. Yes, they're glad to be rid of the muss and fuss, yet they feel a pang of loss, too. "One of my patients stopped menstruating for a while and then started again," recounts therapist Virginia Sadock. "She was so happy to have her old friend return—if only so she could say goodbye." A postmenopausal friend of mine says her life feels more placid these days, but she misses the aura of possibility that each month used to bring.

If the menstrual cycle is, as I've come to believe, a dance of life, most of us are glad to whirl to its rhythm. In the past, unfortunately, this was often the only choreography women knew. Because of this fact of female biology they were shut out of synagogues and schools, libraries and laboratories. Yet despite taboos and prohibitions, menstruating women throughout history have always carried on with the basic business of living. They tilled fields, crossed continents, wove fabrics, worked in factories, taught children, nursed the ill, comforted the dying. The menstrual cycle itself has never been the real barrier in a woman's life. What held us back for far too long were myths and mistaken beliefs about menstruating women.

CHAPTER 8

The Restless Womb

"An animal within an animal." This description of the female uterus by a physician in second-century Rome was neither the first nor the last to depict a woman's womb (and a woman herself) as a strange and wild thing. Centuries before, Plato had declared the uterus so "possessed with the desire to make children" that it careened through the body and attached itself to other vital organs, causing all varieties of disease. For centuries afterward, healers directed women to inhale noxious scents to repel the roving womb downward or to place sweet fragrances beneath them to lure this restless wanderer back to its proper place.

Perhaps more than any other part of the body, the invisible, enigmatic uterus baffled early scientists. Some theorized that it functioned like an oven that provided the heat and fuel to ignite the fire of a new life; others speculated that, like a centrifuge, it spun female and male fluids together until they formed a solid being. According to one widely circulated medieval text, hair lining the inner walls of the uterus grasped a man's semen during intercourse and later held a fetus in place. (Prostitutes, one physician contended, were often sterile because their hairy wombs became clogged with filth.) *Hystera*—Greek for "uterus"—formed the root of a word that was perhaps the most infamous female diagnosis: hysteria, a disease whose vague and debilitating symptoms were blamed on the tyranny of the impetuous, imperious womb.

The utilitarian uterus, the most unerotic of sexual organs, seems an unlikely despot. In a woman who has never had a child, the hollow womb, shaped like an upside-down pear, is only about the size of a fist, approximately three inches long and two inches wide, connected to the vagina at the cervix and suspended from the pelvic walls by ligaments that tend to tilt it either forward or back. Yet it possesses one remarkable and quintessentially female characteristic: an extraordinary capacity for transformation.

Each month, as described in Chapter 7, the innermost lining of the womb, the endometrium, thickens and prepares to nourish a fertilized egg. If none takes up occupancy, the uterus sheds most of the endometrial tissue and begins the process of rebuilding. The uterine walls—the myometrium—consist of longitudinal and circular muscle fibers interwoven like the fibers of a basket. This ingenious design enables the uterus to stretch to twenty-four times its usual size during pregnancy and to contract during labor, creating powerful forces that propel the fetus through the birth canal and into the world.

Outfitted at regular intervals as an embryonic nursery, the womb primarily serves as anteroom of the future. However, as our first home and earliest memory, it also links us to the past. We all, female and male, have floated in its darkness, soothed by the beating of a mother's heart. For us as women, the womb also represents an essential part of our female heritage.

"There is a very long history of female animals with uteruses, going way back in time," says anthropologist Alexander Harcourt, of the University of California, Davis. "They evolved certain behaviors that are different from those of animals without uteruses." Many wombed mammals, given a strange pup, will lick and suckle it; the males of their species will not. As wombed creatures, women too have developed distinctive behaviors: Our pupils dilate at the sight of an infant; our voices automatically rise to a higher pitch when we talk to one; our ears prick up at the sounds of its cries. Are all these instinctive responses signs that we were born to breed?

At a basic evolutionary level, the answer is yes. The species does indeed, as Simone de Beauvoir argued, claw at our innards. The drive to perpetuate life is not uniquely female; males too feel this powerful urge. Yet ours is the sex with the wherewithal to carry life into the future. And so, to a once almost total degree, fertility was the female fate—until women defied it. "As a species, we've evolved brains big and smart enough to refute our evolutionary mandate," says Harcourt. "Our big human brains allow us not to be animals, not to be driven to reproduce unless we choose."

Throughout history, most women—an estimated 70 to 97 percent in various times of peace, war, plague, or prosperity—became mothers, although not by conscious, freely made choice. For most of these eons, a woman's womb, like most aspects of her life, was not hers to control. To whatever extent it was possible to determine if a woman could, should, or would bear a child, that right belonged to her husband, father, or master. Virginity was an essential attribute of a young girl and prospective bride; its loss, whether by rape or seduction, all but destroyed her market value. After marriage, intercourse was a wifely obligation. A woman could refuse only if she was pregnant or nursing.

This does not mean that women did not try to control their fertility. Ancient civilizations used contraceptives—even though they were often forbidden by religious or state edict. Abortion, despite its deadly dangers, also is as old as history. Yet the prospect of childbirth caused even greater dread. "Of all beings who breathe and have intelligence, we women are the most miserable creatures," Medea lamented in Euripides's play, written in the third century B.C. "They say we have a life secure from danger living at home, while they wield their spears in battle. They are mistaken. I would rather stand three times beside a shield than give birth once."

From ancient Greece to the first part of the twentieth century, girls had ample reason for such trepidation. Until modern times, one pregnancy in five was likely to result in the death of the mother. No woman—great lady or peasant girl, beloved wife or bartered bride—was safe from the perils of childbearing. European queens, such as Isabella of Aragon, wife of Philip II, and Jeanne de Bourbon, spouse of Charles V, died after miscarriage or delivery. The same fate befell learned scholars, such as Gabrielle Emilie du Châtelet and Mary Wollstonecraft, and wielders of influence and power, such as Lucrezia Borgia and Beatrice D'Este.

Even today almost 600,000 women around the world die of pregnancy-related complications every year. In the United States, according to in-depth surveys by the Centers for Disease Control and Prevention, the maternal mortality rate may be as high as twenty deaths per 100,000 births—higher than in many industrialized nations. For certain groups of women in the United States, the risks approach those in less developed countries. An African-American, for example, is four times as likely to die in childbirth as a white woman; if she is older than forty, her risk is six times greater, similar to that of women in Vietnam, Tunisia, and Nicaragua.

Even among women who survived childbirth in the past, fertility took a high toll physically and psychologically. Repeated pregnancies, difficult deliveries, heartbreaking miscarriages, and frequent infant deaths, plus the constant demands of a large family, drained women of their energy, robbed them of their youth, and shortened their lives. The fate to which their fertility once led was unenviable. However, it did not prove to be an immutable one.

Although many think of family planning as a recent phenomenon, birth rates in Western nations began their dramatic decline some two hundred years ago. According to historical records, this trend started in France in the 1790s; by 1854 annual deaths outnumbered deliveries. In the United States, the birth rate dropped from an average of 7 children per woman in 1800 to 3.5 by 1900. In England, family size declined from 6.6 children in the early 1800s to an average of about 2 in the 1920s.

Why did women stop having so many babies? The question long has puzzled historians, who cite a complex mix of social, economic, physiological, and psychological forces. Constant revolution and war in nineteenth-century Europe and the Civil War in the United States killed great numbers of men who might otherwise have fathered more children; they also created a climate of uncertainty and social unrest. Many families moved from farms, where every extra hand was welcome, to cities, where a new baby became yet another mouth to feed. There, malnutrition and infectious diseases sickened and killed tens of thousands and undoubtedly sabotaged fertility in many more. Though less vulnerable to these hazards, women of the upper classes were seen as so perilously fragile that they became perpetual patients, their doctors advising against the exertions of sex except for the purpose of planned procreation. And, without doubt, many women and their partners made use of the contraceptives at their disposal, including newly available rubber condoms, spermicides (homemade and commercial products sold for "feminine hygiene"), douches, early models of cervical caps and diaphragms, withdrawal, rhythm, and abstinence. Abortion also became more widespread, particularly in Europe.

However, the "liberation" of the female womb may have owed its greatest debt to the education of the female mind. After centuries of lagging behind, female literacy rates finally caught up with those of males. As still happens, opportunities for girls to study and learn—which spread throughout Western nations in the nineteenth century—led to later marriage, delayed childbearing, and smaller families. In a recent analysis, the U.S. National Center for Health Statistics documented a direct relationship between years of schooling and birth rates. Regardless of her race or economic level, a woman's lifetime fertility declines as her educational level rises. Whenever a woman's window to the world opens, historians note, the door to the nursery tends to close.

Although women, with some feisty exceptions, generally remained second-class citizens well into the twentieth century, increasing numbers began to conceive of a role beyond conception—and to acknowledge the high price of perpetual pregnancy. Even Queen Victoria, pregnant nine times and initially lyrical about the joys of motherhood, came to see her formidable fertility as a burden that strained her marriage and constrained her freedom. Reformers like Margaret Sanger, the pioneer who coined the phrase "birth control," fought to give women the information they needed to take charge of their fertility. The movement she spearheaded would become "the most influential of all time," predicted the futurist H. G. Wells, who wrote that "when the history of our civilization is written, it will be a biological history, and Margaret Sanger will be its heroine."

Thanks to this movement and the development of highly reliable methods of birth control, twentieth-century women have been able to claim their wombs—and their lives—as truly their own. If not for modern birth control techniques, medical experts estimate that a sexually active heterosexual woman would face an average of fourteen births or thirty-one abortions during her reproductive lifetime—truly a mind-boggling prospect.

Yet even though the majority of women in industrialized nations use contraception during their reproductive lives, many still, as the particularly apt Australian idiom puts it, "fall pregnant." In the United States, where 64 percent of women report using contraception, slightly more than half of pregnancies are unplanned. According to the Alan Guttmacher Institute, which monitors population trends, about two thirds of American women have at least one unintended pregnancy in a lifetime. Globally, the World Health Organization estimates that every minute 190 women face an unwanted pregnancy.

In this sense at least, the restless womb still seems to have a life, or at least a history, of its own. When I talk to women, they tell me parallel stories: their childhood, education, careers, marriages, and divorces, the various milestones that accumulate over time. Then they tell another story—of what their wombs have known. They remember not just love and sex, but their not-insignificant overtures and dramatic denouements—the clumsy first fumblings with a diaphragm, the shared sloppy struggle with a broken condom, the decision to go on or off the pill, the sad resignation to abortion.

For an individual woman, fertility is not a purely biological matter. It cuts to our psychological core. Whether or not we ever give birth, we grow up and live with the potential to do so. Our monthly cycles open us up, time and again, to the possibility of conception. In making and ripening an egg, we create the potential for life—and, like it or not, we face a decision.

Whether we decide to try to conceive or not, to continue a pregnancy or not, to become a mother or not, these choices have consequences that profoundly affect our bodies, our minds, and our sense of our personal possibilities. Because of our wombs, we are capable of bringing life into the world. Because of our fertility—and the freedom to express it as we choose—we are capable of filling lives with creativity, love, beauty, and meaning.

"I'll Do Anything"

"There have always been two situations in which women say they will 'do anything,'" observes anthropologist Martha Ward, of the University of New Orleans. "They'll do anything to prevent pregnancy, and they'll do anything to get pregnant." At a certain point in life, because of age, marital status, health, finances, or family obligations, pregnancy may seem unthinkable. With a turn of time's wheel, however, there may be nothing a woman wants more than a baby. (Infertility and women's often desperate quest to overcome it are discussed in the following chapter.)

Most heterosexual women in Western countries devote much more time and energy to preventing pregnancy—roughly 90 percent of their reproductive years—than to trying to become or being pregnant. This is not new. Although many assume that birth control started with the pill, women have long tried anything and seemingly everything to do the same: the foam from a camel's mouth, alligator dung, gunpowder, lead, opium, herbs, alum (applied to the vagina before sex to make the cervix contract). They consulted healers, midwives, priests, practitioners of every form of the black arts and medical sciences. They held very still or stood during intercourse, jumped up and down or sneezed violently afterward, douched with poisons, endured horrible pain, and risked—and occasionally lost—their lives.

Perhaps the oldest form of contraception—though notoriously unreliable—is withdrawal, or coitus interruptus, mentioned and condemned in the Old Testament. Particularly among poorly nourished women, breastfeeding also damped fertility. (Because of the belief that intercourse would interfere with nursing, mothers in many cultures also abstained from sex for prolonged periods of breastfeeding.) Many cultures practiced various forms of rhythm, though their timing was often off. Cherokee women chewed roots of certain plants to prevent conception. Arabic literature and German folklore describe herbal teas that women drank to ensure that pregnancy would not occur or continue.

Women of the past also fashioned the prototypes for many of today's contraceptive devices. With materials similar to those used for menstrual protection—sponges, cotton, wool, silk, seaweed—they formed vaginal suppositories and soaked them in homemade spermicides made with lemons, tannic acid (from the bark or nuts of trees), vinegar, honey, or buttermilk. A plant called silphium, used by the ancient Greeks and Romans, may have been the first oral contraceptive. Centuries before the invention of the diaphragm or cervical cap, women pressed half of a lemon, softened beeswax, or oiled paper around the cervix. Stones, gems, or rings inserted into the womb acted like modern intrauterine devices to prevent implantation.

Men too have long tried to prevent pregnancy. More than two thousand years ago Pliny suggested rubbing sticky cedar gum over the penis before intercourse. When the Crusaders brought protective leather sheaths back from the Middle East, upper-class men in Europe became eager buyers—although they mainly used condoms with mistresses and prostitutes rather than their wives. The import trade thrived for centuries. By the 1700s, fine silk condoms had become a cottage industry in textile towns, such as Leicester in Great Britain, where moonlighting seam-stresses hand-stitched prophylactics for mail-order suppliers.

Yet for most people, contraception remained expensive, unreliable, and largely unattainable until the mid-nineteenth century. With the vul-canization of rubber in 1844, condoms became cheap enough for even the working classes to afford them. The diaphragm, developed at about the same time, required fitting by a physician and the use of expensive spermicidal jelly; because of these costs, its use was more limited. Untold numbers of women just said no, some or all of the time. Demographers report that children born into the smaller families of the nineteenth cen-tury were not more widely spaced than in previous generations. Rather, women tended to have several babies in fairly rapid succession and then just stop—an indication that they may have opted for abstinence, justi-fied perhaps by claims of female fragility and frigidity (the latter a word that first entered the medical lexicon in the nineteenth century, when hysteria and another mysterious female disease, "neurasthenia," were widespread).

Barriers to effective birth control were not just technological, eco-nomic, or medical but legal and political. In the United States, the Com-stock laws, federal antiobscenity statutes of the late nineteenth century, included a ban on birth control information. The prohibition on birth control counseling was overturned in the 1930s, yet it was not until 1965 that the Supreme Court ruled that state bans on dispensing information on contraceptives and their use were unconstitutional.

Today birth control is safer, more effective, and more convenient than in the past—yet none of today's contraceptives is 100 percent safe, 100 percent effective, or 100 percent convenient. And even 95 percent protection (which, some contend, is the best available in real-life use) isn't as good as it may sound. With just a 5 percent failure rate, statistically speaking, seven in ten women who want no more than two children would have to undergo one or more abortions in order to achieve their desired family size.

Nor is the prevention of pregnancy the only reason for precautions. In these sexually perilous times, women also need to protect themselves against sexually transmitted diseases (STDs), many of which—including HIV infection—can be more virulent in females than males. Gynecologists now advise women at risk (a category that includes anyone not in a long-term monogamous relationship with a healthy partner) to use a belt-and-suspenders approach to intercourse: a highly effective means of birth control, such as the pill or a diaphragm, plus a condom to protect against STDs.

"It's not fair," young women often protest when they hear this recommendation. Perhaps. But women, who've long tried anything for the sake of controlling their reproductive lives, have everything to lose if they do nothing.

Contraception and Credibility

"The best advice for a sexually active teenager is to take the pill but not tell her partner," a sex educator tells me. "If a boy knows she's on the pill, he won't wear a condom."

"Are you saying girls should lie?" I ask.

"I don't call it lying. I call it taking care of themselves. And after all the lies men have told women about sex, maybe it's about time."

Her words leave me at a loss. Deception hardly seems a good foundation for an intimate relationship. Yet, knowing what we know about sexual secrets and lies, we can't say that her advice is unwise—or unwarranted. When the Kaiser Family Foundation asked 2,002 Americans the question "Do you think men are responsible enough for preventing unwanted pregnancies?" 73 percent of the women and 66 percent of the men said no. Both sexes agreed that men consider birth control a female's responsibility—an attitude, the researchers calculated, that contributes to 40 percent of each year's unwanted pregnancies.

Perhaps this is why today's women choose birth control methods that don't rely on male cooperation. The most popular form of contraception in the United States is female sterilization. Some 26 percent of women of reproductive age have undergone tubal ligation (cutting) or occlusion (blocking); only 10 percent of American couples rely on male sterilization to prevent pregnancy. The second most popular choice is oral contraception—another form of birth control in which the female assumes all the responsibility and the risks.

Recent innovations in contraceptive technology, such as long-acting hormonal implants and injections, improved intrauterine devices (IUDs), and a female condom, have been designed for exclusively female use. Despite repeated predictions that a male pill is on the horizon, there has not been a significant advance in contraception for men since the condom.

Even though women are the primary users of contraceptives, many remain not just ambivalent but downright dubious about them. Part of the problem is a credibility gap. Time and again, women have put their trust in birth control methods that were later discovered to be unreliable or unsafe. The Dalkon shield, an IUD that at one time was widely used, was taken off the market because of a high incidence of pelvic infection and infertility and some deaths. The advice traditionally given women about rhythm, the only form of birth control sanctioned by the Catholic Church, turned out to be wrong. (As noted in Chapter 3, scientists did not realize until 1995 that fertility peaks before rather than after the temperature spike that accompanies an egg release.) More recently, an analysis from the U.S. Centers for Disease Control revealed that tubal ligation, chosen by so many women because they think of it as the ultimate contraceptive, has a failure rate roughly comparable to that of reversible methods of birth control like the IUD.

But perhaps no contraceptive has made so many women as skeptical as the birth control pill. When it was developed in the 1950s and approved by the FDA in 1960, it sounded almost too good to be true. Within a few years, an estimated 10 million women were "on the pill," and oral contraception became a medical, social, and political phenomenon. Never before had a drug been used so extensively by so many people for a purpose other than the treatment of a disease or the alleviation of symptoms. However, the high-estrogen tablets that women had been assured were completely safe turned out to cause a wide range of potentially serious side effects, including depression, blood clots, gall-bladder disease, and cardiovascular risks.

After repeated reformulations, today's oral contraceptives—a combination pill that releases synthetic estrogen and progestin at constant levels throughout the menstrual cycle, and a multiphasic pill that mimics normal hormonal fluctuations by providing different levels of estrogen and progesterone at different times of the month—contain a fraction of the amount of estrogen in the original birth control pill. A progestin-only mini-pill, with somewhat lower efficacy rates, contains no estrogen at all.

Risks and side effects are fewer with the new pills, but some users still experience spotting between periods, weight gain or loss, nausea, and breast tenderness. And, as the patient package insert states, risks "increase significantly" for women who smoke, have high blood pressure, diabetes, high cholesterol, a history of clotting disorders, heart attacks, stroke, angina, cancer of the breast or other sex organs, jaundice, or liver tumors. Although today's pills are less likely to trigger depression, in certain women multiphasic pills can, as one psychiatrist puts it, "push the button for emotional roller-coasting" and distressing mood swings.

However, birth control pills also have proven to confer unexpected benefits on users: They cut the risk of ovarian cancer in half, lower the danger of colon cancer by 80 percent, safeguard against endometrial cancer, reduce the risk of ectopic pregnancy, pelvic inflammatory disease, and endometriosis, and help maintain bone density.

There is one problem with this good news: Women don't believe it. In one study at Yale University, only 25 percent of women surveyed said birth control pills are very safe; 29 percent said they're unsafe. Some women still think the risks of taking oral contraceptives are greater than those of pregnancy and childbirth. "Women's fears about the pill are based on research that was done ten to twenty years ago on pills that are not even on the market anymore," complains one gynecologist. "There is gross misinformation about oral contraceptives." This may be so, but even women who are up-to-date on the pill's positive effects are uncertain about how to balance potential benefits against possible dangers.

Why is there so much confusion? Some say pharmaceutical companies, wary of high visibility in a litigious society, haven't dared blow their own horn and make the case for the pill's safety and health benefits.

Others think the media do a better job of reporting on bad news than good. Many suspect something else: a lingering puritanical wariness of anything that might encourage or allow greater sexual freedom for women.

This attitude is not exclusively American. Japan, one of the world's most advanced industrialized nations, continues to outlaw the pill, despite evidence of its safety presented by its own scientists. One reason given by Japanese authorities is fear of increased spread of HIV infection and AIDS—even though there is no evidence that pill use increases promiscuity or reduces condom use by those at greatest risk of contracting HIV. With few good contraceptive options, Japanese women have one of the highest abortion rates in the developed world.

Until the late 1990s, American women were also denied access to another birth control option: morning-after, or emergency, contraception. Waking up the morning after unprotected sex, women have long confronted the sick-to-the-stomach realization that they might be pregnant. Remembering the tears and fears of friends in the dorms of my college days, I thought those bad old days were gone—until a friend's daughter phoned a few years ago from her university worrying over a condom that broke during sex. Fortunately, as author of a college health textbook, I was in on the best-kept secret in gynecology: that certain birth control pills, taken for several days after intercourse, can prevent pregnancy.

It is not certain precisely how so-called "morning-after" pills work, but taken in specific doses and sequences within a defined interval, they can prevent 60 to 75 percent of pregnancies that would have occurred without this intervention. Their main side effects are nausea, vomiting, and breast tenderness. This backup method has been available to women in most European countries for many years, yet women in the United States had no idea that this alternative existed. Nor did many realize that the insertion of an IUD after unprotected intercourse can have a similar contraceptive effect.

In 1997, under pressure from population control groups, the Federal Register, in an almost unprecedented move, published information about emergency contraception to make it part of the public record. In 1998, the FDA approved the first emergency birth control kit. Why did it take so long?

Many blame the delay on apprehension that abortion foes, objecting to any postcoital form of contraception, might ignite unwanted political controversy. Others point to the old puritanical reluctance to endorse any option that would give women greater freedom over the consequences of sexual intercourse. If morning-after contraception was widely touted as a fallback, some contend, wouldn't it be just like a woman to be less conscientious about birth control? There is no evidence of this. In one study, only 8 percent of women who'd used postcoital emergency contraception ever sought it again.

Not surprisingly, women wonder if there may be other things that doctors aren't telling them—as well as information that physicians themselves still don't have. Only quite recently did researchers discover that today's birth control pills have unexpected effects on female sexuality. Whereas the initial high-estrogen oral contraceptives suppressed sexual desire (an ironic effect for an alleged sexual emancipator), multiphasic pills—which represent about 40 percent of oral contraceptives prescribed today—seem to enhance a woman's desire, fantasies, and satisfaction. The reason may be that these pills do not suppress a woman's natural sex hormones as much as others.

In a completely unscientific sampling of women I know who are on the pill, I asked if their doctors ever mentioned possible effects on their libido. None had. "Would you believe it's a total turn-off?" I ask. They all concede that this sounds possible. "Would you believe it actually turns up sexual heat?" They shake their heads skeptically. After years of hearing untruths, partial truths, or nothing at all about the pill and its effects, this may be the last thing women are ready to believe.

Abortion and Its Aftermath

Abortion has always been a desperate woman's last option. In one study of four hundred preindustrial societies, each practiced abortion via a variety of techniques: heavy lifting, climbing, starving, placing hot objects on the abdomen, massage, inserting long, sharp objects (such as feather quills) into the womb, eating or drinking toxins, even pulling the pregnant woman through a forked tree to push the fetus from her swollen belly. Sometimes these brutal means worked and ended a pregnancy. In untold numbers of instances, they also ended a woman's life.

For centuries abortion was not generally considered illegal because of the widespread belief that life did not begin until the fourth month of pregnancy, when a baby "quickened." Although neither safe nor sanitary, it became increasingly widespread among married women as well as single girls "in trouble" in nineteenth-century Europe. In cities like Paris, abortion clinics, often conveniently located near train stations, did a bustling business. One group of London abortionists reported ten thousand clients in 1898.

In nineteenth-century America, however, opposition to abortion rose steadily. Antiabortion statutes appeared in state after state in the 1820s; they were significantly amended between 1860 and 1880. In time other Western countries also criminalized and banned abortion. In the United States, it remained illegal until the *Roe v. Wade* Supreme Court decision in 1973; most European countries have since legalized abortion as well. But in some nations, including most of Central and South America, those performing or undergoing abortions still face criminal penalties. Today 50 million women around the world have abortions every year; as many as 20 million may be illegal and unsafe. In Western countries, however, legal abortion has become safer than pregnancy, childbirth, or even a penicillin shot.

Abortion rates vary greatly around the world. The U.S. abortion rate, which has declined to a twenty-year low, still remains higher than that of many Western countries, including Canada, Great Britain, the Netherlands, and Sweden. Although there is no one single or simple explanation for this difference, researchers focus on America's high rate of unintended pregnancies. In many nations with fewer unwanted pregnancies and lower abortion rates, contraceptives are generally easier and cheaper to obtain, and early sex education strongly emphasizes their importance.

No woman in any country ever elects to be in a situation where she has to consider abortion. But if faced with an unwanted pregnancy, she must. Every year three out of every one hundred American women between the ages of fifteen and forty-four choose to terminate a pregnancy. According to federal data, 43 percent of American women undergo an abortion by age forty-five.

These women do not fit neatly into any particular category. Most—

70 percent—intend to have children, but not at this point in time. Many cannot afford a baby; some feel unready for the responsibility; others fear that another child would jeopardize the happiness and security of their existing family.

About 55 percent of women who undergo abortion are under age twenty-five; only 22 percent are older than age thirty. Unmarried pregnant women are six times more likely to have abortions than married ones; poor women are three times more likely to abort a pregnancy than women in higher economic groups. White women account for 63 percent of abortions, yet statistically, nonwhite women (who make up a smaller proportion of the population) are twice as likely to have an abortion as white women. Catholic women are more likely than Protestant women to have abortions, but women with no religious affiliations have a higher abortion rate than those who belong to any particular religion.

More than half of all abortions (54 percent) are performed within the first eight weeks of pregnancy. Only about 1 percent of abortions occur after twenty weeks. The trend to have early abortions is almost certain to continue. Highly sensitive pregnancy tests can now detect pregnancy very soon after fertilization. A new surgical procedure, early manual vacuum aspiration, can be performed as early as eight days after conception. And chemical abortion—by means of mifepristone (RU-486) or a combination of the prescription drugs methotrexate (a drug used primarily to treat cancer, ectopic pregnancies, and rheumatoid arthritis) and misoprostol (Cytotec, an ulcer treatment that causes uterine contractions)—has become increasingly widespread.

Although condemned by right-to-life advocates, abortion medications may in time lower the public profile of pregnancy termination. They are not painless, cheap, or equally available to all, but they do offer women a chance to carry through on their personal choice in greater privacy and safety. This does not mean the decision to end a pregnancy is any easier—in part because of concerns about long-term physical or emotional repercussions. But these legitimate fears have sometimes been exacerbated by the ever-heated politics of abortion.

In the mid-1990s, in large American cities, ads began appearing in buses and subways stating, "Women who choose abortions suffer more and deadlier breast cancer." Abortion's defenders accused the right-to-life groups that had placed the ads of distorting facts to get across their message. The antiabortion groups insisted they were just reporting scientific findings.

What are we to make of each side's claims? The truth is far from clear. In the 1980s several small studies suggested a small increase in breast cancer among women who'd had abortions; several others showed none. In 1996 an epidemiologist at the Harvard School of Public Health reviewed all the available research—nearly fifty studies in all—and concluded that "the quality of the studies was inadequate to permit any conclusion" about a link between induced abortion and breast cancer. Another analysis of twenty-three studies, this time by a declared abortion opponent, showed that risk increased by 30 percent. In yet another study of 6,888 women with breast cancer and 9,529 healthy women, a University of Wisconsin researcher found "a weak positive association" between either miscarriage or abortion and the risk of breast cancer.

Given this array of studies of different sizes, protocols, and varied conclusions, it is no wonder women were confused. Moreover, there was a serious flaw in nearly all these analyses: They relied on women's own reports of abortion, which have proven to be unreliable. (In some surveys, women have admitted to only about half of the abortions performed.) With self-reports as the only source of data, there is no way of knowing whether most, some, or just a few of the women who did *not* develop breast cancer also had abortions but did not admit that they had. Some of the studies also did not take into account whether the abortions occured during the first or second trimester (some researchers believe the risk would be greater with later abortions).

In 1997 Danish researchers, reviewing health registries of more than 1.5 million women, reported no overall increased risk of breast cancer among women who had first-trimester abortions. Because of the use of actual medical records, the large size of the study, the inclusion of Denmark's entire population of women, and adjustments for other aspects of reproductive history, most scientists consider these findings more credible. In assessing all the data to date, a National Cancer Institute official concluded that "a woman need not worry about the risk of breast cancer when facing the difficult decision of whether to terminate a pregnancy."

Whether or not abortion is hazardous to any aspect of physical health, many assume that it must be psychologically devastating, that women who abort a fetus sooner or later develop what some have termed "postabortion trauma syndrome." In her studies at the University of Chicago, psychiatrist Nada Stotland found that there is no such thing. The primary emotion of women who have just had an abortion, she discovered, is relief. Although many women also express feelings of sadness or guilt, their anxiety levels eventually drop until they are lower than they were immediately before the abortion. Even highly religious women are not at greater risk of long-term psychological distress.

Nonetheless, although psychologists consider the mental health risks "minimal" compared to those of bearing an unwanted child, this does not mean women who have abortions never have regrets. As Stotland notes, women have many feelings before, during, and after abortions. But a feeling—even one as painful as loss, sadness, or guilt—is not a syndrome, and a woman's responses to abortion often change with passing days, weeks, months, or years. Anniversaries—of conception, of the date a woman found out she was pregnant, of the abortion, of the delivery date—can trigger memories and a sense of loss, but most women deal with these and move on with their lives.

The best predictor of psychological well-being after abortion is a woman's emotional well-being prior to pregnancy. At highest risk for problems are women who have had a psychiatric illness, such as an anxiety disorder or clinical depression, or whose abortions occurred under complicated circumstances (such as a rape or under coercion by parents or a partner). The vast majority of women remain healthy in mind and body and manage to put the abortion into perspective as one of many life events. "I wish I never had to have an abortion," says a friend who became pregnant at eighteen. "But I've never doubted that I made the right decision. If I hadn't had an abortion, I never would have had the chance to become me."

The Great Escape

In the faux grandeur of a hotel banquet room, men in black tie and women who knew in a blink the price of one another's designer dresses assembled at yet another charity fund-raiser. A vice president of a major brokerage firm, married to a venture capitalist, took her seat at a table of trophy wives. After the usual pleasantries about the good cause du jour, the conversation turned to traditional themes.

"One of the women asked me if I had children," recalls the broker, who had earned her lofty niche in the men's club of major-league investing in a traditionally masculine way—by earning huge profits for her clients. "Suddenly it struck me: I'd just turned forty-three, and I never would have children. I felt so happy, so relieved, and I blurted out: 'I've escaped! I made it through!' Everyone stared at me as if I'd just turned into a creature from outer space."

She is, in fact, part of a global trend. In the United States, one in five women in the postwar baby boom generation has not given birth—many because of a deliberate decision not to. In Europe, as noted earlier, fertility rates in many nations are at an all-time low. Yet women who enthuse about their unbabied state report chilly, if not hostile, responses. Why? "The rejection of parenthood is a delicate and even dangerous topic," says Laurie Lisle, author of *Without Child: Challenging the Stigma of Childlessness*. "It has an element of subversiveness to it."

Indeed, through much of time the out-and-out refusal to reproduce—a uniquely human prerogative—would have been an act of sedition, imperiling the survival of families, dynasties, empires, the species itself. Even today, Lisle points out, "few of us still dare to speak openly about our real reasons for refusing to breed. We are afraid to challenge the view of motherhood as the essential female experience."

So entrenched is the notion of maternity defining women that the medical term for a woman who has never given birth is *nullipara*, from the Latin root *nulla*, meaning "empty, void, nothing, zero." It is a cruelly belittling term—even more disparaging than *childless*, which women without children hope to replace with something more affirmational, like *childfree* or *unchilded* or, as an alternative to *motherhood*, *otherhood*. Above all, "others" want mothers to know that they're doing fine. They don't need children in order to get a life. They have one—and a very good one at that.

According to the limited data available, single childfree women tend to be better-educated, more cosmopolitan, less religious, and more professional than those in the general population. Childless couples are predominantly urban, well-educated, and upper-middle-class, with egalitarian and long-running marriages. In general, childfree women are high achievers, often in demanding careers, who describe their work as exciting and satisfying.

Yet however much money they make, however exhilarating their careers or fulfilled their marriages, these women face a credibility gap of their own: No one believes they truly—deep down in their souls—don't want kids. Parents and in-laws cling to their hopes for grandchildren. Bosses and colleagues speculate that they are canny strategists skirting the dead-end mommy track. Even their friends, gone to marriage and babies and such, suspect that they secretly long to swap their raw-silk love seats for stain-resistant sofas. And if they do take a childless woman at her word when she says she doesn't want babies, most follow up with the blunt question "Why not?" As one woman puts it, "They're really asking, 'What's wrong with you? What terrible thing happened that made you not want to have kids?' "

As women without children note, society deems justifiable only a small number of reasons for not having children: infertility, homosexuality, inability to find a partner, and lack of economic resources. Yet women's reasons for remaining unfettered by children are diverse: a desire to maintain their freedom, more time with their partners, career ambitions, genuine concern about overpopulation and the fate of the earth. Some cite the hostile work environment for mothers and the inadequacy of day care. Others say they're disillusioned with the have-it-all hopes of baby boomers and believe instead in a have-most-of-it philosophy.

The most shocking reason for not having children—and the hardest to admit—is a complete and utter lack of interest. Raising children involves years of messy, monotonous work—and just like any other job, it's not for everyone. This does not mean that childless women do not like children; they do—other people's, that is. They volunteer as Big Sisters, swoop up nieces and nephews on adventurous excursions, delight in watching friends' youngsters blossom. Some are so intensely involved with a child of a friend or relative that trend-spotters have dubbed them "para-moms." "More ice cream, less throw-up," says one friend, summing up the benefits of playing a supporting role in a child's life.

Won't childfree women—as their maternity-minded friends inevitably point out—regret their choice after it's too late to do anything about it? Not necessarily. In a study of ninety childless women over age sixty, a Philadelphia anthropologist found that while the women who believed that a female's primary duty was to have children did express some regret, most women had come up with satisfying alternative ways of living. In another study of nearly seven hundred Canadian women and men over age fifty-five, those who chose childlessness were just as happy as parents who had good relationships with their children— and happier than parents who described their relationships with their children as distant.

"Not everybody needs children to have a full life," says Leslie Lafayette, who founded the ChildFree Network (CFN) to create a sense of belonging among childless people. "We don't want to be defined just by our ovaries. We want to enjoy all the other aspects of being a woman today."

At a day-long seminar for women without children, I listen to tales of unchilded life in a family-sized society. With a jolt, I realize that I am the only woman in the room wondering if the baby-sitter can stay late, the only one with melted Gummi Bears fused into her purse lining and a day planner cluttered with orthodontic assessments and parent-teacher conferences. Among the handouts I grab as I slink to the exit is a bumper sticker with big block letters spelling T.H.I.N.K.E.R.: Two Healthy Incomes, No Kids, Early Retirement. And I wonder: Has the human brain, cleverly calculating the risk-benefit ratio of childbearing and contemplating all the options open to women today, finally put the wayward womb in its place?

CHAPTER 9

To Become a Mother

She never should have gotten pregnant. That's what the specialists at the high-risk pregnancy center told her— not after almost dying twice, once of kidney failure, once when her body rejected a donor transplant. She would have to spend most of her pregnancy in bed and the final weeks in the hospital for round-the-clock monitoring. Tearfully she agreed to everything the doctors ordered. After the room emptied of white coats, I stayed behind. "They don't understand," she cried. "It's like my womb's on fire. I'm just burning to have a baby."

Having sat in on her medical team's conferences, I knew her physicians' concerns were legitimate: She was indeed taking a big risk—with her health and her unborn baby's life. But at an almost molecular level, I understood why. At the time, I too was feeling the same yearning, a gnawing hunger in the very cells of my body. Nothing in my life as an independent working woman had prepared me for this. "It's like hearing a voice," I told my psychiatrist husband, whose patients not uncommonly report out-of-the-ordinary communications. This voice, I assured him, was different, with a single, simple message: "Baby!"

Since we weren't ready for children, I took the journalist's way out: I wrote a book on high-risk pregnancy.

For almost a year I spent my days in the company of perilously pregnant women, all hoping against hope for a healthy child despite diabetes, hypertension, multiple sclerosis, epilepsy—an entire *Merck Manual* of maladies that put them and their unborn children at risk. As we talked, these women would protectively stroke their mounded bellies. Sometimes tearful, often fearful, they were determined to do anything for the sake of the baby they had longed for. What they taught me was something I never again underestimated: the fierce intensity of a woman's drive to become a mother.

Reproduction is, of course, the evolutionary point of living, the oldest, most basic urge on earth. While every species responds to this drive, only humans bring to procreation our unique consciousness and will. We alone become, as some have described us, "obsessed with reproduction." And obsession sometimes defies reason. Thirteen-year-olds barely more than children themselves talk of wanting babies of their own. Couples devote tens of thousands of dollars and years of their lives to infertility treatments that are physically demanding and psychologically degrading. Menopausal women past nature's own point of no return resort to the most drastic of medical interventions to turn back the biological clock and give birth.

"I wasn't trying to make history," said a sixty-three-year-old bank teller in southern California who became the oldest mother on record when she gave birth to a baby girl in 1996. "I just wanted a baby." So did Bobbi McCaughey in Des Moines, Iowa. After treatment with fertility drugs, she gave birth to seven babies—and earned her own place in the annals of reproduction.

These "miracle" births set off both a media frenzy and a firestorm of controversy. Although the two mothers have little in common—indeed, one is old enough to be the other's mother—they both had defied the laws and limits of nature. Amid the hype and hand wringing that followed these high-profile births, the righteous of every persuasion weighed in. Some predicted grave emotional consequences for the innocent babies—the daughter with a mother of grandmotherly age, and each member of the veritable litter. Feminists condemned a culture that still venerates maternity to such an extent that women feel compelled to go to any length for its sake. Psychologists speculated about the unmet needs that had propelled two women to gamble their own health against odds no professional gambler would even consider.

"Mother" Nature certainly had been knocked out of the loop in this woman-made twist on evolution. There was nothing natural about these conceptions and births—except for one thing: the persistent internal voice that drove these women, just as it has driven countless others (myself included) to try anything and risk everything just to become a mother.

Scientists have never been able to trace this procreative urge to any uniquely female gene, chromosome, or hormone. In many species both sexes go to astounding lengths to reproduce. An aphid mother literally explodes to give life to her offspring. As described in Chapter 2, some male spiders sacrifice their bodies for the sake of perpetuating their genes. This primal impulse to reproduce is part of our biological legacy.

For reasons that go beyond reason and stretch beyond imaginable time, many women hear voices—and listen to them. Becoming a mother, now as always, remains too fundamental a drive for many, even most, of us even to want to resist its pull. Regardless of our aspirations and autonomy, we hunger to give life, to feel a fetus move within our flesh, to reach, in this most tangible of ways, into the future and claim part of it as our own.

But if biology primes this reproductive urge, other forces augment it. Psychologists have theorized that a woman craves pregnancy out of desire for the penis she never had (a classic Freudian thought) or a yearning for womanly completion (a more modern view). Historians have shown that the division of sex roles and lack of alternatives for women made motherhood the only choice most women ever had.

Sociologists have documented culture's role in promulgating what some call the "motherhood mandate"—whether in the form of the invention of Mother's Day in 1914 by American politicians alarmed by declining births among native-born women (and rising births among immigrants), the Medals of the French Family that France began awarding in 1920 to married women who had at least five healthy children, or the idealization of childbearing as a noble act of patriotism in Nazi Germany and fascist Italy. Yet motherhood never was in such vogue as in the prosperous, life-hungry years that followed World War II, when a generation of soldiers came marching back home. For them, and for the wives and girlfriends who had grown up in the Depression and through the war years, peacetime brought the first taste of normalcy they had ever known. The craving for family and home, for new beginnings, created a "motherhood mandate" all its own—and gave rise to the largest generation in history.

Curiously, the women born into this baby boom are the ones who have transformed every aspect of conception, pregnancy, and motherhood. Coming of age in the era of the pill and legalized abortion, they could, for the first time in history, delay childbearing for ten to twenty years or even longer. This resetting of the reproductive clock has had unparalleled physiological, psychological, and social consequences.

In the last fifteen years, first births among women older than forty have increased 50 percent. At the same time, age-associated infertility has soared, and the new field of "assisted" reproduction, with its remarkable technological wizardry, has transformed conception from the most natural of acts to the most dazzling (and often emotionally draining) of unnatural feats.

Yet none of these major shifts has changed a woman's fundamental experience of motherhood. Regardless of whether pregnancy is the result of passionate lovemaking or intricate biochemical machinations, the process of becoming a mother changes a woman in body, mind, and spirit. It always has; it always will. Whether a pregnancy progresses normally, runs into complications, or ends in miscarriage or abortion, there is no going back. As with virginity, a woman cannot return to her untouched and intact state. The history of her womb and of her life are forever different.

"A man spends a night by a woman and goes away," the German ethnologist Leo Frobenius once wrote. "His life and body are always the same. The woman conceives. As a mother, she is another person than the woman without the child. She carries the fruit of the night nine months long in her body. Something grows. Something grows into her life that never again departs from it. She is a mother. She is and remains a mother even though her child dies, though all her children die. For at one time she carried the child under her heart. And it does not go out of her heart ever again." Every part of my being, body and mind, changed on a November morning in 1985. I became a mother.

The Empty Womb

When we met, Barbara was at the beginning of her brilliant career in publishing. "She's going to be a star," said the agent who introduced us. Barbara, a dynamo with endless energy, more than lived up to her advance billing. But after we'd gotten better acquainted, I discovered that, just like me, there was one thing Barbara couldn't do: get pregnant. "I have never failed at anything before," she said. "It is the most frustrating situation I ever encountered."

We were both lucky. I, who had learned so much about pregnancy only to find I too couldn't conceive ("I wrote the wrong book!" I wailed to my coauthor, an obstetrician), went through four years of diagnostic dead-ends, insensitive specialists, and state-of-the-science surgeries. Then I got pregnant. After running a similar gauntlet, Barbara, ever the exuberant overachiever, had twins. But for millions of other women every year, the desire for a baby turns into an expensive, exhausting, and heartbreaking quest.

In *Motherhood Deferred*, her soul-searing memoir of her futile struggle to have a child—a book I read with there-but-for-the-grace-of-God-go-I tingles—Anne Taylor Fleming describes a sorority no woman joins voluntarily: the "sisterhood of the infertile." Its membership is large—and growing.

Until 1988 the number of infertile couples was fairly stable, with about 10 percent of couples having difficulty conceiving. From 1988 to 1995, the number of American women with fertility problems jumped from 4.9 million to 6.1 million, a 25 percent increase. The primary culprit is time. As physicians have only recently realized—too late for those baby boomers who put maternity on the back burner for years— a woman's fertility may start to decline earlier than they'd thought. Follicle-stimulating hormone (FSH), the menstrual messenger discussed in Chapter 7, dips, at least slightly, around age twenty-nine, with another decrease at thirty-five. By some estimates, as many as a third of women who try to get pregnant after thirty-five may not be able to; among would-be mothers past age forty, infertility rates rise to half.

The history of "barren" women—and tales of their grief over this fate—dates back to biblical times. Traditionally, only women were held responsible for a couple's failure to reproduce; it was unthinkable that a man might be incapable of siring a child. Because of "female" inadequacy, thrones, fortunes, and lives were lost.

In modern times, a woman's mind was often blamed for her body's reproductive failure. According to various theorists, infertile women were too feminine, or not feminine enough; too maternal, or not maternal enough; too eager to conceive, or not eager enough. Until a decade or so ago, infertility specialists never even "worked up" a woman's partner unless her reproductive health proved indisputably sound. Medical scientists have since learned that, almost always, some very real biological mechanism is at fault in infertility—and the problem is just as likely to be male as female.

As a general rule of thumb—one that may be changing as the age of would-be mothers increases—specialists have estimated that in about 40 percent of cases of infertility the problem lies with the woman; in another 40 percent, with the man. In 10 to 20 percent the causes are unknown or may be the result of female and male "subfertility." About two thirds of all treated infertile couples eventually do have a child, and fewer than 2 percent resort to the most advanced high-tech procedures to accomplish this. Even without treatment, couples with unexplained infertility have a fairly good chance of succeeding if they just keep trying (some researchers report success rates as high as 60 to 70 percent after three years). However, the chances of becoming pregnant and giving birth decline consistently with the mother's increasing age.

This is not news that high-achieving women of the baby boom tend to accept with equanimity. Their usual take-charge ways of coping with challenges don't apply to reproductive physiology. Tough litigators, cool-headed managers, and energetic entrepreneurs find themselves in totally unfamiliar territory. However determined they are, however hard they apply themselves, they cannot will themselves pregnant—nor can they control the intense emotional reactions infertility can trigger.

Infertile women assessed prior to treatment are no more likely to have psychological problems than others. However, this changes during the treatment process. Women undergoing infertility treatments—which are in themselves often embarrassing, dehumanizing, uncomfortable, and disconcerting—are more likely to be depressed than women seeing their gynecologists for regular checkups and minor problems. Over time, their stress levels rise to a point comparable to those of women with cancer or other serious illnesses. And, ironically, stress itself may make their situation worse. The release of stress hormones can inhibit ovulation or cause spasms of the fallopian tubes, blocking the sperm from reaching the egg. In one study of heterosexual women undergoing donor insemination, some women who had previously been ovulatory stopped ovulating after the first several attempts.

Everything about infertility treatment—beginning with the perception of failure implicit in the diagnosis itself—can be psychologically demeaning. A would-be mother may submit to countless scans and undergo delicate microsurgery. Listening to the disparaging diagnoses of the medical lexicon, she may be told that her mucus is hostile, her cervix incompetent, her ovaries sluggish, her hormones insufficient. Month after month, year after year, she has her blood analyzed, her uterine lining snipped and sampled, her ovaries stimulated, her fallopian tubes scoured. As megadoses of hormones course through her veins, a woman may experience a barrage of side effects, including headaches, nausea, bloating, and emotional hypersensitivity. The cryptic acronyms in the high-tech infertility arsenal—IVF, ZIFT, GIFT—become full-length dramas in her life. "After a while, you start to feel defective," says a friend. "You think, 'If I were healthy, I wouldn't be having all these problems.' " In one study, half of women—compared with just 15 percent of men—seeking treatment described infertility as the most upsetting experience of their lives.

Women, as one therapist puts it, "carry" infertility as their problem, regardless of whether the cause lies within their own bodies or their partners'. When they try to get pregnant but find they cannot, they tend to become worried before their mates do. Perhaps because they can't or won't acknowledge a problem that carries an unspoken slur on their own potency, men tend to dismiss a woman's initial concerns as typically female needless fretting. "If I'd said 'You need to relax' one more time, she would have killed me," one husband recalls.

As couples begin the exhausting and invasive process of testing and trying, a woman—much more so than her partner—feels her world shrink. Timing is everything—for hormonal shots to induce ovulation, endometrial biopsies, ovarian scans, "harvesting" of egg follicles. "No one may be more obsessed with motherhood than a woman going through infertility treatments," says a physician. "She thinks of herself only as an egg maker."

Sex, or at least procreative sex, no longer can be entrusted to fallible human lovers. Their gametes—the reproductive cells—are the ones that enter a brave new world of sexless conception. Scientists, choosing from a high-tech Kama Sutra of combinations, can place both sperm and egg in a laboratory petri dish or squirt sperm into the fallopian tube. In a variation called intracytoplasmic sperm injection (ICSI), a single sperm speeds through a fine hollow needle directly into the egg, the obstetric equivalent of opting for the Concorde over a single-engine Cessna. If, despite the route or form of transport, nothing happens (as is the statistical norm, since success rates range between 20 and 30 percent for the high-tech procedures referred to as "assisted reproductive technology," or ART), there are still more alternatives for a couple: another man's sperm, another woman's egg, a surrogate mother who leases out her uterus, transfer of a fertilized donor egg into the uterus of the infertile woman.

Amid all the chemical ado, everyone—from specialists to would-be parents—often focuses so intensively on timing and hormone levels that they lose sight of everything else. Couples may find themselves pulling farther apart at a time when both know they should be moving closer together. Many of the hormones and drugs used in ovulation induction have side effects that leave women feeling overwhelmed, defeated, or depressed.

Success itself can be bittersweet. Many multiple pregnancies—not at all uncommon with infertility treatments—have less than ideal outcomes, with babies who live only briefly or who suffer serious complications as a result of prematurity or other problems. The infant mortality rate for multiples is twelve times that for singletons. A woman who had been prepared for the very real possibility of twins or triplets may be stunned to discover she's carrying five babies—and to hear her doctors suggest "selective abortion" to guarantee that at least some will survive.

But for many women who've spent years trying to conceive, the hardest thing is to give up. "These are women who've never failed at anything," says one psychiatrist. "It's devastating for them to realize that they cannot do something millions of women do without any difficulty at all."

Sometimes a woman's long struggle with infertility takes an intriguing mind-body turn. "I've had women come to see me with major depression after years of infertility treatment," says psychiatrist Kathleen Pajer, of Allegheny Medical Center in Pittsburgh. "I put them on an antidepressant and six months later a good number of them are pregnant. In my desk drawer I have pictures of what I call my Prozac babies." (The women generally discontinue the drug as soon as they learn they're pregnant.)

Stress reduction techniques may have similar benefits. In her research at Harvard University's Mind-Body Institute, psychologist Alice Domar found that women with unexplained infertility benefited from a ten-week stress management program, including training in relaxation, guided imagery, yoga, stretching, and supportive group therapy. The emphasis was not on getting pregnant but on developing a creative, fulfilling life. By the end of the program, 98 percent of the women reported increased well-being and significantly less depression, anxiety, and anger— three of the most common psychological symptoms in infertile women. Follow-up studies found that a significant percentage of women "graduating" from the program had conceived.

No one is suggesting that psychiatric drugs or psychological treatments directly affect fertility. But as with so many aspects of a woman's life, it may be impossible to separate the physiological from the psychological. The uniquely female capacity for giving life involves much more than the manipulation of mechanics. A woman, it seems, still becomes a mother by more than egg alone.

An Altered State

Once a woman's body offered the first clues of pregnancy: an achy heaviness in the breasts, crushing fatigue, a late or scanty period. These days she is more likely to find herself staring anxiously at drops or vials of her own urine, hoping for a plus sign, a change in shade, a double line. The messenger may lack glory, but the message can be glorious nonetheless. Far earlier in gestation than once thought possible, women can find out if they're expecting. But what they won't and don't know—especially not the first time around—is what to expect.

Pregnancy transforms a woman inside and out. The hair on her head ceases its normal shedding and looks and feels thicker. Her feet typically grow by a half or whole size. Her heart speeds up; her pulse races ten beats faster per minute than before. Her body temperature increases.

Her joints loosen, her ribs and pelvis expand. Her center of gravity moves closer to the ground in the later months. Over its nine-month course, pregnancy lifts her diaphragm, shifts the position of her heart, and takes her breath away. It is a physiological tour de force like none other.

Pregnancy confounds the very notion of boundaries. Mother and fetus are linked together in the most intimate of human relationships. The blood pumped by a mother's heart flows into her unborn baby's body. The fetus shares every breath she takes and every meal she eats. Some biologists view this union as the most harmonious on earth. Others, taking a different perspective, describe the fetus as a parasite selfishly leaching nutrients from its selfless host.

At the very least, the fetus is no passive passenger. In humans—along with mice, bats, sloths, and various other species—the placenta surrounding the fetus is "invasive," that is, cells are sent out from the embryo into the blood vessels that supply the uterine lining. These cells destroy the muscular wall of the blood vessels and greatly expand their diameter—the equivalent of replacing a kitchen drain with the Alaska pipeline. This gives the fetus direct access to its mother's blood. A pregnant woman cannot, even if she wanted, constrict the vessels or regulate the flow of nutrients to the placenta. If the placenta does not get an adequate supply of maternal blood, it compensates by increasing maternal blood pressure and blood flow.

A pregnant woman also can do nothing to control the normal physiological changes of pregnancy—a reality made abundantly clear as soon as buttons start popping off her waistband or the zipper on her jeans refuses to connect. In effect, her physiology is commandeered to serve the needs of the fetus. Fortunately mother and fetus share the same goal: the development of a healthy child.

The biology of pregnancy inevitably affects a woman's psychology. Statistically, a woman's likelihood of admission to a psychiatric hospital is lower during gestation than at any other time of life, indicating a lessened risk of severe mental illness such as psychosis. But this doesn't necessarily mean that pregnancy is a state of tranquillity. Emotions invariably push closer to the surface. Tears flow faster. Fears loom larger. A lifetime of feelings may be crammed into nine intense months.

"You can't show me a pregnant woman who isn't at least a little bit anxious and tired and worried," says psychiatrist Vivien Burt. "There aren't any. But women don't like to talk about their negative feelings because they know they're supposed to be happy."

Since pregnancy is a time of great psychological adjustment and potential growth, some growing pains are to be expected. So is a mix of many emotions, sometimes all seeming to hit at once. A pregnant woman may be laughing one moment and burst into tears the next. Rather than being annoyed with a rude salesclerk, she may fly into a fury. Instead of being touched by a sappy commercial, she sobs. Such emotional volatility—or, as therapists put it, "lability"—comes with the territory. A pregnant woman's rapidly changing moods reflect the nonstop changes within her and the constant adjustments she has to make.

Most women move through certain predictable stages from the time that they first learn they're pregnant until delivery. In the first three months, when rising hormones bring on fatigue and morning sickness, they may feel weepy, irritable, or intensely emotional—as if, in one woman's words, they're "feeling for two." It's also not uncommon for them to feel ambivalent about having gotten pregnant in the first place.

Once quickening occurs, in the second trimester, and they feel the baby moving within them, women typically become more committed and positive. They also become more physically comfortable, as morning sickness and fatigue lessen. As their bodies adjust to higher hormone levels, many feel more serene than before. This is a time of quiet excitement, of anticipation and planning.

The last, long stretch of the third trimester can be the hardest, physically and psychologically. In addition to the discomforts of being very pregnant, many women experience a certain letdown. They may feel that they've been pregnant forever; the novelty has long since worn off. As they look toward labor and delivery, they may become more apprehensive about how painful birth will be, how they'll respond, how their partners will react. Many an expectant mother, back aching, bladder always full, too uncomfortable to sleep, mumbles, "This kid had better be worth it"—and immediately feels guilty at the very thought.

If complications develop—as they do in 15 percent of pregnancies— the normal anxieties of pregnancy intensify. If women have to devote more time to tests and monitoring, if they have to spend weeks or even months on bed rest, they're likely to register at least occasional pangs of resentment. Women, high-risk or not, find themselves caught between the idealized stereotypes of what they are supposed to feel and do and the often-less-than-perfect realities of daily life. The conflicted feelings that virtually all pregnant women have—although to differing extents and intensities—may remain unspoken simply because they seem too unlike the stereotype to put into words.

Unspeakable Feelings

She had never faced a tougher audience. As one of the world's few perinatal psychiatrists specializing in psychological issues related to pregnancy, birth, and the postpartum period, Vivien Burt had been asked to give a lecture to couples expecting their first babies. "My job was to prepare them emotionally. I talked about all the nice wonderful things, then a little about maternity blues, and finally I brought up the subject of depression before and after delivery. They said, 'Why are you telling us this? We're so looking forward to having a baby, and you're telling us to be alert for these terrible things. We don't want to hear it.'"

A few months later Burt got a phone call from one of the women in the group. "She told me that during my lecture, she'd kept thinking, 'What the hell are you talking about?' She was thrilled to be pregnant and couldn't imagine ever being depressed about it. But she wrote down my number, and when she called, she said, 'I know I need to come to see you and I need to see you quickly. Something is not right.' She came in; I treated her for depression, and she responded beautifully."

The women who make their way to a therapist during pregnancy—usually after weeks of anguish—are different from those riding the usual highs and lows of pregnancy. "They're not just tired; they haven't slept in weeks," says Burt. "They're not just tearful; they can't stop crying. They're not just anxious about the pregnancy or the baby; they're profoundly distressed." Adding to their turmoil is the sense that such emotions are utterly inappropriate. Trying to be reassuring, friends, family members, and obstetricians may dismiss their fears and feelings. But doing so can make matters worse.

As many as 10 percent of expectant mothers may develop clinical depression during pregnancy. They're less likely to eat well or to seek prenatal care. They're more likely to use alcohol, drugs, or nicotine, all of which can have adverse effects on the fetus. If they are diagnosed early with a mild to moderate depression, standard forms of "talking therapy," such as interpersonal therapy (which focuses on relationships) and cognitive-behavioral techniques (which help a person change the way she thinks and acts) can make a big difference. In more severe cases, obstetricians and psychiatrists carefully weigh the risks and benefits of medications.

Little research has been done on the use of psychiatric drugs in women, and even less on their use in pregnancy. "In many cases, the risks of not treating clinical depression or severe anxiety disorders in pregnancy can be greater than using an effective medication," says Burt. If a woman doesn't get help, not only does she suffer, but the whole family suffers. There is an increased possibility of obstetrical complications, and the woman's psychological problems are likely to worsen after delivery.

This is not the only unfortunate outcome in pregnancy. Sometimes, despite the most ardent hopes, the most conscientious prenatal care, and the most advanced obstetrical treatments, the unthinkable happens, and a pregnancy ends in miscarriage or stillbirth. Few medical events are more emotionally devastating than the loss of a long-wished-for, deeply wanted pregnancy. The end of a brief life before it even begins leaves an indelible mark on would-be parents.

An estimated 10 to 15 percent of women with confirmed pregnancies—300,000 women in the United States every year—miscarry at some point after eight weeks of gestation. Yet, as any woman who's gone through the experience can testify, there is no comfort in numbers. "You grieve for the baby you never knew and the child—beautiful, perfect, wondrous—who might have been," says one woman. Women also grieve a loss that remains forever invisible to all but their closest loved ones.

Some women feel the loss in an extremely intense, almost physical way. Many who miscarry had not reached the point in pregnancy where the fetus seems separate. "His flesh was my flesh; his blood was my blood," one woman explains. "Losing him was like losing part of me." Typically women feel both vulnerable and responsible, as if they had done something to cause the loss or should have, could have, done something to prevent it. They tend to blame themselves, trying to iden-tify what they did wrong: exercising or not exercising, working or not working, eating too much or not eating enough.

Guilt, that ugly little intruder, preys on grieving mothers. And if, like many women, they felt any ambivalence about being pregnant, they may think that somehow their negative feelings led to the miscarriage or stillbirth. Some women interpret a loss as a punishment for past sins, imagined or real. Such self-inflicted guilt, allowed to fester, can lead to depression.

Fathers, of course, also grieve, but in different ways and at different times. At first their greatest pain is their helplessness. They see their part-ners hurting so badly that they cannot find the words to console them. Not knowing what to do or say, some men pull away, burying themselves in work or drowning their sorrow in alcohol. Others strive to put the loss behind them and get on with their lives as quickly as possible—a reaction their wives may interpret as uncaring or insensitive.

Some women need at least a year to work through their feelings of loss; others want nothing more than to try again to have a baby as soon as possible. "I lay on the table in the emergency room, bleeding and doubled over with pain, and all I could think of was getting pregnant again and doing it right the next time," says a woman who had an ectopic pregnancy. This is understandable, yet most physicians and therapists advise waiting at least several months for physical and psychological healing to take place.

Postpartum Problems

Miscarriage, as everyone realizes, is a heartbreaking loss. Birth, in comparison, represents the essence of joy. Yet the reality of life after delivery can be quite different than what many women expect. The months after childbirth are, in fact, the time of a woman's greatest psy-chological vulnerability. An estimated 10 to 15 percent of women who have never before suffered from a mental disorder become depressed after childbirth. If they've had previous depressions, they face a 25 per-cent risk of a recurrence. If they've had a prior postpartum depression, the likelihood of another such episode rises to 50 percent. Women who have had high-risk pregnancies, who conceived only after a very long period of trying, or who do not feel they are getting adequate spousal and social support also are more vulnerable.

Of course, almost all new mothers—eight or nine of every ten—undergo some emotional turmoil. Three or four days after the high of delivery, they may feel sad, anxious, irritable, weepy, restless, unable to sleep. Since so many women feel this way, doctors now consider the "baby blues" a perfectly normal phenomenon. But it doesn't *feel* normal to find yourself—as I did—bursting into tears when the weather forecast calls for rain.

Considering the hormonal hurricane that occurs before, during, and after delivery, emotional repercussions shouldn't be surprising. Estrogen and progesterone plummet after childbirth; prolactin and oxytocin increase. These changes serve many practical purposes, from contracting uterine blood vessels (lessening the risk of hemorrhage) to stimulating milk production to reinforcing a mother's protective instincts. But the psychological effects can be disconcerting.

The vast majority of new mothers regain their bearings after the first ten or twelve days. But in others—perhaps because of the speed or severity of the hormonal upheaval—negative feelings intensify rather than dissipate. In addition to the classic symptoms of major depression—sadness, hopelessness, changes in appetite and sleep, lack of interest and enjoyment in favorite activities—they may become very anxious and ruminate over the health and well-being of the baby.

Postpartum—or, as the British prefer, postnatal—depression can and often does come out of the blue, striking women of every social class and educational level. It has been recognized for centuries in countries around the world and is as common in rural Africa as in Frankfurt, Paris, Chicago, or Sydney. In all these places, many women do not seek help or get effective treatment for months, if at all. They may sense something is wrong but not guess what it is. Even obstetricians and pediatricians, the health professionals new mothers see routinely, may assume that it's just like a new mother to be exhausted or emotional, and so they ignore or dismiss very real symptoms of depression.

Recognizing women at risk can make an enormous difference in preventing postpartum depression and its long-term effects. Sometimes simply stabilizing hormone levels in vulnerable new mothers can help. In a double-blind, placebo-controlled British study of sixty-one women who'd had previous postpartum depressions, estradiol patches—like those worn by menopausal women for hormone replacement therapy—significantly reduced their depressive symptoms after subsequent deliveries.

Treatment with antidepressant medications, beginning immediately after delivery, also is effective. However, many women are reluctant to take an antidepressant for fear they will not be able to breastfeed their babies. Although data are limited, it does seem that medications given a mother, and their active metabolites, can make their way via breast milk to her baby. "There is no evidence that they are harmful," notes Burt. "But we don't have studies that have followed children for five, ten, twenty years."

Sometimes postpartum depression develops six to twelve weeks after delivery or when mothers wean their babies or begin menstruating again. While hormones may also be involved in these cases, psychosocial stressors, such as a lack of support from a partner or family or a baby's illness, seem to play a large role. Again, recognition and treatment can help both mother and child.

Without professional help, a depressed new mother is likely to get worse rather than better—and she is not the only one who suffers. Unable to bond with her infant, she is much more likely to express dislike or indifference and to be less responsive to her baby's needs. By the age of nine months, a depressed woman's baby, who may either cry a lot or become listless, may perform less well on developmental tasks—and these patterns persist for years. Fortunately, this bleak fate is far from inevitable. "New mothers usually respond rapidly to treatment," says Burt. "You can literally see the difference—not just in how they feel, but in how they care for their babies. As a therapist, it's particularly gratifying because you're helping two lives, not just one."

Depression isn't the only postpartum problem. Anxiety disorders, which are the most common of all mental disorders, affecting as many as 30 percent of women at some point in life, also can occur for the first time after delivery. Some new mothers develop panic attacks. Others begin having repetitive, intrusive thoughts about harming their babies. To block these from their minds, they may try counting, repeating a certain behavior, following various rituals—all symptoms of obsessive-compulsive disorder (OCD). The drop in estrogen at delivery, which may affect levels of the neurotransmitter serotonin, and prolonged sleep deprivation may be contributing factors. Treatment, usually with a combination of medication and behavioral therapy, is highly effective.

Much more rarely, in an estimated one or two of every thousand births, a new mother develops the most severe form of mental disorder: psychosis. Generally within the first two or three days of delivery, she experiences mood swings, confusion, disorientation, agitation, bizarre behavior, delusions, paranoia, or auditory hallucinations. Some women harm themselves or take their own lives. In about one of every fifty thousand cases, women with postpartum psychosis kill their babies.

With treatment with antipsychotic and other medications and hospitalization, most women suffering from postpartum psychosis never again lose touch with reality. However, they remain at increased risk of depressive disorders, not just after subsequent births but throughout their lives. Sadly, women who experience dark and unspeakable urges often are too afraid and too sick to seek help. The stigma is indeed enormous, since nothing may be more horrifying even to contemplate than the possibility that a mother might take her child's life.

The Making of a Mother

Large primates like gorillas and orangutans, with spacious vaginas and chutelike birth canals, have an easy time giving birth. "It's practically a nonevent," sniffs one biologist. "The baby just slides out." Human mothers have a harder time. However, the problem is not just the size of the fetus or the shape of the mother's pelvis, but the fact that only human infants emerge from the birth canal upside down and facing backward. Regardless of whether she is squatting or lying down, a woman cannot— at least not without great difficulty—reach down, as nonhuman primate mothers do, to clear a breathing passage for the infant or to remove the umbilical cord from around its neck. If she tries to tug at her baby, she risks damaging its spinal cord and central nervous system.

"Is this an evolutionary mistake?" I ask anthropologist Wenda Trevathan, who has studied human birth from prehistory to today. Not necessarily, she responds, noting that long ago—perhaps at about the time that our hominid ancestors became bipedal—our foremothers found a social adaptation to this obstetrical dilemma: seeking assistance during birth.

Females of most other species go off to give birth in solitude; women don't. "Human birth," Trevathan observes, "is a social rather than a solitary event." In a survey of 296 cultural groups, she found that having birth attendants—be they sisters, neighbors, friends, midwives, or obstetricians—is almost a cultural universal. A need for other women at the time of birth, for their emotional support as well as their physical assistance, may be part of our hard-wired female identity. So deep is the urge to reach out to others, so great is its importance to the survival of mother and child, that it may have given rise to our seemingly instinctive need to connect. Even today the support of others directly affects a new mother and her new baby. In a study of pregnant African-American teens, who as a group are at high risk of delivering low-birth-weight infants, those who received strong social support throughout pregnancy were more likely to give birth to bigger and healthier babies.

Nature has other ways of ensuring the well-being of a helpless newborn. An astounding change occurs in a new mother's brain, in two groups of cells located within the hypothalamus: the supraoptic nucleus and the paraventricular nucleus. Usually the neurons within these nuclei are separated from one another by a type of brain cell called glial cells. A few hours after birth the "veil" of glial cells moves away, bringing the cells that secrete oxytocin, a hormone that promotes bonding as well as milk secretion, into direct contact with one another. This activates the cells and stimulates oxytocin release to reinforce the bond between mother and newborn. As a result, the brain of the new mother becomes so exquisitely sensitive that the very sight, sound, and smell of her baby releases oxytocin. Some new mothers say their milk "lets down" and their breasts leak even when they hear their baby whimper over a telephone line or intercom.

Thus, just as it did in the womb, the newborn interacts directly with its mother's biology to ensure that its needs are met. At the same time, the process of feeding and holding her baby is so rewarding that a new mother will do so despite her own exhaustion. When nursing mothers wean, the glial cells move back into place between the oxytocin-producing neurons in the hypothalamus, creating a physiological as well as psychological distance between mother and child. But by this stage, the mother is smitten, and the infant has learned other ways, such as smiling at the sight of her, to catch and hold her attention.

But biology alone does not create mothers. Motherhood brings together all the aspects of a woman's life: our reproductive biology, evolutionary instincts, deepest feelings, social conditioning, cultural heritage. But there is one ingredient in the making of a mother that scientists rarely mention or study: love. Maybe it too comes from body, mind, and soul, a blend of hormones, genes, neurotransmitters, emotions, beliefs. A mother falls in love with a child, as the writer Anne Roiphe describes it, "not sanely, not rationally, but wholly and completely, the way people get up on an airplane and give control to the pilot, to the currents of wind, and let themselves be lifted up and taken away."

For many of us, this lack of control is new and disturbing. With a daily pill we can control our menstrual cycles. With a diaphragm or condom we can block sperm from fertilizing our eggs. With access to abortion we can end a pregnancy almost as soon as it starts. Yet as would-be, expectant, and new mothers discover, control over reproduction is elusive, if not impossible. We cannot compel an egg to ripen and make its way to the right place at the right time. We cannot command the thousands of precisely timed stages of fetal development to occur in the right order at the right moment. We cannot wish away labor contractions, nor can we negotiate with a hungry newborn for just five minutes more of desperately needed sleep.

And so, as we throw the reproductive dice, even the most sophisticated and tough-minded of women may find themselves bargaining with whatever gods may be: "Don't let my period start. Let the pregnancy test be positive. Make this the month." Once pregnant, the pleas intensify: "Whatever you do, wipe that worried look from the sonographer's face. Let the heartbeat be strong. Make the amniocentesis normal." During birth, we inhale, belly-breathe, exhale, pant, and pray: "Get me through this. Make it stop. Make the pain go away." Then, in those tense first moments: "Let me hear my baby cry. Don't let the cord be around its neck. Make it breathe." Yet it isn't until a mother holds her newborn that the real petitioning begins—and it never ends. All of her life a mother will lobby and rail and plead, imploring the fates to hold safe her precious child.

To become a mother, some say, is to put your soul on the block, to open yourself up to bartering and blackmail, to discover yourself—sometimes much to your own amazement—acting just as mothers always have. Your baby cries, and you seem to respond at a cellular level. Your toddler disappears momentarily in a crowd, and your heart stops. The phone rings in the night, and it's your child—off at camp or school or even a grown-up, independent life—that you fear for first.

This is not politically correct behavior for the twenty-first century. It violates conventional premises of feminist autonomy and invincibility. But it is the way many of us are, part of the psychobiology that makes us female, and it does no good to deny or ignore this reality. However, while the rationale for motherhood may stretch beyond the rational, while mothers may always react with their hearts rather than with their heads, there is every reason to bring reason into the decision to become mothers.

As we enhance our fertility, extend our reproductive lives, create zygotes in laboratories, and freeze embryos for future use, we need to rethink what it can and should mean to bring life into the world. When does infertility treatment exact too high a cost? Should a mother defy age—and the ageless wisdom of the body? What should we make of the relationship between a zygote and its parents? Is an egg donor a mother? What about the woman who leases out her womb for a child biologically unrelated to her? To what extent does biology ever define what it means to be a mother? Where will we draw the line between physiology and psychology, the rights written in blood and the love given in hugs? We may not have the answers, but the questions are too important not to ask and consider very carefully.

Of all the aspects of brave new motherhood that may warrant trepidation, there is one that does not—the capacity of the human heart to embrace a child with a completely different genetic makeup. This is something that happens every day, a triumph of selfless love over the selfish genes that allegedly direct evolution. A few years ago, at a birthday party on a postcard-perfect day, families gathered near a sunny pool. I had just joined a group of women when a faint splash vaguely registered in my consciousness. Instantly one of the women turned and dove into the pool. The rest of us—realizing belatedly that a small child had fallen into the deep end—stood by in mute horror. With strong strokes, the woman swooped up the little girl and carried her from the pool. "It's okay," she crooned. "Mommy's got you. Mommy's here. You're safe. You're going to be all right."

We formed a circle around this sopping wet pair, tears of fear and relief streaming down both their faces. The little girl finally relaxed against her mother's shoulder. The mom flashed a reassuring smile as her hand cradled her daughter's head. Watching from the sidelines, I realized only then that the mother's hair was red, her child's dark. Everything about them—eyes, noses, faces, skin color—was different. As I later learned, they shared not a single gene. The child was born thousands of miles away from the woman she calls Mommy, in a different culture, a different environment, almost a different world. Biology contributed not one whit to the bond these two had forged. But no one who witnessed this mother's instant, unthinking response to her child in danger could doubt an essential fact: that she, through an alchemy science probably never will fully explain, was utterly and wholly a mother.

C H A P T E R   1 0

Second Puberty

It is neither the best of times nor the worst of times, but somewhere right smack in the middle. No longer the girls they once were, women at midlife are smarter and savvier than they've ever been. For many, the whirlwind years of breathless juggling are winding down. Ahead lie the wisdom years, when all that they've learned comes into flower. The tricky part is the passage from one stage to the other.

As with the other biological transitions in a woman's life, the time around menopause—the last of the female "blood mysteries"—can be a rocky one. Once again women find themselves doing what they're meant to do, what they do so often throughout their lives: They change. In the process, they grow—not physically (at least they try not to), but in understanding and insight. Once again they stand poised at the brink of something new—and it's not surprising that they may be knocked temporarily off balance. Just as teen limbs and torsos lurch ahead of cognitive development, middle-aged bodies and minds may swing out of synch. But like puberty, the climacteric—the medical term for the time during which a woman's ability to conceive declines—doesn't go on forever. Within a few years most women return to a new hormonal equilibrium, and some report the highest satisfaction levels of their lives.

Evolutionary theorists now laud menopause as "among the biological traits essential for making us distinctively human—something qualitatively different from, and more than, an ape." Menopause is virtually unheard-of in the wild; in captivity the females of only a few species stop reproducing late in life. But, as discussed in Chapter 3, anthropologists recently have recognized the significance of postmenopausal grandmothers.

Throughout history relatively few women outlived their ovaries. Even at the turn of the twentieth century, the average life span for Western women was about fifty. Today almost one third of the women in the United States are fifty-plus, with three or more decades of postmenopausal life stretching before them. In the next decade more women—some fifty million by the year 2010—will enter menopause than at any other time in history. This generation, the baby boomers— veterans of the sexual revolution, natural childbirth, and the women's movement—is redefining what it means to be a woman "of a certain age."

"We're not going over the hill," one forty-something feminist declares. "We're taking the hill." While I admire her spirit, I doubt if moxie alone will get us where we want to go. The end of a woman's reproductive life, like menarche, menstruation, and childbirth, is an intricate psychobiological process that defies conscious control.

A woman's ovaries follow a timetable of their own. An estimated 1 percent of women naturally experience "premature ovarian failure," or early menopause, prior to age forty. Women who smoke, are extremely thin or malnourished, or have certain medical conditions, such as diabetes or thyroid disease, typically enter menopause before their age peers. About one in four plunges into early menopause as the result of surgical menopause (removal of the ovaries) or as a consequence of cancer therapy.

In most women the ovaries start to "sputter," as my gynecologist puts it, in their mid- to late forties. The transition stage known as "perimenopause"—a general term used for the changes that occur during the climacteric—begins at a median age of 47.5 years. The ovaries' gradual shift from reproductive readiness to postreproductive repose takes an average of four years. However, this varies from a matter of months in women who undergo chemical or surgical menopause to as long as a decade.

Usually a woman's reproductive hormones do not diminish slowly and steadily, like a man's, but in a series of plunges and plateaus. Estrogen, the prototypical female hormone, isn't the only one to drop, but—as Chapter 4 discusses—it is so ubiquitous, so involved in the functioning of almost every organ system, that we register the impact of its decline throughout our bodies. Menstrual periods become erratic. Skin may turn dry, itchy, sensitive to pressure. In some women, the dip in estrogen causes their hearts to race or skip a beat. The brain, rich in estrogen receptors, may respond in various ways: headaches, mood shifts, memory lapses, fragmented sleep. "It's like the Joni Mitchell song," says a friend. "You don't know what you've got till it's gone."

The final shutdown of the ovarian estrogen production line comes at about age fifty-one to fifty-two—a figure that is remarkably consistent around the world and over time (even in reports from ancient Greece). As temperature controls go awry, as many as nine in ten menopausal women experience hot flashes that may make them sizzle one minute and shiver the next. Other changes, less noticeable but nonetheless momentous, occur within the heart, blood vessels, brain, and bones.

Along with the timing, the degree of these changes varies with each woman. An estimated 10 to 15 percent of women sail through menopause without any significant complaints. At the other end of the spectrum, a similar percentage develop symptoms that make it impossible for them to function as usual. The majority of women, 70 to 80 percent, are somewhere in between, managing, despite temporary discomforts, to get on with their busy lives. "Menopause is not life-threatening," says one woman in a support group for the "hormonally challenged," "but it certainly can be life-disrupting."

According to the old stereotypes, women who survived past menopause lost all value as their youth, fertility, and sexual attractiveness faded away. In effect, they became invisible, and so they long remained, especially in the area that long ignored our entire gender: medical research. However, because women today matter more—before and after menopause—science has finally begun to take seriously a process once considered even more taboo than menstruation itself.

"Thirty years ago menopause research involved about a half dozen experts around the world," says gynecologist Wulf Utian, founder of the North American Menopause Society. "I would go to meetings, and no one was talking about it. I felt I was a lone voice in the wilderness." Now annual NAMS meetings draw thousands of attendees from around the world for a news-making array of renowned speakers, heated debates, and hot research findings.

The new scientific appreciation of "the change" has given rise to new attitudes. In a recent NAMS poll, more than half of women between forty-five and sixty viewed menopause as a positive phase in their lives. Of those who had completed menopause, eight in ten expressed relief to be done with menstruation; six in ten did not associate menopause with a lessened willingness to try new things or with becoming less attractive.

While attitudes have become more positive, menopause, with its temperature spikes and memory warps, its edgy nerves and itchy skin, still can hit today's busy women where it hurts most—in their hectic, hassled, not-a-second-to-spare lifestyles. This reproductive transition, as this chapter discusses, need not bring a productive woman to a screeching halt. Nonetheless, it may indeed call for a pause—at least long enough for her to look both back and ahead, to draw on what she's learned and to make plans for where she wants to go.

The endlessly changing female body has important lessons to teach at midlife—about acknowledging needs, recognizing susceptibilities, celebrating strengths, and living both long and well. Much like the girl-about-to-become-a-woman at first puberty, what the midlife woman discovers in "second puberty" is the headiness of realizing that she too still has a great deal of living to do. But this time she has an added advantage: the wisdom, born of experience, of knowing how to go about it.

Starting in the Middle

A male gerontologist I know once described the forties as "the last great decade." While these years certainly have their moments, I'm not sure most women would agree—or they might just be too busy to notice. For women today, the forties can bring almost anything. Some fall in love, marry, and have babies; others send youngsters off to college, pack their own bags, and head across the country in an RV. Many, tugged between the demands of a toddler, a teenager, or both and the needs of aging or ill parents, feel the squeeze of being part of the "sandwich" generation. After decades of climbing corporate ladders, a growing number finally glimpse the view from the top; others find themselves downsized out of a job or passed over for a long-sought promotion. Some settle, cozily or not, into second or third marriages; others, whether by divorce or death, find themselves suddenly on their own.

The threads of happiness and grief, exhilaration and exhaustion, triumph and failure are tightly interwoven at midlife. Some women are forming new families as their own parents' health declines. Children speeding toward adulthood and independence may slam the door on the way out of their parents' lives, either staying away for years or boomeranging back to take up uneasy residence under the same roof. A husband's career and self-image may go into a tailspin, threatening to drag down a marriage. Moves, mergers, financial setbacks, accidents, serious illnesses—the stuff of sleepless nights and stressful days—can stealthily sabotage a woman's sense of well-being. Then, just as their lives are popping at the seams with the thousand-and-two details of dailiness, women's bodies may start springing some surprises of their own.

When they do, most forty-something women don't have a clue as to what's happening or why. A forty-four-year-old travel agent found herself wrenched from sleep, plagued by headaches, and so cotton-headed she would show up at her son's soccer field when she should have been at her daughter's guitar class. She blamed stress, the business, the brain tumor she was sure she had. "When my doctor used the word *perimenopause*, I didn't know whether to feel relieved that I wasn't dying or upset that my days as a babe were numbered," she says.

Even for the most liberated of women, aging can be an unnerving prospect. In our mind's eye, if not our mirrors, we're still just kids. Yet we can start to feel like strangers in the bodies that we'd settled into comfortably over four decades. Some women say it's like the "tween-age" years all over again—complete with pimples and sweaty palms. With no small amount of apprehension, they start to ask, "What's happening to me?"

The best way to think of it may be as a change in seasons. Like trees silently unleaving in the fall, the egg cells, or oocytes, in a woman's ovaries start to senesce, or die off, at a faster rate in her late thirties. Eventually the number of egg cells drops to a tiny fraction of the estimated two million packed into her ovaries at birth. Trying to coax some of the remaining oocytes to ripen, the pituitary gland churns out extra follicle-stimulating hormone (FSH). This surge is the earliest harbinger of menopause, occurring six to ten years before a woman's final periods. Eventually the other menstrual messenger, luteinizing hormone (LH), also increases, but at a slower rate.

These frustrated signalers, like New York City taxis trapped in gridlock and honking their horns, keep blaring louder and louder. Sometimes the ovaries respond with a surge in estrogen even higher than the usual levels during a woman's peak reproductive years. However, in an increasing number of cycles, ovulation does not occur. Without a corpus luteum to produce progesterone, the lining of the uterus may not be fully shed each month. The result may be spotting throughout the month or very heavy flow during the woman's next period. Among women in their late forties, 70 percent report irregular bleeding.

The follicular or ripening stage of the menstrual cycle grows shorter in perimenopause, with cycle lengths typically decreasing from a median of twenty-eight days in a woman's twenties to twenty-six days in her forties. Menses may stop for months on end, then return with a sudden gush or a slow dribble. In a longitudinal study that followed sixteen women through perimenopause and beyond, psychologist Norma McCoy, of San Francisco State University, found that the year before their periods stopped altogether was the time of greatest irregularity. Women's cycles ran alternately early or late, short or long, heavy or light. They had fewer "good" days every month, reported more psychological symptoms, had sex less often—and enjoyed it much less.

A woman's concentration of estradiol remains in the normal range until approximately three years before menopause, when it gradually begins to decline. Estrone, a weaker estrogen produced primarily from conversion of adrenal and ovarian androstenedione (an androgen) by fat cells, becomes a woman's primary estrogen. Women with higher levels of body fat may experience fewer menopausal symptoms, such as hot flashes, because their bodies produce more estrone.

These hormonal shifts can trigger an array of symptoms. The most common are nighttime awakenings, caused by a spike in temperature (a subdromal hot flash, in medical terms) that is just intense enough to disrupt sleep. A woman may sit bolt upright, the back of her neck damp, her heart pounding, and not be able to get back to sleep for hours. About 10 to 20 percent of perimenopausal women also experience daytime hot flashes—a symptom that becomes more prevalent with the more drastic hormonal changes of menopause itself.

Even in women who have never suffered from premenstrual syndrome (PMS), perimenopause can trigger its classic symptoms: irritability, tearfulness, fatigue, migraines, mood swings, anxiety. The suspected culprits are changes both in reproductive hormones and in neurochemistry. Some women also report headaches, heart palpitations, dizziness, insomnia, tingling sensations in the skin, chills, restlessness, listlessness, headaches, or stress incontinence (release of urine when running, laughing, or sneezing).

While many women feel no need to seek help with such perimenopausal problems, an array of options can ease the way through this physiological prelude to menopause. More and more women are trying herbal and nutritional remedies, such as plant-based estrogens (phytoestrogens), including those found in soy products like tofu and soy milk, and lifestyle changes, like exercise and relaxation, to promote better health. Physicians often suggest low-dose oral contraceptives, which relieve symptoms like night sweats and offer protection from pregnancy—a not-insignificant benefit. Among women in their forties, the rate of unplanned pregnancies is almost as high as among teenagers.

But for many women the primary concern of perimenopause is what lies ahead. In various surveys, these women—unlike those who have already made it through—register the most negative attitudes, including anxiety and apprehension, about menopause itself. These views can turn into a self-fulfilling prophecy. In several studies, the perimenopausal women who had anticipated the most difficulty during menopause did indeed suffer the greatest distress.

What women often fear most is that "the change" heralds the beginning of the end—not just of fertility, but of sexuality, desirability, professional achievement, and importance in the lives of those they care about most. Not so, say counselors and health professionals. As they see it, while perimenopause and menopause end reproductive functioning, they also can mark the beginning of new and rewarding chapters in a woman's life.

The Neurobiology of the Change

It starts in a woman's head. As reproductive hormones dip, the reaction of the brain's temperature-regulating center is to fool the body into thinking it is overheated. Trying to dissipate this excess warmth as quickly as possible, the body dilates blood vessels near the surface of the skin, causing a hot flash or flush—a wave of heat that originates in the head and neck and spreads to the upper torso, arms, and ultimately the whole body. Sweat pours over a woman's face and neck and trickles down her chest and spine. During the night she may rip off a sopping wet nightgown. During the day she may open a window or fling off her jacket. Her heart may beat rapidly; she may find it hard to breathe. Some women feel weak or anxious as perspiration evaporates and their bodies begin to shiver.

During each hot flash, a woman lurches from hot to cold, sweat to chills, in an on-off, back-forth cycle that can last up to thirty minutes and occur once a month, once a day, or—in a small percentage of women— once an hour. Hot flashes tend to occur most frequently in the first year after surgical menopause or the first two years after natural menopause. Women who experience menopause at an earlier age than usual, who undergo medical or surgical menopause, who smoked during their perimenopausal years, or who drink alcohol report more hot flashes than others. Women with a short perimenopause of six months or less are not as prone to hot flashes.

Medical science has yet to figure out why hot flashes strike certain women more than others or why they begin before menopause in some and persist for years after in others. Subtle and not-so-subtle changes in the thermoregulatory system or in interactions among estrogen, other hormones, and brain neurotransmitters almost certainly play a role. Yet although hot flashes have been linked with decreases in estrogen and increases in epinephrine, cortisol, and other hormones, no single factor has been definitively identified as the trigger.

Hot flashes signal less visible but equally dramatic changes within a woman's body. Throughout her reproductive years, a chart of a woman's ovarian production of estradiol and progesterone resembles the peaks and valleys of a mountain range. By the end of her cycling, estradiol·

levels drop by 85 to 90 percent, progesterone by 99 percent. Following menopause—defined as an entire year without a menstrual period—these key hormones "flatline," that is, the levels stay low and unchanging.

FSH, in contrast, keeps rising to a level ten to twenty times that of earlier years, reaching its maximum about one to three years after menopause. LH increases threefold. These two messenger hormones may remain elevated for decades. What purpose do they serve? Although there has been little research, some speculate that they may prime the brain to work in different ways. One psychologist theorizes they may be "wise woman" hormones that may somehow feed the greater insight and intuition that come with age.

A woman's androgens—the first reproductive hormones to stimulate growth in girlhood—are the last ones to decline. The cells of the ovaries that manufacture androgens typically outlive estrogen-making cells by several years, and the adrenal glands continue their androgen production throughout a woman's life. As a result, a woman's levels of testosterone, androstenedione, dehydroepiandrosterone (DHEA), and other androgens decline much less than those of other sex hormones—by about 50 percent from age forty to sixty. Since less estrogen is available to counter their effects, these "male" hormones may give women the boost in energy—and, some find, feistiness—that's been dubbed "postmenopausal zest." They are also responsible for less desirable effects, such as the thinning of scalp hair and the sprouting of facial hair.

After its years of constantly gearing up for pregnancy, a woman's entire reproductive system, densely supplied with estrogen receptors, changes dramatically with menopause. The vulva and vagina become less elastic; the vaginal opening becomes narrower; the vagina itself shortens (this is called vaginal atrophy). It takes longer for lubrication to occur during sexual arousal. The vulva, labia, and pubic mound lose collagen and subcutaneous fat. Membranes in the vagina become thinner and drier, making them more susceptible to tears during intercourse. The result can be itching, infection, and pain during sex. Muscle control diminishes in the urethra, bladder, and vagina, often resulting in stress incontinence.

The reproductive system is far from the only target of menopausal changes. Another—only recently recognized—is the estrogen-hungry

brain. Sleep patterns change dramatically, as sleep becomes more fragmented and dream, or REM sleep, which is crucial to sleep's restorative
effects, diminishes. Even though women's memories tend to hold up
better and longer than men's, as discussed in Chapter 11, as they move
through menopause women often complain of feeling "fuzzy-minded."
They forget the word for the whatchamacallit in the kitchen drawer or
the name of the person who taught their children piano for years.

Even though they may not create as much immediate angst as hot
flashes, disrupted sleep, and memory meltdowns, the long-term effects of
menopause are no less significant—especially for a woman's cardiovascular system. Throughout her reproductive years, as Chapter 5 notes,
estrogen keeps her arteries supple, prevents blood clots, boosts levels of
beneficial high-density lipoprotein (HDL), and decreases harmful low-
density lipoprotein (LDL). As estrogen falls, a woman's heart becomes as
vulnerable as a man's. Her HDL slumps; LDL increases; her risk of blood
clots grows; atherosclerotic plaque builds up in her arteries.

Also at risk are a woman's bones. Although the process of bone loss
begins in the thirties, it speeds up to as much as 2 to 5 percent annually in
the first five years after menopause. Women with small bones, smokers,
and those with a family history of bone problems are at increased risk of
fractures and the bone-thinning disease known as osteoporosis.

Menopause itself, however mild or intense, is what physicians call
"time-limited." In more than 80 percent of women, symptoms persist for
longer than one year, but they generally abate within five years. However, women need to take a much longer view. Because some changes,
such as the buildup of atherosclerotic plaque and the weakening of bone
tissue, can develop and progress silently over the years, women need to
educate themselves about what can happen to their bodies and minds
both during and after the change.

Mood at Midlife

"I just don't feel like me anymore." This is a phrase therapists and
physicians hear often from middle-aged women, who may describe themselves as inexplicably blue, lonely, hopeless, fearful, shaky, restless,
apprehensive. Some feel that something has gone out of their souls.

"When I lecture, I show a cartoon of a dejected-looking dog whose owner says, 'He's lost his will to fetch,'" says psychiatrist Barbara Parry. "That's how a lot of the women I see feel. Nothing seems worth getting up and going after."

When you consider the dramatic changes occurring in women's bodies and lives, it's not surprising that their minds and moods register their impact. As noted above, hormonal shifts, particularly the decline of estrogen, have profound effects on brain chemistry. The mood-regulating neurotransmitter serotonin and energy-boosting beta endorphins fall. As a result, some women feel, as one psychiatrist puts it, "as if they've had the rug pulled out from them."

What some call the "domino effect" can have a similar effect: Over the course of weeks, months, or even years, troublesome physical symptoms—hot flashes, insomnia, urinary tract infections, vaginal itching and burning—can undermine equanimity. Not surprisingly, the women who "flash" most tend to register the greatest emotional distress. Some medical disorders that often develop at midlife, such as hypothyroidism, as well as common medications, such as certain cholesterol-lowering drugs and antihypertensives, may themselves sabotage emotional well-being.

Almost any woman making her way through midlife may come down with what counselors sometimes call "the gloomies." "These women get up every day, do their jobs, and take care of their families, but a lot of them feel less competent than they want to be," says psychiatrist Vivien Burt. "They can't sleep. They're tired and tearful and overwhelmed. And they're frightened. What they're experiencing may not be a severe, disabling psychiatric disorder, but it is real, and it makes them miserable." She has found that estrogen replacement (discussed later in this chapter) often can help these women sleep better, feel more energetic, and function on an even keel once more.

At any age, stressful events take a toll. But according to several studies, the emptying of the nest and the death of parents—the stereotyped female heartbreakers of middle age—do not in themselves bring on emotional problems. However, when they are added to other stressors, such as a career setback or marital conflict, a woman may develop mild depression that, if unrecognized, can deepen and become more difficult to treat.

Reports of women becoming bleak and bitter after menopause date back to the ancient Greeks, who considered aging into a crone yet another example of female inferiority. More recent theorists have been no kinder—and no more accurate. In 1896, just as more women began to survive beyond their reproductive years, the famed psychiatrist Emil Kraepelin coined the term "involutional melancholia," a syndrome of middle age characterized by depression, hypochondria, and nihilistic thoughts. For decades so many midlife women were diagnosed with— and often hospitalized for—this problem that it became known as "meno- pausal depression," and it seemed unavoidable. Indeed, twentieth-century psychiatrists and psychologists—female as well as male—assumed that it was inevitable for a woman to become depressed as she turned into a stereotypical hag with shriveled ovaries, withered breasts, and creased skin. They described menopause as a physiological disaster, a time of decline, partial death, and "justified" grief and sadness.

Once again the assumptions about women were wrong. As it turns out, while menopause is indeed inevitable, depression is not. Epidemio- logical studies of depression rates around the world have found that women who have never had clinical depression (serious enough to war- rant professional treatment) are *not* significantly more likely to develop it at menopause itself.

Yet this good news should not obscure some more-sobering statis- tics. Women are more vulnerable to first-time episodes of depression *before* menopause, in the perimenopausal years of greatest hormonal upheaval. According to the National Institute of Mental Health's large-scale Epi- demiologic Catchment Area Survey, the rates of first-time episodes of clinical depression for American women peak at two points in the life span: between ages twenty-five and twenty-nine and again between the ages of forty-five and forty-nine.

Are hormonal changes responsible? There is no conclusive evi- dence, but they do seem to play a role. Hormone replacement therapy, some studies suggest, can improve women's moods and ease the symp- toms of mild depression. In women with more severe or persistent depression, it does not have the same benefits. However, it may quicken the helpful effects of antidepressant medications and possibly may even boost their efficacy. In preliminary research comparing the effects of estrogen replacement, antidepressants, and placebos on depressed menopausal women, the combination of antidepressants and estrogen replacement yielded the greatest improvement. (See Chapter 13 for a comprehensive discussion of depression in women.)

Unfortunately, many women who develop depression at midlife assume their symptoms are a normal part of aging or simply try to tough them out. "Even though the majority of women go through menopause without too many problems, there are women—a small percentage, granted—who do get depressed," notes Parry. "For them, the situation is the same as for men with heart disease. If they deny that there's something wrong and call whatever they're feeling heartburn, they really end up in trouble. If they recognize that what's happening isn't normal, they can get treatment and go back to their high-functioning lives."

Midlife Sex: From Joy to "Oy!"

A sex therapist I was interviewing told me the most surprising thing she'd learned about sex in the middle years: For women especially, it can be, as she put it, "unbelievably hot." Women in their late thirties and early forties—more confident than ever and more comfortable with their own sexuality—may discover pleasures they never guessed at when they were younger. Yet this sexual surge tends to fade with time. One psychologist who studied women's progress through their forties describes it as "the last bloom of the rose before the frost."

Women certainly remain sexual and sexy long past midlife, but their sexual responses go through some changes. Because they don't ovulate in every cycle in their late forties, women no longer consistently experience the usual midcycle surge in sexual interest. They may notice a decrease in vaginal secretions during sexual excitement. Without adequate stimulation and lubrication, intercourse can be painful—a problem they may blame on an inept partner or a souring relationship, rather than their aging bodies.

The loss of estrogen at menopause affects other aspects of female sexuality, from sensory responses to blood flow. Skin may become so sensitive that even tender touches, such as caressing of their breasts, may feel extremely irritating. Orgasms may be less intense. In addition to these age-related changes, medications that women may start to take at midlife—including antidepressants and antihypertensives—can blunt sexual response.

A woman's own sense of her body and beauty also may affect her sexuality. In a society that idolizes the young and the taut, the physical signs of age—wrinkles, bulges, squishy thighs, saggy breasts, blue-veined legs—may make even the most enlightened woman feel less desirable than she once did. The classic symptoms of menopause also take a toll. "It's hard to feel sexy when you're drenched in sweat and can't stand anyone touching you," says one woman. Serious illnesses, such as breast cancer and heart disease, also invariably affect the way women view their sexual potential.

Even so, baby boomers may not be as willing as women in the past to resign themselves to sexless or sexually unfulfilling lives. "I'm fifty, and I've always enjoyed sex," says one woman. "Why should that change now?" In one survey of five hundred midlife women, more than half said sex is better than at age twenty-five; most of them anticipated remaining sexually active well into old age. "If they've had a rich, wonderful, exciting sex life, women are not eager to give it up, especially if they have a man in their lives who wants a sexual relationship," says McCoy.

Women in long-term relationships are most likely to engage in regular sex, which—perhaps because it spurs changes in hormones or vaginal secretions—may itself prime their sexual interest (this use-it-or-lose-it philosophy also applies to brains, muscles, and other systems). Women who continue to be sexually active, whether through intercourse with a partner or self-stimulation, have better vaginal health and fewer difficulties during sexual intercourse compared with women who rarely have sex.

As with so many aspects of lesbian women's lives, virtually nothing is known about their experience of menopause or its effects on their sexuality. While there are anecdotal reports that some women first seek out same-sex partners at midlife or beyond, there has been virtually no scientific research into such changes in sexual preference.

In an estimated one in five heterosexual postmenopausal women, sexual desire diminishes or dies away completely. The reasons are complex. A woman without a regular partner—or whose partner may have health or sexual problems—may resign herself to self-stimulation or abstinence. Other women, who never considered sex a special pleasure, may be relieved not to have to feign any interest in it. "I think of sex as something I used to do, like wearing a bikini or drinking tequila shooters," says one woman I know. "None of them seems appealing to me anymore."

Yet for others, a mysterious midlife disappearance of any and all interest in sex can be distressing. "My sex drive just up and left," an office manager told a support group of midlife women. "I was in the same loving relationship I'd been in for ten years. I still cared for my partner. I felt just as healthy as ever. I'd been through menopause without too many problems. Then one day I realized I'd rather do my nails or fold the laundry than have sex."

Although psychological factors always play a role, there may be a hormonal underpinning for a midlife loss of interest in sex. As researchers now understand it, it is not the well-known drop in estrogen that diminishes desire, but the smaller decline in androgens. In decades of research on women who experienced surgical menopause, psychologist Barbara Sherwin, of McGill University, found that many reported decreased sexual fantasies, desire, and arousal. While replacing estrogen had little effect on their sexual interest (although it did seem to enhance sexual response), the use of testosterone or a combination of estrogen and testosterone did.

"Low-dose testosterone can help with lack of desire, problems with arousal, absence of sexual fantasy, and lack of sexual gratification," says Sherwin, who reports that she has had women—and their husbands—come to her office begging for this treatment. An Australian study, in which women took testosterone supplements over a two-year period, also documented enhanced libido. However, other researchers have noted that women who take testosterone supplements start making less of their own natural androgens—a consequence with unknown physiological and psychological repercussions.

Particularly in the United States, many women remain wary of androgen replacement. Some fear masculinization (about 5 percent of women develop facial hair; others report acne, oily skin, and a deepening of their voices) and still-unknown long-term complications. Others doubt that hormones alone can restore something as elusive and subjective as a libido. In a sense, they're right. As Sherwin and other researchers have found, testosterone cannot instill passion in a relationship in which love died long before desire.

However, when love endures and hormones remain or are kept in healthy ranges, sexuality may take on new meaning after midlife. "Sex truly is wasted on the young," says sex therapist Lonnie Barbach, author of *The Pause*. "They may have the equipment and the energy, but they don't have the experience. If couples have had a really good, caring relationship over a long period of time, they talk about sex in a way that a twenty-five-year-old couldn't begin to understand. For women at midlife and beyond, sex has a real depth that you just can't know when you're younger."

Not Your Mother's Menopause

I was in my twenties when I wrote my first magazine article on hormone replacement after menopause. After plowing through scientific studies, interviewing dozens of experts, and talking to real women about their experiences, I was astounded by the confusion and controversy. "At least they'll have this figured out by the time we hit fifty," I told my friends. I was wrong. We're almost there, and questions about the best approach to menopausal changes still outweigh answers.

Even so, we have far more choices than our mothers—and their mothers before them—ever imagined. Once women simply endured. Then, in the late 1960s, as the first women who gave birth to baby boomers began to move into midlife, they were told something that, as so often has happened, sounded too good to believe: They could remain "feminine forever." A best-selling book with this title argued that estrogen loss was the cause of the "disease" of menopause, and estrogen replacement was its cure. Millions of middle-aged women started taking estrogen. However, within a decade they discovered that they were at increased risk of endometrial cancer—a danger that, as scientists subsequently found, can be averted by adding progesterone.

"There was a tendency to think that because menopause happens to all women, one treatment should be right for all women," observes gynecologist Morris Notelovitz, founder of the National Menopause Foundation. "The good news for women today is there is a wide range of options so every woman can receive individualized care during menopause and beyond." Hormone replacement therapy, or HRT, now comes in different combinations, forms, and doses. Many regimens use much lower doses of estrogen; some use plant-based phytoestrogens or substitute natural progesterone for synthetic progestins; special formulations add testosterone to estrogen and progesterone.

However, HRT still entails side effects and risks: Some women who try HRT become depressed (particularly if they had a similar reaction to birth control pills), develop gallstones, or experience a worsening of breast tenderness, migraines, fibroids, or endometriosis. These problems may explain why, at least in the past, as many as half of women who began HRT stopped within two years. Others find that the progestin component of combination treatment is most problematic. Although there are few hard data to confirm this, switching to a natural progesterone or a different dosing schedule may help.

The biggest concern for women—and the primary reason they refuse or discontinue HRT—is the threat of breast cancer. Is this fear justified? It's not clear. Research studies, using different forms and doses of estrogen in different groups of women over differing periods of time, have produced contradictory findings. Breast cancer rates generally increase among women who have taken replacement hormones for prolonged periods (five, seven, or ten or more years in various studies). However, it is not certain if mortality rates from breast cancer also increase, or if every formulation presents an equal risk.

Countering HRT's risk of breast cancer are some major health benefits, including a greater than 50 percent reduction in heart disease, the number-one killer of women. Because of this potentially life-saving advantage, in statistical analyses, the presence of a single risk factor for heart disease, such as a family history of cardiovascular problems or hypertension, even among women at high risk for breast cancer, tips the risk-benefit balance in favor of HRT. "Women are ten times more likely to die of heart disease than breast cancer," notes Columbia's Marianne Legato. "For many, the risks of not taking HRT are far greater than with its use."

HRT also prevents the dramatic loss of bone density that begins after menopause and that can lead to osteoporosis. Women who start HRT within five years of menopause decrease their risk of hip, wrist, and other nonspinal fractures when compared with women who have never used estrogen. Yet once they stop HRT, bone loss proceeds at the same rate as in early menopause. However, traditional hormone replacement is no longer a woman's only option for strengthening bones. New treatments include raloxifene (Evista), a new "designer" estrogen that targets the bones but does not stimulate estrogen receptors in the breast; two drugs in the class known as bisphosphonates, alendronate (Fosamax) and risedronate; and calcitonin-salmon, a synthetic version of a natural hormone administered as a nasal spray.

In addition to its benefits for heart and skeleton, HRT may also benefit the brain. Some studies suggest that HRT users score higher on tests of verbal and spatial memory, language, and attention (although the insomnia and fatigue caused by hot flashes in women not on HRT may in themselves lower their scores). Estrogen may increase production of acetylcholine, a neurotransmitter that regulates memory, learning, and other cognitive functions. As discussed in Chapter 11, small studies indicate that HRT may offer some protection against Alzheimer's disease and may alleviate symptoms in women who have already developed some memory loss as a result of mild to moderate dementia. However, according to a recent analysis of the limited and sometimes less-than-rigorous research to date, there is not yet sufficient evidence to warrant HRT's use solely for this purpose.

HRT does clearly provide many short-term quality-of-life benefits that make living in a menopausal body more comfortable, although many women report that plant-based estrogens and herbal and nutritional remedies, though scientifically untested and unproven, can do the same. HRT relieves hot flashes, improves sleep, alleviates sexual symptoms, makes intercourse more enjoyable, and lessens urinary tract problems. Women on HRT report that they think better, remember more, and feel more energetic. They're also less prone to many age-related problems, such as tooth loss and driving accidents (possibly a consequence of improved concentration).

For these varied reasons, an increasing number of women are trying HRT. According to current estimates, 25 percent of all postmenopausal American women use HRT (up from 16 percent a decade ago); among those age fifty to fifty-four, the rate approaches 50 percent. Many feel they couldn't get by without it. "If my brain isn't working or if I can't sleep, I am in bad shape," says one teacher. "A woman can tolerate a few bad nights or foggy days, but not a lot." Physicians are still debating the controversial question of how long a woman should take HRT, whose benefits generally end when a woman discontinues its use. At least with the traditional formulations, the risk of long-term use (primarily of breast cancer) has to be weighed—and reweighed—against the likelihood of heart disease or osteoporosis if a woman stops HRT.

The recent advent of new treatment options, particularly the designer estrogens, or selective estrogen receptor modulators (SERMs), may greatly expand women's options. In clinical trials, the first two SERMs to be introduced in the United States—the anticancer drug tamoxifen and the osteoporosis preventive raloxifene—have significantly reduced the risk of breast cancer. Other SERMs, currently in use in Europe, may offer the benefits of estrogen, progesterone, and testosterone with few of their drawbacks. However, these new agents, like all medications, have side effects of their own, some of which will take time to discover, and they may not relieve the full array of menopausal symptoms (such as hot flashes). Sorting out which ones are likely to be most helpful to which women may take years.

Even so, the baby boomers moving through midlife need not try to tough out debilitating symptoms or make do with a one-for-all menopause remedy. Today's choices are not always simple; the alternatives may be less than ideal. However, we are fortunate to have them. And because of research now under way, our daughters will have even more options. By the time they reach menopause, "the change" may be just that—a change in menstrual cycling, not in a woman's current or future well-being.

"Big Woman" Time

The Lusi people of Papua New Guinea have no words for middle age or menopause. When a woman stops having children and becomes a grandmother, she becomes a *tamparonga*. This term, which means "big woman," is an expression of honor and respect. Other cultures, including some in the Caribbean, also refer to respected elders as "big women." I, a little woman, like the notion of women growing large with wisdom and compassion as they age. And I wonder: Why are things so different here?

Certainly the biology of menopause is universal. But if menopause were simply a physiological event, all women everywhere would experience it in essentially the same ways. This is far from what actually occurs. The only universal truths about menopause are that it happens to all women and that it brings fertility to an end. Beyond this, its signs, symptoms, and meanings vary from culture to culture. Rather than being "a thing unto itself," menopause is a different phenomenon in different places.

Is the experience of menopause easier for women in societies in which this passage enhances their status? Because so many factors affect the psychobiology of menopause, this is hard to say. In Finland, where women have long taken menopause in stride as a natural process, they report fewer menopausal symptoms. In Japan, where women traditionally gained power as mothers-in-law in charge of extended households, women rarely complain of hot flashes or psychological symptoms. However, it may be that the Japanese diet, rich in tofu and other soy products that contain phytoestrogens, may prevent many symptoms. It also may be that cultural conditioning silences women from discussing them.

When two friends, both family therapists, headed to Kyoto to train Japanese counselors, I asked for their firsthand observations. The women they met, mostly of menopausal age, confirmed that hot flashes or other menopausal symptoms were indeed rare. "But all through the seminar," my friends reported, "so many women would break into a sweat that we had to put out boxes of tissues so they could mop their foreheads."

I asked a Japanese woman, born in Tokyo but now living in the United States, what she thought. "Japanese women never talk about their bodies, and there isn't even a word that means 'hot flash,'" she says. "When I came to this country and heard women talking about menopause, I thought, 'American women are very strange. This will never happen to me.' But it did. Yet when I asked my own mother, who is still in Japan, she refuses even to talk about it."

Western thinking about menopause can be just as muddled. Most research has studied white women seeking help for problems, not a cross-section of healthy women from various ethnic and racial groups. Because the focus has been on patients and problems, the image that long dominated thinking about menopause has been of a depressed, sexless, sweating, fretting, suffering woman.

The "postmodern" view, which emerged from the feminist movement of the 1970s, looked at menopause as similar to menarche: a natural reproductive event, rather than an illness, with benefits as well as drawbacks. A woman loses fertility but gains freedom from pregnancy. Her "nest" empties, but she gets to enjoy a quieter, tidier, more serene environment.

As liberating as this perspective is, it may not take into account the very real discomfort some women experience. "For my fiftieth birthday, I got a T-shirt that reads Real Women Don't Get Hot Flashes—They Get Power Surges," says a friend who subsequently discovered that even liberated, feminist, assertive, successful, and self-confident women like herself can and do get hot flashes. "I turned into a human blast furnace," she says. "But what are you supposed to do when you live and work in a culture that believes you should never let them see you sweat?"

In her stigma-shattering best-seller, *The Silent Passage*, published in 1991, Gail Sheehy predicted that as baby boomers hit menopause, corporate boardrooms would soon be lighting up with hot flashes. However, the glow has been decidedly dim. Many midlife women, sweaty foreheads pressed against the glass ceiling, fear that any admission of female frailty may sabotage their careers. Rather than whipping out pocket fans or flinging off the jackets of their power suits, they're attending seminars on "strategizing menopause" and downloading coping tips for working women (for example, switch from silks to breathable cottons; wear thigh-high stockings rather than pantyhose).

"If you announce you're menopausal, you'll be discounted," lectures one corporate consultant. "Your boss and your colleagues will think of you as over the hill, even if you're younger than most of the men at your level." She suggests that women executives, regardless of age or menstrual status, keep a box of tampons semidiscreetly in their desks—just so people don't think they are past any prime, reproductive or productive.

This does not seem the way "big women" might act and react. And as aging baby boomers transform yet another life phase, this may well change—if only because of this generation's propensity for sharing experiences and telling even painful truths. Although there are still some social circles in which menopause remains what one editor calls "a room-emptier," women are filling up rooms—at women's health centers, in community auditoriums, and in each other's homes—to learn more about their changing bodies and changing lives.

The Toronto Hospital's women's health center reports a constant demand for additional educational programs on menopause. In the Netherlands, a group called Vrouwen in de Overgang (VIDO) has grown from a small support group of menopausal women to a nationwide program that maintains a house in the country—a latter-day equivalent of the menstrual huts of tribal nations—where midlife women can go to escape the stresses of family and work. Newsletters for midlife women make their way into mailboxes and modems around the world. On the Internet, dozens of websites provide information on everything from clinical trials of new estrogens to the potential benefits of acupuncture.

The women I know who've participated in midlife groups—some as leaders, some as members—report a common transformation. The newcomers are typically the most anxious. They don't like what's happening to their bodies, and they expect to feel worse rather than better. Many want nothing more than to short-circuit the years-long process of changing, just do it, and be done with it.

The senior women in the group are far more positive, and eager to reassure younger women that it is not, as they worry, so very dreadful in this new stage of life. "If women only knew what lay on the other side, they wouldn't fear fifty," Germaine Greer once observed. "On the other side of all that turmoil, there is the most wonderful moment in one's whole life—really the most golden, the most extraordinary, luminous instant that will last forever."

In survey after survey, women's happiness soars after menopause, even though not all enjoy advantages such as good health, financial independence, and gratifying relationships. Self-esteem strengthens. Energy increases. In one study at Sweden's Karolinska Institute in Stockholm, postmenopausal women, particularly those with jobs they enjoyed, were less bored, less lonely, more in control of their inner needs and outer environment. Many felt much better about themselves than ever before in their lives.

Rather than shriveling in spirit, shrinking in value, and disintegrating in body, many more women may well discover that they too can become "big women." Just as girls emerge from puberty into the fullness of womanhood, their mothers and grandmothers can move into new territory and begin to claim it as their own. A birthday card I recently received read, "Not everything in life comes with a 'use-by' date." To the list of items that get better with age—cheese, red wine, homemade preserves, rich plum puddings—the sender had inked in an important addition: women. My sense is that she's right. Time may in fact be on our side.

PART THREE

The Woman Within

I was always looking outside myself
for strength and confidence,
but it comes from within
It is there all the time.

Anna Freud

CHAPTER 11

Is There a
Female Brain?

First they took away her candle, then they put out the fire in her hearth. Finally they made her strip off her nightclothes before getting into bed. But despite their fears that she would ruin her health with her endless reading, the parents of Marie-Sophie Germain could not stop their determined daughter. In the black cold of the night, she would wrap herself in a blanket and read by the light of candles she'd smuggled into her room.

Born in Paris in 1776, Germain, like most French girls of her time, received little formal education. Confined to her home for safety's sake during the violent years of the French Revolution, she immersed herself in mathematics, teaching herself from books in her father's library. Later she used a pseudonym (M. LeBlanc) to obtain lecture notes and exchange ideas with noted mathematicians. Despite her lack of formal education, Germain tackled some of the thorniest mathematical challenges of her time and developed the modern theory of elasticity (the mathematical representation of stress and strain in materials such as steel beams)—work that contributed to the theoretical bases for modern construction.

Dismissed by many academicians simply because she was a woman, Germain eventually won recognition from the prestigious Institut de France, which invited her to attend its sessions—an invitation historians describe as "the highest honor that this famous body ever conferred on a woman." But Germain never earned a living from her work, and when she died of breast cancer at age fifty-five, her death certificate listed her not as a scholar or scientist but simply as a *rentier*, or property holder. Her little-known life story bears witness to a basic fact about the female brain: Its history is largely an untold tale of what might have been.

One of the classic arguments of men in the endless debate over female intelligence is why, if women are so smart, they haven't written more books, painted more masterpieces, made more scientific discoveries, garnered more intellectual prizes. "Every genius born a woman is lost to the world," Stendhal once wrote. Not so, Simone de Beauvoir pointed out, for geniuses are made, not born. Even brilliant minds need not just the requisite amounts of neurons and neurotransmitters but education and opportunity.

If not for luck and sheer determination, Marie-Sophie Germain's indisputably excellent brain might never have flickered with the glow of inspiration. Yet for centuries, many dismissed women as the gender of "fruitful wombs and barren brains." Female intelligence was ranked only slightly above that of an ape—and considerably below a man's. One nineteenth-century French intellectual conceded that some women—the Marie-Sophie Germains of the world—possess outstanding brains, but considered them as rare as "a gorilla with two heads; consequently, we may neglect them entirely."

Neglect them they did. Most girls through history learned only what their mothers could teach them—cooking, weaving, gardening, perhaps some simple prayers and songs. For centuries even aristocratic girls, literate and well-schooled in womanly arts like needlework, rarely learned Latin, the language of scholarly discourse. The great ages of intellectual innovation, such as the Renaissance and the Enlightenment, were male triumphs that barely touched most women's lives. It wasn't until the late nineteenth century that the doors to advanced education finally opened to women, and even then only to a small and select group.

In 1898 one of these women, the pioneering feminist and economist Charlotte Perkins Gilman, objected to the very notion of a gender difference in intelligence. "The brain is not an organ of sex," she protested. "As well speak of the female liver." These days, as we saw in Chapter 4, gender biologists do indeed speak of the female liver, describing it as one of the most sexually distinctive of organs. What, then, of the brain? Is the spongy, three-pound organ within my skull any less female than my liver or other assorted body parts? Do the effects of the sex hormones somehow stop at the neck?

Of course not, but the very phrase "female brain"—with its implied assertion that all women, regardless of age, race, or culture, think alike—has an unsettling ring. "Why do you never hear anyone talk of 'the male brain'?" asks psychologist Carol Tavris, author of *The Mismeasure of Woman*. "Because it's considered the 'normal' one." The male brain—like the male body in human physiology—has served as the sole model of human intelligence, logic, rationality, and creativity.

In the past, much brain research simply reinforced this view. When nineteenth-century scientists—mostly white European males—measured, weighed, palpated, and probed brains from human cadavers, they invariably found the brains of white European males superior. Their discovery that a woman's brain, on average, weighs 10 to 15 percent less than that of a man was interpreted as indisputable proof of female intellectual inferiority. Further investigations eventually revealed that the size difference was relative to overall body weight—and that some women have bigger brains than many men.

These days the tools for comparing brains have become more sophisticated. Some, such as sensory tests, provide straightforward information about sex differences in light and sound perception. Men, for instance, are more sensitive to bright light, can detect more subtle differences in light, and retain their ability to see well at long distances longer in life. On the other hand, women hear a much broader range of sounds, use both ears more equally in listening to words, and are better at detecting "pure" tones (those of a single frequency). Their hearing begins to deteriorate later in life, at about age thirty-eight, compared to age thirty-two in men.

Neuroimaging techniques like high-speed functional magnetic resonance imaging (fMRI) and positron emission tomography (PET), which allow scientists to study brains as they think, feel, or remember, have

revealed other differences in female and male brains—in the cells activated as they rhyme or read, for instance, and in their responses to emotional memories and expressions (discussed in the following chapter). Yet
despite all sorts of speculation about what these headline-making differences might mean, no one is really sure. Although we have learned more
than ever about the brain's form and functions, this knowledge has yet to
translate into fuller understanding of how any of us learns, loves, imag-
ines, or ponders—let alone how women and men may go about these
things differently.

More traditional ways of assessing brains, such as tests of performance, also have their limitations. They show that female and male skills
are more alike than not, with the sexes' scores often overlapping on most
cognitive tests. The differences between any two women—or, for that
matter, any two men—tend to be as big or bigger than those between a
particular woman and a particular man or than the averages of all female
and all male scores.

Where does this leave us? With far more questions than answers—
and, for some, lingering suspicion of any research that categorizes brains
by sex. "I have been asked, even by women studying for their M.D.-
Ph.D.'s, to stop our research or at least stop publicizing it," says neuropsychiatrist Raquel Gur, of the University of Pennsylvania (an M.D.-Ph.D.
herself). "They are afraid that women will lose twenty years of gains if
word gets out that the sexes aren't the same. I disagree. I think of the differences between male and female brains not in terms of strength or weakness but as something that is important to recognize."

The differences, nonetheless, are small—as might be expected. We
are two different sexes, after all, not two species. "Male and female brains
do the same things, but they do them differently," says Gur. In time the
subtleties within these differences may lead to new ways of thinking
about our organ of thought—and of fully appreciating its potential. As
for now, the bottom line on the female brain is this: Never underestimate
what it can do.

Consider a contemporary woman very much in the tradition of
Marie-Sophie Germain—an American university student from Romania
named Ioana Dumitriu. In 1997, at age twenty, she became the first
woman to win the Olympics of college math, the William Lowell Putnam
Mathematical Competition, a test so difficult that a third of the select

group who take it score 0 of a possible 120, and about half score 2 or less. (The scores of Dumitriu and the other winners are not known, but they ranged from 76 to 98.)

"I didn't ever tell myself that I was unlikely to win, that no woman before had ever won and therefore I couldn't," she said afterward. "It's not that I forget that I'm a woman. It's just that the mathematics community is made up of persons, and that is what I am primarily." Indeed. And as a person and as a woman, Dumitriu challenged age-old notions about the limitations of the female brain. "What is happening now is that the stereotype is defied," she told an interviewer. "It starts breaking." It's about time.

The Inside Story

During his residency training in neurology, my husband sometimes kept slices of brain for dissection in our refrigerator. Fumbling for breakfast provisions, I'd wonder whether the owners had ever anticipated taking up afterlife residence next to the strawberry jam, just down from the milk and a shelf above the cheese. The pale samples were an unappetizing sight, reeking of formaldehyde, offering no hint of the living brain's wondrous abilities. Yet dead brains have taught neuroscientists much of what we know about differences and similarities in the structure of the two genders' brains.

Brain size alone—the main focus of centuries of study and speculation—seems fairly unimportant. The brains of geniuses have turned out to be no bigger and sometimes smaller than those of lesser intellectual lights. If size did matter (and a few diehards continue to insist it does), its impact seems minimal—probably no more than two to three ounces and three or four IQ points. And size isn't constant. As discussed later in this chapter, male brains may shrink so much more over time that by middle age, the all-important frontal lobes become about equal in size in both genders.

According to a different measurement, that of nerve cells per unit volume, certain regions of the female brain may be denser. By meticulously counting neurons in samples of the brains of nine cadavers— five women and four men—psychologist Sandra Witelson, of McMaster

University in Canada, found about 11 to 14 percent more neurons in two layers of part of the cerebral cortex, the outer layer of the brain, in women. What does this increased density mean? No one knows for sure. However, since the layers that Witelson studied are linked to language and recognition of speech tones, she speculates that the greater number of neurons may be an advantage in skills such as learning to read.

One of the first sex differences discovered in brain physiology was in cerebral blood flow. Raquel Gur and her husband, neuropsychologist Ruben Gur, conducted an experiment to determine if blood flow increased to either hemisphere for specific tasks. To their surprise, the flow of blood to one or the other hemisphere was almost 20 percent higher in women than in men.

"Nobody had described anything like that before," says Ruben Gur, who viewed their findings as good news for and about women. "But every time we'd give a presentation of our data, a man would inevitably stand up and say, 'Doesn't that mean women have to work harder when they think and that's why their blood flow is higher?' We had to point out that women's brains have a higher rate of blood flow at rest, and the increase in blood flow induced by thinking is the same as for men."

Since then, more sophisticated neuroimaging techniques have provided intriguing but still inconclusive glimpses into how female and male brains work. "Whatever they do—even just wiggling their thumbs—women activate more neurons in the brain," reports neuropsychiatrist Mark George, of the Medical University of South Carolina. When a male puts his mind to work, brain scans show neurons turning on in highly specific areas. When females set their minds on similar tasks, so many brain cells light up that their bright-colored scans glow like Las Vegas at night.

This observation supports the theory, initially based on animal research, that the male brain tends to be more "lateral" and divides tasks between its two hemispheres, while the female brain draws more equally on both sides. The compartmentalization of the male brain, researchers theorize, may enhance the ability to focus intensely—an evolutionary essential in many species.

"A male's main function is to find territory, find food, find a female," explains neuroanatomist Marian Diamond, of the University of California, Berkeley. "He has to be able to focus in order to survive. What the female needs as a mother is to be ready to go in all directions in order to protect her young."

In humans, neurologists had long suspected that the sexes processed language differently in the brain. "In medicine, we'd observed that women who have strokes tend to regain more of their verbal abilities than men," explains George. "Their use of neurons in both hemispheres may be why. Because women activate a larger number of neurons when they speak or read, they're less vulnerable if part of the brain is damaged."

The most well-publicized confirmation of this theory was a study by Yale University professors Sally and Bennett Shaywitz. With detailed MRI scans, they showed that in men, neurons in the region called the inferior frontal gyrus, a small area behind the eyebrows, lit up on the left side of their brains while they performed a rhyming task. In women, neurons in this same area generally lit up in both the left and right hemispheres. Such differences, which have also shown up in tests of electrical brain activity, have not emerged consistently in neuroimaging research. For instance, a Washington University study that also compared female and male brains during a language task—in this case, a word association test—showed no significant differences in regionalization.

Other researchers have zeroed in on the corpus callosum, the fibers running down the center of the brain and linking the two hemispheres. Some theorize that certain parts of this bridge are thicker in females, possibly allowing more "cross talk" between right and left hemispheres. Here again, however, conclusive anatomic evidence has proven elusive. Some studies have confirmed size differences in females; others have disputed or refuted these findings.

One of the difficulties in pinpointing sex differences is the fact— recognized only in recent decades—that the brain is a moving target, constantly changing and adapting. Diamond first demonstrated this "plasticity" in pioneering studies in the 1960s that compared rats of various ages placed in plain cages with those in "enriched" cages filled with mazes, wheels, and companions. Regardless of the animals' age, the neurons in the cortex, the brain's outer layer, grew when the rats were placed in a stimulating environment. (As discussed in Chapter 2, similar changes in female rats' brains occur during pregnancy.) Other research has confirmed that enriching experiences can have a similar effect on human brains—again, throughout life.

Because the brain is a work in progress, no one knows—nor may ever know—whether any sex differences are hard-wired at birth or a consequence of experience and education. Even with today's high-tech imaging techniques, studying the human brain remains, as Deborah Blum writes in *Sex on the Brain*, "like peering down at Manhattan through an airplane window at night, seeing that fantastical rise and fall of light, and trying to know—from that distance, in the dark—who lives there, who's talking to whom, and what they might be saying." This is not to say the view isn't worth contemplating, but we're a long way from knowing what's really going on.

Which Sex Is Smarter?

Three men walking on a beach come upon a magic lamp. They rub it, and a genie appears and promises each of them one wish. "I want to be ten times smarter," says the first man. *Poof!* goes the genie, and the man becomes ten times smarter. "I want to be a hundred times smarter," says the second man. *Poof!* goes the genie, and he becomes a hundred times smarter. "I want to be a million times smarter," says the third man. And with a final *poof!* the genie turns him into a woman.

My daughter, who learned this joke at summer camp, delights in its telling—as do other girls and women who feel overdue for a positive punch line that varies from the age-old theme that "female intelligence" is an oxymoron. Yet there is no simple answer to the question of which gender truly is "smarter." The best one may have been that of Samuel Johnson, who, when asked whether man or woman is more intelligent, responded: "Which man? Which woman?"

Intelligence per se appears equal in both sexes. Average IQ in both sexes is about 100, and cognitive skills generally overlap. However, women tend to underestimate their intelligence—possibly, various theorists have long argued, because they lack self-confidence or are socialized to be modest. Recent research shows that women most consistently underestimate or misjudge their abilities at tasks considered typically masculine. In one study, for instance, when 160 British undergraduates assessed various abilities, there were no sex differences in the self-ratings of linguistic or musical skills. But the women rated themselves significantly lower than the men in logic-math, spatial, and kinesthetic ability—all realms our culture portrays as male strengths.

In actual performance, the sexes are strikingly similar. In a recent analysis of standardized academic test scores from more than 150,000 students age thirteen to seventeen, two education researchers found sex differences only in highly specific skills. Boys score a little better on math, science, and social studies, while girls are slightly stronger in reading comprehension, perceptual speed, and remembering associated concepts. Girls do better at anagrams, boys at analogies. But boys have a wider spread of scores, with more boys scoring higher and more boys scoring lower, while girls' scores are less variable. At the very top of the math scale, boys outnumber girls by a remarkable seven to one. However, in writing skills, girls showed an even more marked superiority.

This verbal advantage starts early. Girls generally speak sooner, learn to read more easily, and are less prone to learning disorders. Researchers Sally and Bennett Shaywitz, based on their neuroimaging studies of the brain, speculate that the female's bilateral approach may allow her to draw on the experiences of the right brain as well as the reasoning powers of the left brain. In youth, this may translate into a two-year edge in verbal skills. In adulthood, women, whose vocabularies are no larger than men's, are nevertheless more verbally adept: In timed tests, they think of more words that start with the same letter, list more synonyms, and come up with names for colors or shapes more quickly than men. They even memorize letters of the alphabet faster.

Women also excel in perceptual speed and at a cognitive skill known as "disembedding." Give them a task such as finding every *a* in a paragraph, and they'll do it faster. Show them a group of objects, switch things around, and they will notice more of what's been changed. (This may explain why I can zero in on the mustard after my husband has been staring at the open refrigerator for five minutes.)

On the road, women again notice more, paying greater attention to landmarks like the coffee shop on the corner or the church across from the playground. When retracing a route or giving directions, women rely on such landmarks—unlike men, who think in terms of direction and distance. "Half a mile west, then north two miles and take the proximal turnoff," my husband will say. "Past the McDonald's to the purple house with all the flowers out front, then turn by the gas station," I'll translate.

This gender difference isn't limited to humans. In laboratory experiments, female rats will map their routes through a maze according to the placement of blocks of various colors and shapes along the way. If these cues are removed, they get confused. Male rats, by comparison, seem to have some inner sense that allows them to calculate how far they've gone in one direction; they become disoriented when ramps in a maze are shortened or lengthened.

But the most dramatic gender differences appear in another spatial skill: mental rotation of three-dimensional figures. Shown drawings of a three-dimensional target figure, rotated at different angles, males can find its match with greater speed and accuracy than females. Some have argued that such three-dimensionality is an innate benefit of the male brain's superspecialization or an evolutionary trait honed through millions of years of chucking spears at fast-moving game. However, even this seemingly hard-wired ability may not be as immutable as has been thought.

In one experiment, when middle-school children made drawings from various angles, including corners, of structures they had built with small cubes, they dramatically boosted their performance on spatial tests—and the girls improved just as much as the boys. In another study, both female and male high-school students increased their scores when allowed to go back to work on problems of mental rotation that they had failed to solve during a timed test—and the girls improved more. Even the wording of instructions for spatial tests can make a difference. In one study of college students, men performed better than women when the instructions emphasized the spatial character of the task. When they did not, there were no differences in the sexes' scores. These findings do not rule out or refute the possibility of a biologically based difference, but they do testify to the impact education, experience, and context can have.

Is the Math Gap a Myth?

Of all the red-hot controversies that have swirled around the subject of gender differences in brain abilities, none has stirred greater furor in the United States than the infamous gender gap in scores on the Scholastic Assessment Test, or SAT (formerly the Scholastic Aptitude Test). Among high-school seniors graduating in 1997, the average math score for women was 494—thirty-six points below the average male score of 530. On verbal scores, the gender balance shifted: The average for women was 530, for men 507.

What's behind these differences? Some contend that they stem from basic differences in brain development and biology. Others blame a one-approach-for-all-minds educational philosophy that shortchanges both genders in different ways. And then there are those who believe the real problem is the SAT itself, which they contend is not a good predictor of college math grades, especially for girls.

Whenever the loaded subject of math and gender slips into the conversation, I remain uncharacteristically mute. Much to my chagrin, I have never, ever gotten my checkbook to balance. At times I have closed a bank account and opened a new one simply because my bookkeeping had become so hopelessly muddled. Unlike my husband, I cannot convert dollars into pounds, marks, francs, or lire in my head; I'm sometimes stumped by sixth-grade math homework. Yet when anyone—especially anyone male—tells me it's just like a woman not to have a head for numbers, I bristle.

Part of me would love to pin the rap on my female brain or the Catholic-school nuns who made math such a mind-numbing learning experience—or both. Yet my sister—my closest biological relative and a graduate of the very same parochial schools—is a whiz with numbers. Vice president at a major bank, she manages multimillion-dollar accounts, calculates compound interest in her head, and has a checkbook suitable for framing in a basic bookkeeping class. I have female friends who flit nimbly through spreadsheets, fine-tune figures for due-diligence reports, and set up international loan programs. Nothing in their brains—nor, even more dramatically, in Ioana Dumitriu's—interferes with their ability to figure out figures. My limited math literacy, I've had to conclude, is my personal inadequacy, not my gender's.

If it were otherwise, the performance gap would exist in all times and places. This is not the case. In the United States in 1947, boys scored higher than girls in verbal and abstract reasoning and ability to deal with numbers. In 1980 the reasoning differences between the sexes had been virtually eliminated, and girls were performing as well, if not better, in numerical skills. Similarly, the male superiority in mechanical skills in 1947 had been cut in half by 1980.

There also are geographic and cultural variations. Japanese school-girls score better than American boys on items in which American boys outperform American girls, such as word problems. The difference between Japanese girls and American boys is much greater than the difference between Japanese girls and boys or between American girls and boys. Could culture be an even greater influence than gender? This is yet another question to be answered.

For decades in Great Britain, more girls than boys have passed secondary-school entrance examinations. ("Girls Brainier than Boys," declared one newspaper headline in 1954.) In order to ensure that girls didn't take up two thirds of the seats, the schools set quotas, explaining that girls outperformed boys at age eleven, the time of the exam, simply because they matured earlier. And in fact, on the General Certificate of Education tests given to sixteen-year-olds, girls in the 1950s did do more poorly than boys, especially in math and science.

In 1992, when school administrators in one district reviewed the GCE results, they discovered that boys were no longer outperforming girls. In fact, many were failing badly in language-based subjects, such as English and history. Even more surprisingly, girls were doing about as well in math as boys. Nationwide, the Department of Education of Great Britain reported similar findings. Yet neither gender was necessarily thriving. Even though the girls achieved higher scores, they consistently undervalued their intelligence.

Educators all over the world have come to wonder whether coed schools, or at least a teaching philosophy that assumes that girls and boys learn in similar ways, are at fault. In Barbados, single-sex schools were the norm until fifteen years ago. "Boys did well, and girls did well," reports psychiatrist Sharon Harvey, a native of the Caribbean island. "In today's coed schools, the girls are doing very well—much better than the boys— and are becoming the leaders in every way. There's a whole debate about what is happening to the boys of Barbados." In Great Britain, too, some educators are advocating a return to more single-sex classes and schools to help boys focus on classwork and overcome what some see as a "resistance to learning."

In the United States, enrollments at single-sex schools are soaring, and even coed schools, public and private, are setting up all-girl and all-boy classes in math and science. Although a 1998 report by the American Association of University Women found no evidence that single-sex education is in itself better for girls than coeducation, there is growing recognition of gender differences in learning styles. As early as first grade, girls approach arithmetic problems in different ways from boys. In middle and high school, girls' math smarts (and scores) improve when they get frequent feedback, engage in collaborative group work, and learn connections between abstract concepts and practical applications.

Issues of gender inequity in education may go beyond teaching approaches. As researchers have documented, social dynamics are different in same-sex and mixed-sex classrooms. In elementary grades, boys are more active and assertive. They shout out an answer—any answer—before the teacher has finished a question; girls wait until they're sure they know the right response. And even teachers with gender-equity training report that they still devote more attention to the high-spirited hijinks of boys than to the quieter academic difficulties of girls.

As noted in Chapter 6, often girls' academic confidence and grades start to slump just at the time when their bodies develop, their periods begin, and their self-confidence grows shaky. Small classes and caring teachers may make a bigger difference, but it is also true that at least some girls speak up more and perform better without the distractions and disruptions boys can bring, especially in challenging subjects like math.

Despite the furor over test scores among the young, few know or note that any gender gap all but disappears with time and experience. By midlife, both math and spatial scores are generally equal. By old age, women score higher. Why? As discussed later in this chapter, the reason may be partly biological, since parts of the male brain may shrink more over time. But practical experience may also teach the remarkably plastic female brain a thing or two about space.

Take parallel parking, a skill that I'd always thought of as a guy thing. My inherent lack of spatial sense, I rationalized, explained my inability to squeeze my car into a space smaller than a bus-stop zone. But when I tried this excuse on a female friend, she immediately countered by asking if I'd ridden a bicycle as a child. No, I never had. "That explains it," she said blithely, adding that she used to ride miles every day. "I'd weave between cars, race down alleys, cut through trees. Today I can drive anything and park anywhere."

Her point was well taken. If I am dimensionally challenged, I can't blame nature; nurture too had something to do with it. But as I discovered, it's never too late to tackle new tricks. Since our daughter started attending an urban school, I've had to parallel park far more often than in the malled suburbs. By trial, error, and with an occasional scrape or dent, I've gotten better. These days as I maneuver my car, with more deliberateness than deftness, into position on the streets of San Francisco, I can almost feel neurons lighting up in what had once been a dark place in my brain.

The Aging Brain

Grow fast. Get big. Run hard. Die early. This may sound like an epitaph for a macho punk, but what it really describes is the hard-wiring for the male brain. Sculpted by prenatal testosterone, conditioned by an active, exploratory childhood, it seems designed for an early prime—and, at least from today's perspective on the human male, a premature decline.

From the ages of eighteen to forty-five, in MRI studies conducted by the Gurs, neurons in the male brain died at a rate three times faster than in the female. By middle age, the frontal lobes and hippocampus in the men had shrunk so much that they reached approximately the same size as the women's. "If you look at men from young adulthood to middle age, you see a steady decline in abilities, particularly attention, as well as a decline in brain volume," says Ruben Gur. "You don't even see a trend in women the same age toward any deterioration of abilities or volume."

This discrepancy continues after midlife. In one recent study at Henry Ford Hospital in Detroit, researchers found that between the ages of sixty-five and ninety-five, the men experienced an average 30 percent increase in cerebrospinal fluid around the outside of the brain, an indication of shrinkage within the brain. Women over the same period showed just a 1 percent increase in fluid. The consequences of the shrinkage in male brains may include poorer verbal memory, diminished ability to pay attention, and increased irritability.

Such changes are not inevitable, however. Dissections of the brains of healthy seniors generally do not reveal a significant loss of brain cells. The real culprits may be variables such as disease, isolation, alcohol use, and depression. A lack of novelty and challenge—an unfortunate consequence of age or illness for many of the elderly—can weaken mental abilities, just as lack of exercise or inadequate nutrition undermines physical well-being. Stimulation, whether in the form of a challenging crossword puzzle or a spirited discussion, may help preserve brain health throughout life.

However, there may also be physiological gender differences in the ways in which brains, like bodies, age. Recently, German scientists documented a decline in cerebrovascular reactivity—the ability of vessels in the brain to maintain optimal blood flow—in women in their fifties, sixties, and seventies, compared to women in their thirties and forties, but no such changes in men as they aged. This gender difference, they theorize, may provide a clue to the increased incidence of fatal strokes in older women.

In other ways, women may be at an advantage. A woman's brain, Ruben Gur speculates, adjusts its metabolic rate—its utilization of brain glucose—as it loses tissue with aging, whereas the brains of older men continue to metabolize glucose at the same rate as when they were younger. Women, in other words, may gear down to a more fuel-efficient cruising speed, while male brains keep revving the engine—possibly because of testosterone's influence. "Even though women too lose tissue as they age, they seem to be riding herd on what's left," says Gur. The fact that men "overdrive" their neurons, at least in theory, may cause earlier burnout.

Neither women nor men are usually aware of subtle changes in their cognitive abilities over time. What we do notice—with a mix of anxiety and frustration—is that our memories aren't as reliable as they used to be. We see a somewhat familiar face across a crowded airport but can't think of the person's name. We dash down to the basement to retrieve something but forget what we wanted by the time we get there. Standing in front of the ATM, our access code evaporates from our minds.

This is the bane all brains are prone to, says psychologist Thomas

Crook, whose research firm has tested the memories of more than fifty thousand women and men. Yet even though both genders suffer age-associated memory loss, women's memories outperform men's at every age. "Anytime we see a difference, it always favors females," says Crook. "Women have a greater ability to associate names with faces than men, and they're better at recalling lists of things and details of personal experiences."

One reason that we remember certain people and places better may be our unique way of filing information in our memory banks. "The events that we remember best—like Kennedy's assassination or the explosion of the Challenger space shuttle—are those that we 'tag' [associate] with an emotion," Crook explains. "Women may do this more automatically." If Crook is correct, a wife is more likely than her husband to remember their anniversary. To him, it's just another date; to her, it's one of life's emotional highlights.

Throughout life, estrogen seems to strengthen a woman's mind and memory by building and maintaining the densest possible network of neuronal connections. As estrogen drops at menopause, her brain becomes increasingly vulnerable. Some middle-aged women complain of "fuzzy thinking" and memory problems. The reason may be that estrogen's decline reduces production of acetylcholine, which allows messages to leap from one neuron to the next.

These changes may explain why women's brains, though more durable in many ways, eventually become more prone to Alzheimer's disease. Of the four million Americans with this illness, an estimated 75 percent are female. Males, in yet another hormonal irony, may be protected by their brain's conversion of testosterone, which declines more gradually than estrogen, into neuroprotective estradiol. Alzheimer's disease also seems to strike women harder, and those with this form of dementia perform significantly worse than men with Alzheimer's in various visual, spatial, and memory tests.

Hormone replacement therapy, discussed in Chapter 10, has shown promise in keeping women's brains healthy as they age. Postmenopausal women often report that their memories and thinking improve after taking replacement hormones. In several small studies, the risk of Alzheimer's disease declined by 40 percent among women on HRT.

Other reports have noted some cognitive improvement in women with Alzheimer's when they begin estrogen replacement therapy. However, a recent analysis of twenty-seven studies of estrogen and its effect on intellectual function and Alzheimer's disease concluded that many of these investigations had not been well done in terms of scientific rigor. Before estrogen can be recommended as a means of protecting the postmenopausal brain, large-scale clinical trials will have to provide more convincing proof of its benefits.

As with other dimensions of human behavior, hormones never seem to hold all the answers. In longitudinal studies that have followed thousands of individuals from middle age into their nineties, the women and men who maintained the sharpest memories and mental abilities benefited most from three factors: an above-average level of education, the pursuit of stimulating interests, and marriage to a smart spouse. No hormone alone, it seems, could ever match the meaning any or all of these three can add to the life of the mind.

Thinking Like a Woman

In 1972 Polly Matzinger was working as a cocktail waitress in Davis, California. When two professors from the local university started talking about animal mimicry, she couldn't resist asking: "Why has no animal ever mimicked a skunk?" Her question, original and intriguing, so impressed one of the professors that he spent months bringing her articles and convincing her to study science.

Now a medical researcher at the National Institutes of Health, Matzinger is still asking questions—ones so provocative that they are challenging the conventional view of immunity. She gets her ideas not just in the laboratory but at home, in the bath, on walks. One day, while watching a field of grazing sheep with her Border collie, the dog jumped up to protect the sheep when they were startled by a sudden sound. At that moment it occurred to her that almost every organ of the body has a few sentinel cells that, much like sleeping watchdogs, leap into action at any sign of danger.

Is such thinking distinctively female or simply creative? Certainly inspiration takes spark in many ways in both sexes, but the female brain may bring a unique perspective to problem solving. Women, observes cultural anthropologist Mary Catherine Bateson, are "peripheral visionaries," capable of simultaneously following several trains of thought (or, in the case of a busy mother, several children). Perhaps this propensity for operating on several channels at the same time leads females to make connections that might never have occurred to a man.

Although little research has been done on creative thinking and gender, the process of discovery may take distinctive turns in women. The geneticist Barbara McClintock, who won a Nobel prize for her identification of "transposable" or "jumping" genes, which move from one cell to another, in corn kernels, described her work with words rarely associated with the hard sciences, such as *affinity* and *attraction*. Rather than observing molecules at arm's length, she used her powers of empathy to broaden her insight into genetic mutations. "Things are much more marvelous than the scientific method allows us to conceive," she once commented.

The ability to see with more than eyes alone is often referred to as intuition—which some see as an innately female trait and others as a survival skill cultivated by the powerless of either sex. "Some say that women developed intuition because they were weak and subjected, that if they were liberated they wouldn't need to pay so much attention to men," observes psychologist Judith Hall, of Northeastern University, an expert in nonverbal communication. "Yet it is a true asset. Women should see their intuition as a gold star rather than a black mark."

Psychiatrist and neuroscientist Mona Lisa Schulz, a self-described "medical intuitive," regularly calls upon her sixth sense in diagnosing and assessing patients. Based on her personal experience and professional research, she believes that women may tune in to intuition more easily than men. "We've learned that people use multiple areas of the brain when making decisions—intuitive or otherwise," she says. "And because women's brains are less lateralized, they may have better access to both sides of the brain. They usually don't see things as cut-and-dried, the way men do."

This "and-but" perspective, contrasted with a more classically male "either-or" viewpoint, can be a real advantage in every part of a woman's life. Some business analysts speculate, stretching far beyond any hard data, that because of the fundamentally holistic organization of the female brain, women tend to look at the totality of what they do—not just at one particular task, but at where it fits into the overall scheme of things. And because of their sensitivity to unspoken messages (as discussed in the following chapter), they often are adept at figuring out intricate situations—why a young child seems anxious, for instance, or why office morale has slumped. "Because they're so good at seeing nuances," says Raquel Gur, "women can read what's happening quickly and ask: 'What should I do now?' "

This also may be why women are often particularly effective at motivating others—a skill mothers hone whenever they're faced with three kids, two cookies, and an urgent need to get everyone in the car immediately. In studies of female management styles, women in business often display similar savvy in motivating staff members. Rather than pitting sales representatives in different regions against each other in competition for a Hawaiian vacation (as her predecessor had done), an executive I know organized teams, set goals, and offered incentive bonuses for all. "We beat the old records because people weren't competing against each other," she says. "They were focusing on doing their best."

Unfortunately, through much of history, few women got a chance to demonstrate their best. Many ended up as "lost brains"—inventors and innovators whose ideas were never taken seriously simply because of their gender. Only a few women, exceptional in talent, luck, and perseverance, were able to break through the barriers and show what a female brain might do.

Helen Taussig, born in 1898, was one of these exceptions. The daughter of a renowned Harvard University economist and a frail mother who died when Taussig was eleven, she grew up determined to become a physician. Rejected by Harvard because of her gender, Taussig became one of the few women admitted to the Johns Hopkins School of Medicine. On graduation in 1927, she applied to Harvard for an internship. Again she was refused. Hopkins offered her a position—but only if she went into pediatrics. Because the faculty assumed she'd be naturally good with babies, Taussig was given responsibility for the most difficult and hopeless of infants, the "blue" babies whose color indicated a mysterious disease that would inevitably kill them.

As she cared for these doomed infants in a dark room in the hospital basement, Taussig did more than comfort and console: She meticulously observed the mysterious babies she called her "little crossword puzzles." Through years of research into cardiac physiology, she eventually figured out what was wrong with them—a blood vessel in the heart called the ductus arteriosus, which normally closes at birth, remained open and blocked the flow of blood to their lungs. She came up with an idea for a cure: an operation on the heart to create an artificial shunt to redirect blood. Even though cardiac surgery was unheard-of at the time, Taussig didn't give up. However, since she had neither the training nor the experience to devise a surgical procedure, she visited a famed vascular surgeon at Harvard Medical School to suggest a collaboration. He laughed at her idea as a ridiculous female notion.

Back at Hopkins, Taussig presented her idea to a vascular surgeon named Alfred Blalock. Although he was skeptical, her persistent arguments won him over, and he agreed to work with her. In 1944 their innovation, the Blalock-Taussig operation, not only ushered in the era of surgery for congenital heart defects and saved the lives of thousands of babies, but paved the way for all open-heart surgery.

Taussig, considered the creator of pediatric cardiology, eventually won many awards, including a Presidential Medal of Freedom and something she'd long craved: a degree from Harvard Medical School. In her acceptance speech, she told of the three times before that she had come knocking at Harvard's doors and been rejected because she was a woman with a woman's seemingly far-fetched ideas. Her audience enthusiastically applauded her—and Harvard's belated acknowledgment of the outstanding contributions a female brain can make.

C H A P T E R   1 2

Gender and Emotion

The people of Grey Rock Harbour, a wind-scoured fishing village in Newfoundland, used to say that only women have nerves. The men of the town—ocean fishermen who sailed small boats in rough seas—never complained of problems with their nerves. The women did. All the while their men were out fishing, the women would worry. They'd blame their "nerves" for making them so edgy, for their checking the sky a dozen times when the winds blew hard, for their restlessness when night fell and still there was no sign of the returning fleet.

In the late 1970s everything changed. The fishing industry collapsed. The men no longer went to sea; their women no longer waited anxiously at home. Both wives and husbands found jobs at local processing factories. Many of the land-bound sailors became, as the women described them, "ruined men," who worked too little and drank too much. There were more extramarital affairs, more divorces, more single mothers. Yet even though the women's lives were, by some measures, harder than in the past, they no longer complained about their nerves.

In almost every place and time, just as in Grey Rock Harbour, ours has been the sensitive sex, prone to tears and fears, jangly nerves, endless fretting. It was always just like a woman to *feel* more, to act—and, more often, react—with an emotional intensity that reverberated throughout body, mind, and spirit. If a man, echoing Descartes, could declare, "I think; therefore I am," women throughout time could have said, "We feel; therefore we are."

Some contend that women are born this way and that evolution fine-tuned their psychological antennae to bind them to their ever-needy infants or alert them to potential threats. Others argue that in societies where they had little control over their fate (most societies, that is, through most of history), worry became women's work. "We are," one anthropologist quips, "women the worriers."

However, as the women of Grey Rock Harbour demonstrate, female "nerves" are capable of extraordinary change—and of holding up to extraordinary challenge. Despite the stereotypes of fragile and fearful females going to pieces, women are made of sturdier stuff. In World War II, psychologists studied the impact of Hitler's Blitz on families in blacked-out, bomb-battered London. Much to their surprise, the number of male psychiatric casualties outnumbered the females by 70 percent. "It may be that women are more emotional than men in romance," the researchers concluded, "but they are less so in air raids."

Sex, in fact, may have less to do with emotion than another rarely studied variable: power. "Many personality characteristics associated with women—being intuitive, emotional, nurturant, collaborative—are associated with differences in access to power," observes psychologist Jacquelyn James, of the Murray Research Center at Radcliffe College, who notes that any "out" group tends to develop such traits to a greater extent than an "in" group. And women were outsiders for a long, long time.

Not allowed to do "manly" things in the worlds of ideas and commerce, women could at least claim their feelings as their own. Barred from so many places, they cultivated the inner territory of the emotions, and the soul-deep sense and sensibility we've come to think of as female became a source of immense satisfaction in their lives. Only recently have scientists come to recognize the significance of the emotions for personal fulfillment and true self-understanding in *both* sexes.

"The place of feeling in mental life has been surprisingly slighted by research over the years, leaving the emotions a largely unexplored continent for scientific psychology," observes psychologist Daniel Goleman, author of *Emotional Intelligence*. "There is real strength in what has been a feminine preserve in this culture, but women felt powerless to bring up the idea of emotions as a serious topic."

This does not mean women did not or do not take them seriously. The capacity for emotional experience and expressiveness is one of the things the women I interviewed said they appreciate most about being female. "If I had been a man, I would have had more options," a woman from Chile tells me. "But women have a way of looking at the world, of being aware of subjective experience, of knowing the importance and validity of feelings, of being aware of others and of aspects of reality, that men do not recognize. This is what enriches our lives." An American friend, a talented musician, echoes this sentiment: "I can't imagine being a man," she says. "It would be like going from conducting a symphony to playing the bassoon. Think of all the notes you'd never get to play."

Are Women More Emotional?

I sniffle at sad movies, get weepy at Christmas pageants, choke up when beautiful, betrayed Butterfly hugs her son for the last time. I cry in anger and frustration, at times of greatest joy and deepest pain—and, I must admit, at totally trivial things. My husband calls me the family's emotional barometer. When schedules get too overcrowded, tensions too high, time together too scarce, I'm the one who senses that something is amiss and starts making adjustments.

This comes as no surprise. Emotions have long been a woman's turf and trademark. "Women *do* emotion," says psychologist Stephanie Shields, of Pennsylvania State University, noting that according to long-entrenched stereotypes, "a woman experiences more emotion than a man, experiences it more often than he does, and has less control of her emotions."

The reality isn't as simplistic as these stereotypes. Emotions know no gender. Men grieve; women rage; both sexes sigh in despair and crow with delight. Asked to record their feelings in diaries, females and males report the same beliefs about emotion and describe their experiences of emotion similarly. However, as Goleman observes, "women, on average, experience the entire range of emotions with greater intensity and more volatility than men—in this sense, women *are* more 'emotional' than men." When volunteers in a University of Illinois study logged their moods for forty-two days, for instance, women reported more intense emotional experiences—positive and negative, pleasant and unpleasant. The exception was anger, which men reported feeling more frequently and fiercely.

Other researchers challenge this difference. "The gender stereotype that males express more anger than females is largely inaccurate," contends psychologist Leslie Brody, of Boston University, who has reviewed and analyzed the research on sex differences in emotion. She notes that while men may more often express anger in the form of aggression, women (as discussed later in this chapter) express anger equally often in other forms.

With other emotions, too, women and men differ more in the expression than in the actual feeling—and the reasons are complex, even when it comes to the most classically female form of emotional release: crying. Women do indeed weep more than men. In one survey, 80 percent of women said they cry; the same percentage of men said they don't. Societal norms and stereotypes (beginning with the big-boys-don't-cry messages that bombard even the littlest tykes) account for much of this difference. However, research into the biochemistry of tears reveals that, microscopically, female and male tears are different, and women's higher levels of prolactin, which fluctuate throughout the menstrual cycle, may lower their threshold for weeping. A man may feel just as emotionally moved as a woman, but tears are less likely to well up in his eyes.

Women and men may also become emotional for different reasons. In general, relationships with friends and families and occasions such as births, reunions, separations, and deaths elicit the strongest reactions in women. Men's emotions are more likely to be triggered by world events, achievements, and illnesses. Perhaps, Brody theorizes, women's traditional roles as caretakers highlight the emotional importance of family milestones, while men's long-standing roles as providers and protectors underscore the significance of events related to achievement and control.

Starting very young, women may be "schooled" in emotional expressivity. As infants, girls are more likely to clap and smile in response to a human face, look into caregivers' eyes for longer times, and babble more in the singsong pidgin of preverbal conversation. As noted in Chapter 6, we don't know how much of this is innate and how much is encouraged by parents who may cuddle girls and coo to them more. Whatever its origin, their early knack for emotional engagement provides girls with a crucial building block for developing other social skills.

As they grow, girls and boys learn very different lessons about emotions. In general, parents discuss feelings (except anger) more with daughters than sons. Even when mothers are playing with their young daughters or telling them stories, they discuss emotional states in greater detail. And since girls tend to develop language skills earlier than boys, they may become more adept at verbalizing feelings and using words instead of fists to settle conflicts.

Boys, on the other hand, are encouraged to minimize or deny feelings of vulnerability, fear, or hurt. As they proceed through the elementary-school years, Goleman observes, boys' faces—once as openly emotional as girls'—become less expressive; girls' become more so. Interestingly, though, not all boys learn to shut down emotionally. In cross-cultural studies, both boys and girls who interacted frequently with younger children scored higher on measures of nurturance and displayed greater affection.

Even in adulthood, caring for a child may have a similar impact. Men who take primary responsibility for raising their children are more nurturing and affectionate and disclose more feelings than others. "Their emotional expressiveness resembles what we stereotypically associate with women," says Brody. In her studies, men (and women) who do more "female" household tasks, including child care, also report greater nervousness than others. Taking care of a young child—certainly one of the most heartwarming and nerve-wracking experiences I've ever had— seems to elicit feelings that have less to do with being female or male than with the nature of nurturing.

The emotional reactions of parents to work and family issues also may be less tied to gender than traditionally assumed. In studies of two-career couples, psychologists at Radcliffe College's Murray Research Center have found that husbands are as emotionally sensitive as wives to issues related to the marital relationship or the family—and their physical health is equally likely to be affected by problems in their private lives.

The Neurobiology of Emotion

In a laboratory at the National Institute of Mental Health, volunteers lay quietly in a brain-imaging machine and thought about the saddest moments of their lives. As old sorrows washed over them, blood flow in certain brain regions increased, revealing the coordinates of the places sorrow calls home.

In both women and men, these melancholy regions lie at the front of the brain, in the left dorsal lateral prefrontal cortex, and deeper down, in the region of the so-called emotional brain known as the anterior paralimbic loop. But as psychiatrist Mark George discovered, there is a dramatic gender difference: Sadness saturates an area eight times larger in women than in men.

"We took the PET scans of thirty-one psychologically superhealthy women and thirty-one comparably superhealthy men," George explains. "The computer morphed the scans for each sex and squished them together so we could develop mean activity maps for men and women and see the areas that differ." At least in this small sample, these differences were far greater than anyone had anticipated—but not for all emotions.

Happiness, for instance, seems a unisex brain experience, one that involves a turning down rather than a speeding up of brain activity. Neurologically, it involves different places and patterns in the brain than sadness. This may explain why it is possible to be both happy and sad at the same time, to feel the poignancy of bittersweet emotions on the occasion of a child's marriage or a friend's departure for an exciting new destination. Other emotions, such as anger and anxiety, though still under study, also seem to show few differences in female and male brains.

Why does sadness single out women? Perhaps it is the nature of what makes us feel sad, George speculates. "The memories that people recalled to evoke sadness all involved family, friends, and loved ones; they were rarely about work or achievement." Because relationships are so central in our lives, women seem to have expanded the capacity to react to their loss. When our link with a loved one breaks, it seems, even our brains may register the pain.

As discussed in Chapter 13, the extent of this sadness may also make women more susceptible to depression. Some theorize that women may react so intensely to sad experiences that, over an extended period of time or with frequent recurrences, they "burn out" or overwork neuronal networks in the emotional brain, which may shut down completely. This may be why many depressed women describe themselves not as sad but rather as numb or incapable of feeling. On brain scans, the lack of activity in certain areas shows up, fittingly enough, as a dark, deep blue.

Neuroimaging studies also have revealed a gender difference in reading others' emotions. In their work at the University of Pennsylvania, Raquel and Ruben Gur studied the brains of volunteers looking at photographs of female and male actors depicting various emotions. Both sexes could tell a happy face when they saw it; they scored almost perfectly in happiness recognition. Both women and men correctly picked out a sad male face 90 percent of the time, but men recognized sadness on women's faces only 70 percent of the time.

"A woman's face had to be really sad for a man to see it," Gur notes. "The subtle expressions went right by them." It could be that men's brains evolved to pay more attention to other men, who posed a potential danger, than to women, or that they never acquired the same education in reading faces that girls receive.

Men's brains also had to work harder to evaluate emotion. According to the PET scans, a woman's limbic system exerted much less effort than a man's—even though the women did a far better job at identifying emotion than the men. "The men's brains were working overtime, but the extra effort didn't do them any good," observes Gur. "They just didn't get it." This may be one reason why men are slower in recognizing emotional problems in an intimate relationship. Regardless of how upset his partner looks, a man may not notice—or, if he does, may not make the connection between her expression and her emotional state.

A man's relative lack of literacy in emotional expressions may not just make it harder for him to recognize others' feelings. Beginning in childhood, many boys and men, struggling to maintain the tough mask of masculinity, may learn to tune out emotional messages so successfully that they lose touch with their own feelings. Curiously, as the following section shows, this is the opposite of what tends to happen in girls and women.

The "Externality" of Women

The wives of the prosperous burghers of Holland long favored the ruff, a pleated collar of stiff white linen that encircled the neck and framed the face. Over time, however, ruffs became so large that they effectively cut off a woman's head from her body. A stylish woman couldn't eat in public for fear of staining her immaculate outfit; unable to see her own feet, she had to tread cautiously along Amsterdam's cobbled streets.

Although the disembodied-head look went out of style long ago, what has persisted is a different type of disconnection between a woman's brain and body. In years of research on individuals' ability to assess internal signals from their own bodies, such as blood pressure, heart rate, and blood sugar levels, psychologist James Pennebaker, of the University of Texas, discovered that in controlled laboratory settings, men are much better at tuning in to physiological processes than women.

"When subjects have no source of information other than internal cues, men have a much greater sense of what is going on inside their bodies," he explains. "Even when making an external observation, they generally rely more on internal judgments." In tests of what is called field independence, for instance, men, looking at an upright rod in a frame, rely on the vestibular system of the inner ear to determine whether a rod is straight or crooked. Women are typically more influenced by the frame: If it's off center, they're likely to say the rod is slanted; if it's straight, they'll conclude the rod is straight.

A woman, Pennebaker notes, tends to look at the overall picture, not only taking the context into consideration but ignoring internal cues and reacting to external ones. In fact, women become so skillful at gathering information in this way that they can often compensate for tuning out their own body signals. In a stark laboratory setting without clocks or other cues, diabetic men are much more accurate in estimating their levels of blood glucose. In the real world, women do just as well by relying on external indicators, such as scheduled appointments or time of day.

What makes women more external and men more internal in assessing physiological states? Brain differences, as discussed in Chapter 11, may be at least partly involved. "People whose brains are highly lateralized, as are most men's, are better at focusing on body sensations," says Pennebaker. "Women's entire brains are constantly taking in and integrating information from everything that's going on around them." This in itself may distract them from what's going on inside.

Social conditioning, as mentioned above, also plays a role. By preschool, little girls are particularly adept at sizing up a situation and intuiting what's going on. In research at Wellesley College, the girls in a group of preschoolers did better in listening to a story and matching the child's feelings in the story to a photograph. Not only were they on the whole correct more often, but the three-year-old girls performed as well as five-year-old boys. Yet stereotypes also start young. In another study, preschoolers were presented with images of girls and boys expressing an emotion and were later asked to recall what emotion was being expressed and whether the person was a girl or boy. The children were three times more likely to make mistakes in recalling the sex of a person expressing a counterstereotypic emotion (e.g., a crying boy) rather than an emotion usually linked with that sex (e.g., an angry boy).

The feminine advantage in reading emotions grows stronger over time. In an analysis of more than 125 studies in various cultures, psychologist Judith Hall, of Northeastern University, found that, beginning in third grade, girls and women are consistently more accurate than men at interpreting unspoken messages in gestures, facial expressions, and tone of voice. Whether looking at photographs or watching videotapes or actual interactions, women show significantly greater skill than men in figuring out how the people they observe are feeling. Even in experiments in which words are deliberately garbled or do not betray any feelings, women can intuit the emotional content of a conversation.

Their traditional lack of power and status may well have contributed to women's evolution of such acute powers of observation. It also may be no coincidence that differences in externality emerge at puberty, when girls, as therapists observe, "move into their heads." Their bodies, with budding breasts, flaring hips, and bleeding cycles, may no longer seem trustworthy to them. And in order to achieve what they think of as the cultural ideal—which these days too often translates into a state of buffed emaciation—they may deliberately ignore the frantic signals of hunger or exhaustion that their bodies are sending them.

The implications of being the more "external" sex are many. In long-running marriages, wives, but not husbands, respond to marital tiffs with higher levels of stress hormones and lower immune responses. An argument that seemed nothing more than a fleeting squall to a husband may echo like thunder through a woman's psyche. Externality may even be one reason why a popular stop-smoking approach, the nicotine patch, generally works better in men. "The patch does away with the internal craving, which is what drives men to smoke," Pennebaker explains. "But women tend to be more sensitive to social cues. Most smoke because of where they are or who they're with."

Is a man's physical self-awareness an advantage? Not necessarily. Men around the world are less likely to report medical symptoms or seek help for them. "Men are good at detecting what's going on in their bodies and terrible at doing anything about it," says Pennebaker. Here too, social conditioning and stereotypes are a handicap: Tough guys think they're supposed to tough out physical symptoms—even when they're chronically painful or potentially life-threatening.

Women's Words

Eve's words, as the Bible tells the story, got the entire human race in trouble. The first dialogue on record, her discussion with Adam of the apple from the forbidden tree, led to their expulsion from paradise. Men have always been wary of what women have to say—so much so that in many times and places, women were not even allowed to speak in public. And when they did open their mouths, women had to choose their words carefully. Their fate could depend on what they said and how they said it.

Perhaps this is one reason why women remain so exquisitely sensitive to words. The childhood rhyme "Sticks and stones may break my bones, but words cannot hurt me" doesn't apply equally to the genders. At any age, words get to women—a reality that still surprises men when an offhand sarcasm wounds their wives or a casual vulgarity offends female coworkers.

Only recently have scientists begun to explore gender differences in the way women and men use language. In ongoing research, psychologist Pennebaker developed a computer program to analyze four 450-word essays by more than nine hundred university students. The preliminary findings suggest that sex differences in written language are huge—larger, in fact, than many other psychological and personality characteristics.

In writing, women use more words overall; more words related to emotion (positive and negative); more idea words; more hearing, feeling, and sensing words; more causal words, such as *because*; and more modal words (*would, should, could*). Women use fewer numbers, fewer prepositions, and fewer articles, such as *an* and *the*, that, Pennebaker notes, "make language more concrete." Women use more question marks, more pronouns (especially *I*), and more references to other people. Men use more body words and, even in an academic assignment, twice as many swear words. Women write more about the past and present; men mention the future more often. Women use more motion words and more occupational words related to either school or work, and they write more about home. Men write more about sports, TV, and money.

When speaking, other gender differences emerge. In her insightful studies of language, linguist Deborah Tannen has noted that men speak more often and for longer periods in public, often as a way of putting themselves in a "one-up" situation; women speak more in private, usually to build better connections to others. In a male's hierarchical social order, she explains, conversations "are negotiations in which people try to achieve and maintain the upper hand if they can and protect themselves from others' attempts to put them down and push them around." To women, who see the world as a network of connectedness, conversations are something else entirely: "negotiations for closeness in which people try to seek and give confirmation and support, and to reach consensus." While men use words to preserve independence, women talk to draw others closer.

Perhaps this is why, in public and private, women, again like classic outsiders lacking in power of their own, generally are better listeners, facilitating conversation by nodding, asking questions, and signaling interest by saying "uh-huh" or "yes." Men interrupt more, breaking in on another's monologue if they aren't getting the information they need. Women are more likely to wait for the speaker to finish. "There's more than one interpretation for why a woman is less likely to interrupt," says psychologist Hall. "It could show that she's being submissive and not playing the aggressive role. But it also could mean that she is less of a social blunderer and is more adept at reading the other person's signals."

Sex differences also appear in nonverbal language. Beginning in their preteen and teen years, women consistently outsmile men in all sorts of situations—with children, other women, or men, whether or not they're in positions of authority or power. They even manage to grin under stress. "If you put a man and a woman in an equally nerve-wracking situation, the woman will laugh and smile," notes Hall. In hospitals, for instance, female physicians smile considerably more than their male colleagues.

Women also look more at others' faces. In experimental studies that measure gaze, females of all ages consistently look at others more than males do. When engaged in conversation, a woman's gaze typically shifts in a predictable way: She glances at her companion as she starts to speak and looks away when nearing the end of her comment; then she glances back to check the effect of her words.

In social interactions, two white women talking together look into each other's eyes far more often than two men; African-American women are less likely to do so than white women. When a man and a woman are together, the man gazes into the woman's eyes more often than he would a man's, while a woman makes eye contact less than if she were with another woman—a nice exercise in reciprocity. "A man talking with a woman will act more like a woman, and a woman will act more like a man," observes Hall. "It's as if they're adjusting to accommodate each other's cultural norm."

Women's eyes display another sex-specific response. When they look at babies, their pupils dilate, whether or not they themselves are mothers. This opening up, also seen among courting couples, is so universal that some anthropologists call it the "look of love." Men's pupils usually don't dilate at the sight of an infant—unless they are fathers. Somehow becoming a dad causes a man's eyes to respond to a baby just like a woman's.

Grumpy Men, Guilty Women

In the early years of our marriage, when my husband was serving in the military, we regularly crisscrossed the country, driving east to west, west to east, north to south, south to north. On the road again and again, we'd spend fourteen-hour days in our car, crooning along to the radio, counting dead frogs and squished armadillos along the highways. By evening, with the fierce summer heat rising in waves above the pavement, the tedium took its toll. Bob would get testy; I'd get teary—and then I'd feel guilty about being so emotional. Fortunately, we realized that our weary bodies were signaling our brains to make us stop. Once we rested, our good spirits returned.

Nonetheless, I've wondered if there are gender-specific emotional default states. Neuroimaging studies suggest this may be so. When the Gurs studied women and men in a state of relaxation (to whatever extent it's possible to relax with one's head in the hollow bore of a brain scanner), they discovered a sex difference in the limbic system, a ring of structures within the brain that process the entire spectrum of human emotion.

Most male brains "idle" in an evolutionarily ancient region of this system—sometimes called the "reptilian brain"—that gives rise to unsubtle, active expressions of emotion, such as aggression. The resting gear for the female brain, in comparison, lies in a different region—the cingulate gyrus, a more recently evolved part of the limbic system related to symbolic forms of expression, such as gestures, facial expressions, and words.

Does this mean that men are emotionally more primitive and women more evolved? "The logical conclusion is yes," says Ruben Gur. "At the very least, this difference may explain why men are more prone to physical action, while women opt for verbal tactics. You could argue that women are half a step ahead of men in evolution in the sense that they use the newer part of the brain more in dealing with emotion."

These brain differences do not characterize all women and men, however. In the Gurs' study, 35 percent of the men displayed the limbic activity typical of women, whereas about 17 percent of the women exhibited malelike patterns. This shouldn't be a surprise. As we all know from personal experience, some extraordinary men do indeed seem more highly evolved than others—and some mean-spirited women may lag woefully behind the rest of their gender.

An even more powerful influence in real-life responses, I believe, is a social double standard. Anger remains an acceptable emotion for a male to express; for women, it's okay to pout but not to shout. Both sexes recognize this: Men rate themselves higher on scales of anger and contempt, and women see themselves as having a greater number of both positive emotions and inwardly directed negative emotions, such as shame and guilt.

This does not mean that rage is exclusively male. In her studies, British psychologist Anne Campbell has found that women and men get angry at equal intervals—six or seven times a week—but respond quite differently. Men are more likely to yell or pound their fists, without any apparent embarrassment. When women let loose with such a display, their response is quite different. "After an outburst, women tell themselves, 'Whoa! Get a grip,' while men say, 'That ought to show them,'" Campbell notes. The more classic female response is to keep their anger bottled up but always simmering. "Women have cornered the market on the seething, unspoken fury that is always threatening to explode."

Sometimes female rage does indeed explode—physically as well as verbally. In a recent review of dozens of studies of aggressive behavior in heterosexual couples in Canada, Great Britain, New Zealand, and the United States, British psychologist John Archer, of the University of Central Lancashire, found that during an argument with a partner, women were as or even more likely to slap, kick, bite, choke, or use a weapon as men. However, male violence had more serious consequences: Women accounted for 65 to 70 percent of those requiring medical care for injuries inflicted during a quarrel.

What makes women angry? In many cases, the causes are the same ones that enrage men—and women's responses are similar, if less intense. However, women more often report anger because of a violation within a relationship, an action (or lack of action) that makes them feel ignored, rejected, jealous, or as if they've been treated disrespectfully or unjustly. Sometimes such anger is not only justified but useful: It can signal something ominous in a situation and alert a woman to make necessary changes. (Male anger, psychologist Brody reports, is more likely to erupt because of a threat to their autonomy, such as not being allowed, for whatever reason, to do what they want to do.)

The healthiest way for a woman to deal with anger is neither to bottle it up (the classically feminine response) nor to let it erupt (the typically masculine reaction) but rather to heed it as a warning of issues in urgent need of resolution. "Venting" by shouting or throwing things typically makes women feel bad because it hurts innocent bystanders and damages relationships they value. Ruminating over what made them angry does little more than keep feelings of rage at a constant simmer. What works best is a strategy associated with women with high self-esteem: talking over the situation with the person who provoked the anger or a trusted confidante and then trying to solve the underlying problem.

Of all the occasions for anger, women may be most upset when they get angry at their children—something that, sooner or later, all mothers do. When researchers have looked at life experiences associated with anger, they discovered that parenthood greatly increases the emotion's incidence—and much more so in mothers. This is understandable. Even in egalitarian families, fathers are less likely to ride the emotional ups and downs of children's crises, demands, and needs. Mothers are the ones children wail for when hurt or frightened, the ones they cling to for comfort. The more children in the family, the more often mothers may find themselves pushed to the boiling point. And whether they spank, sulk, or scream in anger, they end up feeling guilty. Some think they've failed to live up to their standard for maternal perfection; others may feel shame, even self-revulsion, at the thought that they might have hurt their child—psychologically, if not physically.

Regardless of whether anger is an issue, mothering is closely linked to what has long seemed a particularly female emotion: guilt. It's not surprising that the two are so intertwined. After all, no responsibility is greater than giving life. Cradling a newborn, a woman knows that her child will encounter pain as well as pleasure, illness as well as health, sorrow as well as joy. Yet we think somehow we can protect our children from any and all misfortunes. When we don't, we feel guilty.

"The flip side of guilt is a certain grandiosity," says Constance Buxer, a psychoanalyst in New York City. "A working mother will say, 'If I were home, my kid wouldn't have gotten sick.' I can't interview the bacteria that caused her kid's fever, but I know her absence didn't put them in his body. Women think that their love alone can protect a child, but it can't." Her advice: Start dealing with guilt the way a man would.

When men feel guilty, they focus on a specific act, such as an impetuous affair or a few drinks too many, and they don't brood about it. "There is a definite gender difference in how we react to acts of omission and commission," says Buxer. "Women are, as a breed, trained almost from infancy to be more reflective, to acknowledge and internalize our feelings. We feel guilty about not measuring up to whatever criteria we think we should. Men are more likely to think it's the other guy's fault. They tend not to be so introspective or self-judgmental."

Freud speculated that, by their very femaleness, women may be naturally prone to such self-condemnation. Psychiatrists thereafter traced the origins of women's guilt to cultural rather than biological factors, especially to what's called the "tyranny of the shoulds." Traditionally women learned that they *should* be nurturers, selfless givers of life and love. These days we face a whole new set of shoulds—as supermothers, sensuous lovers, feminine feminists, working Wonder Women. When we don't live up to them, we feel guilty.

The real problem isn't guilt, however; it's our sky-high self-expectations. The famed psychiatrist Karl Menninger once remarked that one of the goals of psychotherapy is not to eliminate guilt but to make sure it's "attached to the right things." As women, our biggest challenge may be making sure it's not attached to everything.

Women and the Pursuit of Happiness

"Did Freud really have a clue as to what women wanted?" I ask psychiatrist Ethel Person, of Columbia University's Center for Psychoanalytic Training. "You're missing the point," she tells me. "At least he asked. Hardly anyone had ever done that before."

Through most of history, the pursuit of emotional happiness—written into the American constitution as an inalienable human right—was a male quest. Women's domestic burdens were so great, their health so seemingly precarious, their opinions so seemingly inconsequential, that their wishes seemed beneath notice or beyond comprehension. Why even ask? Fathers, husbands, brothers knew what was best. A female's status was so subordinate that it may never even have occurred to them that women might want what they took for granted: respect, autonomy, opportunity—and the right to pursue happiness as they defined it.

From a man's perspective, American middle- and upper-class women in the peaceful and prosperous 1950s seemingly had everything they could need to make them happy: houses in safe suburban subdivisions, newfangled appliances to take the drudgery out of housekeeping, children they could build their lives around, husbands who were reliable providers. Yet these were the women, neither sick nor well, neither happy nor miserable, who developed what Betty Friedan called "the problem that had no name." Squeezed into stereotyped roles, they suffocated.

The exceptions were the women who defied social pressures and expanded their worlds by volunteering, maintaining active social ties, and taking paid or unpaid jobs. A major longitudinal study that tracked 427 married women (age twenty-five to fifty) with children from 1956 to 1986 found that those who took on multiple roles beyond those of home-maker were most likely to remain in vibrant good health, with fewer major illnesses, better mental health, and greater longevity.

Today's women, according to a recent metanalysis of national surveys on happiness by University of Michigan researchers, are generally as happy as men. Happiest of all are those who feel in control of their lives, and these are mainly working women. This is not what anyone expected.

In the 1970s, when women entered the workforce in greater numbers than ever before, many experts predicted they would pay a high emotional price for leaving behind their sheltered lives and trying to live and work like men. Yet on almost every measure of physical and psychological well-being, working women score as high, if not higher, than those who do not work outside the home. Even more than marriages (which can crumble) and children (whose needs can overwhelm), a job—as long as it's not a stifling, dead-end, low-status position that offers no gratification—boosts women's self-confidence and helps them through the rougher passages of their lives.

One of work's most obvious dividends is a greater sense of financial security. In a poll by the *Ms.* Foundation for Women and the Center for Policy Alternatives, the more economic security women reported, the happier they tended to be. And for today's woman, security rests on her own employment outlook, health insurance, and retirement savings—not on a spouse with a steady income.

However, it's not just the money that matters. With the exception of so-called "pink-collar" workers in spirit-numbing positions, most women derive great emotional satisfaction from their jobs. As they see them, work-related benefits go far beyond financial compensation: deep emotional bonds with coworkers, mutual interest and respect, a shared commitment to common goals, emotional support in times of crises. Compared with men, women report higher levels of intimacy in their workplace relationships and talk more with coworkers about non-work-related subjects, including family and spiritual matters.

Women also tend to pursue interests beyond work and home, particularly after the breathlessly busy years when their children are young. More than a million women over age forty are enrolled in college—twice the number of male midlife students. Many more are flocking into evening and weekend classes to learn new languages, master new skills, develop new hobbies, prepare for new careers. Others have transformed "adventure travel" into one of the hottest segments of the travel industry; women make up 60 percent of customers for excursions such as wind-surfing in the Gulf of Mexico, sailing on women-crewed boats, or trekking across Montana's mountains.

At the same time that new interests are drawing them farther into the world, many women are savoring the traditional pleasures of home. They garden, collect, decorate, design, sew, or simply daydream over magazine spreads of elegant interiors and picture-perfect table settings. "Women don't see any contradictions between having jobs and enjoying doing things at home," observes Myrna Blyth, editor of *Ladies' Home Journal*. "When all women did or could do was fold napkins, it drove them to drink. These days, when they prepare only a few special meals a year, a beautifully folded napkin is part of the pleasure."

In general, women with multiple sources of pleasure, small and large, report better health, less psychological distress, and a greater sense of self-esteem and life satisfaction. Why is busier better for women? "Multiplicity," as researchers refer to the life spice of variety, gives a woman a greater sense of purpose and a more positive view of herself. Women who see themselves in many ways—as mothers, workers, wives, tap dancers, gardeners, potters, political activists, bowlers, hikers, French students, choir members—derive satisfaction from very different parts of themselves: their creativity as well as their competence, their dramatic flair as well as their diligence.

With women doing so many different things for fun and profit these days, it's easy to overlook the pursuit that once represented a woman's sole source of happiness: love. "Love is the whole history of a woman's life, but only an episode in a man's," wrote the eighteenth-century French author Mme. de Staël. Nothing could fill a woman's sensitive soul, touch her heart, fulfill her life more than love.

It's still the same old story, but not to the same extent. Biology, evolution, history, and culture have imbued all humans with a deep desire and capacity for love. We crave such attachment—males just as much as females. "In love the genders are more alike than different," says analyst Person. Neither sex loves better, longer, deeper. What does differ is the meaning of love in their life experiences.

As Person explains, each of us, female and male, faces the same existential problems in life—loneliness, mortality, a yearning for meaning—but each sex attempts to solve these problems in different ways, with what she calls "a passionate quest" for meaning and fulfillment. For women the passionate quest has usually been a search for emotional connection and romantic love. Men, despite the loves in their lives, have more often defined themselves by the pursuit of achievement or power.

Today the pursuits of women and men are more similar. Women have become passionate achievers. And men—some men, at least—are looking beyond status and success for greater emotional fulfillment. Again, Freud may have been right in his succinct definition of happiness and psychological maturity: "to work and to love." Personally, I prefer Tolstoy's variation on this theme: "One can live magnificently in this world, if one knows how to work and how to love, to work for the person one loves and to love one's work." This may not be all that a woman (or man) wants, but it is a mighty good beginning.

Men Are Like Wallets, Women Are Like Purses

Some women therapists I know ask female patients to empty out their handbags as a way of getting a sense of their lives. Often the contents form a small mountain on their desktop or carpet. "I never cease to be amazed by what women carry around with them," says one. "Just by looking, I can find out more than I might have in weeks of therapy."

Counselors never do the same with a man and his wallet. What, other than telltale hints of financial status, could this most boring of accessories reveal? Men's wallets are flat and functional, available solely in shades of tan, brown, black, or burgundy, and tend to bulge in the middle over time. There may be a photograph or two, usually years out of date, and perhaps, among the young and ever-ready, a condom.

Men's wallets are a necessity; women's purses are an industry. Some of the most fashionable women I know dress in understated clothes but carry a chic handbag. But what's most intriguing about a woman's purse is inside: We can pull more surprises from the depths of our handbags than magicians from their top hats: lipstick, blusher, hairbrush, tissues, tampons, pens, keys, checkbook, candy bars, cough drops, gum, breath spray, nail file, dry cleaners' tickets, movie stubs, photos, grocery lists, calendar, calculator, screwdriver, and, if the owner has young children in her life, an array of treats, toys, and trash (where else can a kid dump a half-licked lollipop?). To a man, the contents of a purse may look like a mess. To us, there's meaning in the muddle.

Emotions are not entirely different. A woman's life is packed with feelings, and however many there are, however much they change, she always tries to make room for them. If occasionally they spill over, if a seam holding them together sometimes threatens to break, this too is to be expected. She picks everything up and moves on with her life.

Men, who've long had to keep their hands free and minds uncluttered and ready for action, still tend to fold their feelings into unobtrusive compartments and tuck them out of sight. However, as discussed further in Chapter 15, there are signs that the emotional lives of the sexes are coming closer together—a change with potentially enormous implications.

In a study of ninety-five school-aged youngsters from mostly middle-class families in New England, psychologist Brody discovered that fathers who are more involved with their children have daughters and sons who express fewer gender-stereotyped emotions. "These findings," she notes, "imply, at the very least, that gender differences in emotional expression are not invariant, nor are they largely biological in origin: we seem to be doing something as a culture to bring them about."

If this trend toward more active, hands-on fathering continues to spread through the culture, more stereotypes about emotions and gender may topple—now and for generations to come. Children raised by two caring, emotionally involved parents may yet teach us that there is an alternative to both the male wallet and the female purse (and their emotional equivalents): the ubiquitous, unisex, far larger and more accommodating backpack.

C H A P T E R   1 3

Vulnerable Women

Highway 1, which soars and spins above the rocky coast of northern California, may be one of the world's most spectacularly scenic roadways. But in a house above the dunes north of the Monterey peninsula, the fourteen women gathered for therapist Ruth McClendon's annual women's retreat pay no heed to the summer traffic, the cawing gulls, or the glimmering seascapes. Their focus is not out far, but in deep.

"There is a storm in my heart," says a woman from Japan who crossed the ocean in search of peace. The other women nod in empathy. They too have known their share of heavy weather. Many have struggled with depression that chilled their souls and darkened their spirits. Some tried to blot out anxiety and dread with food, alcohol, drugs, or sex. Several survived nightmarish childhoods or the traumas of rape and abuse. A few had found themselves, in black nights of despair, swallowing pills by the bottleful, jumping out of a car, fingering a loaded gun.

Despite such harrowing passages to and from a private hell, these women are, in psychological terms, "high-functioning": capable, competent, coping. Or so they seem. Prior to the retreat, each filled out a questionnaire that included the query "What is your biggest bluff?" Almost all zeroed in on the gap between the people others thought they were—devoted mothers, loving wives, "together" women—and the reality of who they really are—scared little girls who cry in the night and wonder how they'll make it through the day. "I'm like a swan," one woman wrote. "I may look calm, but underneath the surface I'm paddling like mad just to stay afloat."

It's a feeling many women know—even those with far more placid pasts and unclouded presents. We try to be so good, to perform so well, to give so much without ever letting the effort show. Most of us, most of the time, pull it off. But if stresses build, if biological vulnerability gives way, if unhealed wounds reopen, any woman may feel pushed to a personal breaking point. What happens then often depends on what else is going on in her life.

"Women come in and say, 'I'm tearful. I feel empty. I can't sleep. I sleep too much. My appetite is up. My appetite is down. I've gained weight. I've lost weight,'" reports UCLA psychiatrist Vivien Burt. "But almost invariably, there's a second part to what they have to say: 'I wonder if this has something to do with this time of my life or with this time of the month, with being pregnant or wanting to be pregnant, with going through menopause or with getting older.' We used to listen to a woman's symptoms and treat her in the same generic way we'd treat a man. But the second half of what women say, the part about what's going on in their lives, is just as important."

As I listen to the women at the retreat, I can see what she means. Some do indeed suffer from depression and anxiety disorders, the most common mental disorders among women. Others have troubling emotional symptoms: They're jumpy, irritable, chronically tired, obsessed with food. All are struggling with wrenching life issues: A stunning, long-legged former model, aching from the cold rejection of a mother who never loved her, fears that her deep rage will explode against her own children. A powerfully muscled young woman, who bulked up to fight off her abusive stepfather, has learned that the man she thought of as her dad, the only steadfast figure in her tumultuous life, is not her biological father. A twenty-year-old, the ne'er-do-well in an accomplished family, pregnant with her second child, weighs her desire to do "the one thing I do really well" with the demanding realities of single motherhood.

A young scientist with a blossoming career and radiant good looks still feels the emptiness of always being "the ugliest and stupidest" among her dazzling sisters. A successful executive who'd decided to be "just like my dad, a real hard-ass who did whatever he wanted," came to hate the hard-drinking, drug-taking, fast-living woman she became. "I decided to kill myself by swallowing an entire bottle of Valium. I slept for days, woke up, went to work,and never told a soul," she tells the group. Now she wonders what will happen if ever there is a next time.

As the tides rise and fall on the beach outside, the women cry, rage, laugh, hug, hold each other's hands. At times the only sound is a soft sobbing. At others, curses and angry yells—the screech of emotions long denied—echo through the room. Time and again, just as it seems that one of the women will go over some invisible edge, McClendon reaches out to catch her. She gives some of the women padded bats to pound out their anger. She asks others to put their arms around those who yearn for the comfort their mothers never gave them. Some she challenges; some she consoles. As they "work," as they push through the easy lies to the hard truths, the women seem to shed years along with tears. "I want to go back to being the little girl who kept climbing higher and higher in a tree to see how far she could jump," one woman says. "I want to know what it's like to like myself again."

Midway through the second day, journalistic objectivity falls away. My eyes brim over as I listen to stories of childhood abandonment. I cringe at accounts of soul-scarring cruelty. And I wonder if maybe Bob Dylan was right: that someone who looks and talks and makes love just like a woman does indeed break just like a little girl. But by the end of the retreat, I change my mind. The women, though pushed almost to the brink, manage to find a way back.

"I'm tired of being angry; what good does it do?" asks a woman who'd started off saying she'd "need a lobotomy to get rid of all my anger." "I'm not going to worry anymore that if I get too strong my husband will leave me," says another; "I can't change him; I can only change me." "I've been an alcoholic, an addict, a bulimic," says yet another. "I'm finally ready to be a grown-up."

Months later I check back with McClendon. Some of the women have continued in therapy in her Los Gatos practice. A few are taking medication for underlying psychiatric problems. But almost all, having confronted the issues that were keeping them down, have moved on. The "swans," who once had to paddle so frantically just to stay above water, have learned how to ride with the tide.

Tears on Earth

I was waiting for a friend in a hotel lobby when Eric Clapton's soulful tune "Tears in Heaven" started to play. "I'll tell you," a woman nearby said to her companion, "if there are tears in heaven, you can be sure a woman is crying them." Yet sorrow is not reserved for either sex. No one, female or male, negotiates life's twists and turns without an occasional scrape or more, internal as well as external. According to the 1993 U.S. National Comorbidity Study, one of the most comprehensive mental health surveys ever done, about one in every two individuals—48 percent of the American population—experiences a mental disorder at some point in life.

In this study, rates of mental disorders were about equal in both sexes. In other countries, the balance tips toward women. A comprehensive review of gender and mental health in Western Europe found a consistently higher prevalence of such disorders among women than men, with only one exception—the Netherlands, where, as in the United States, the sexes were equally vulnerable. Other research suggests that developing countries also tend to have fewer gender differences but higher overall rates of mental illnesses such as depression.

In general, though, these disorders manifest themselves differently in women and men. Each sex is prone to different problems, develops different symptoms at different times in life, and responds to different treatments. Early in life, as noted in Chapter 6, boys are at greater risk. In childhood boys outnumber girls with infantile autism, learning disabilities, attention deficits, hyperactivity, and conduct disorders. As many as two thirds of young adults with serious mental disorders are male. Throughout life, many more men abuse drugs, explode into uncontrollable violence, or engage in sexual deviations, such as pedophilia and fetishism. Men also drink more heavily and dangerously than women; male alcoholics outnumber females by as much as five to one.

Men also face a greater risk of suicide. Although women attempt to kill themselves four times more often, men—who frequently choose guns as their weapons of self-destruction—are three times more likely to succeed. Teenage boys are twice as likely to take their own lives as teenage girls; the suicide rate among elderly men is ten times that of elderly women.

Schizophrenia, perhaps the most devastating mental disorder, occurs equally in both sexes, but develops at an earlier age in men than women. Women with schizophrenia undergo shorter and fewer hospitalizations and are more likely to return to a reasonably normal life. Gender variations in brain anatomy may explain such differences. Both women and men with schizophrenia, for example, have the same pattern of abnormalities in brain structures, such as enlargement of the fluid-filled ventricles in the brain, but in men they are more severe.

The affective disorders—depression and anxiety disorders—generally single out women far more often than men. The exception is bipolar disorder (manic-depression), a potentially fatal illness that is characterized by mood swings that include depression and the state of intense energy and impulsiveness called mania. Although it strikes both sexes equally, women tend to have more depressive episodes, to feel worse before or during their menstrual periods, and to "cycle" more rapidly from one mood to another. Yet this mental illness is deadlier in men, who usually have more manic episodes and are much more likely to take their own lives.

The Sadder Sex

"Maybe what we need is a ribbon—a pale blue one," says a fundraiser for an advocacy group for research into depression. AIDS has its ubiquitous red ribbons, sported by celebrities at the most glittering events. Breast cancer has its delicate pink ribbons, worn by women during charity functions, marches, and lobbying efforts. Depression, still cloaked in stigma, stays out of sight. Yet this illness strikes more women than any physical disease and, in both sexes, accounts for more lost days of productivity, higher hospitalization rates, and more disabling complications than heart disease, the number-one killer in the Western world. By the year 2020, the World Health Organization predicts, depression will be the second-greatest cause of disability worldwide.

Like many other illnesses, depression is a thief. While it does not steal sight or mobility, it robs individuals of their joy in living, their pleasure in the people and things they love most, their energy and enthusiasm, their sexuality, and their sociability. For a woman who finds meaning and fulfillment in the webs of connections, depression tugs at strand after strand until the delicate threads of her life start to unravel. This is an illness that hits women where it hurts.

And it hits a lot of us. In Paris, luminous City of Light, about one in every five women—21.9 percent of those surveyed by epidemiologists—lives under depression's cloud. In Italy, the depression rate among women is 18.1 percent; in New Zealand, 15.5 percent; in Germany, 13.5 percent; in the United States, 7 percent. In each of these countries, these rates are generally two to three times those of men.

This gender gap has long stirred debate and denial. Some critics charge that women may simply be more willing than men to admit that they're depressed or more likely to seek medical care. But even when these factors are weighed, the sex difference persists. Others contend that men in distress drown their problems in alcohol rather than becoming sad, tearful, and hopeless. In studies of the Amish population in the United States, who prohibit alcohol use, and of Jewish Americans, who also drink less than other groups, women and men are equally likely to develop depression. Yet these data do not mean that fewer women among teetotalers become depressed, but that more men do so.

Depression also seems more equitably distributed on college campuses, but again the reasons are unclear. "It may be that certain women in certain settings—such as students with more advantages and opportunities than others—aren't as vulnerable," comments psychiatrist Barbara Parry, of the University of California, San Diego. "But you can't generalize from specific populations. Saying that women don't get depressed more often than men is like saying women don't get pregnant. They do—and it happens everywhere." Even in Asian countries, which report very low rates of depression and other psychological disorders—largely because of the great stigma attached to mental illness—the gender gap still favors women.

In the United States, Canada, and Sweden, however, the sex difference in depression seems to be narrowing. Men born since World War II appear more prone to depression than older generations, while women's depression rates seem to be holding steady. In 1994 the U.S. National

Comorbidity Survey found the depression rate among American females to be 1.7 times higher than males'—down from the 2.4 times found by the Epidemiologic Catchment Area survey in the mid-1980s.

Does this imply that men's lives are getting worse or women's better? It isn't clear. However, it may be that as women and men's lives become more similar, the protective forces that may have kept depression at bay for the traditionally dominant gender are breaking down. Today's men must deal with rapid change, economic insecurity, tenuous relationships, increased mobility, fewer entitlements, constricted opportunities—challenges women have long faced. And perhaps, just like women, they are discovering that depression often comes with this less privileged territory.

The Biology of Depression

At therapist Ruth McClendon's summer retreat, the participants share pictures of themselves as children. A woman I'll call Carly, one of the quietest in the group, shows me photographs of herself as a little girl with curly hair and saucer-wide brown eyes. "I looked through all the albums," she says plaintively, "but I couldn't find a single one of me smiling. Even as a baby, I never smiled. I was born sad. It's in my genes."

Although modern science has found a genetic basis for many illnesses, including some mood disorders, the biology of depression is more complex than she suggests. Depression does not "run" in families as infallibly as genetically determined diseases like hemophilia or Huntington's chorea do. However, many individuals do inherit a greater susceptibility to its downward tug. In a study of more than a thousand pairs of female twins, the risk of an identical twin's developing depression if her sister had the disease was 66 percent higher than the risk in the general population. Close relatives of depressed individuals, such as siblings, are 25 percent more likely than others to develop the same problem.

Brain chemistry also may contribute to female vulnerability. The neurotransmitter serotonin or its metabolites (particularly one known to scientists by its molecular designation of 5-hydroxytryptophan, or 5-HTP) is most closely linked with depression. According to recent research by McGill University researchers, women produce less of this crucial mood-regulating chemical. As a result, they may be especially vulnerable to its fluctuations during stress, hormonal changes, or seasonal variations. Whenever a woman's serotonin drops too low, her risk increases not only for depression but also for eating disorders and impulse disorders (such as trichotillomania, or hair pulling, and repetitive self-mutilation).

"We don't know enough yet about serotonin to explain its precise role in women's mental health," says psychiatrist Donna Stewart, of The Toronto Hospital. "But I think we're going to discover a complex interaction between serotonin, brain function, and reproductive hormones." Scientists, exploring the effects of estrogen on serotonin receptors, have already identified some clear relationships. After childbirth, for instance, as estrogen and progesterone plummet, levels of tryptophan, a precursor of 5-HTP, drop dramatically—and may thereby trigger the almost universal state of sadness known as "baby blues" (described in Chapter 9). In most women, tryptophan rebounds by the second to fifth day after delivery, and serotonin levels rise. If they don't, new mothers face increased risk of postpartum depression.

Yet reproductive hormones, whether stable or fluctuating, do not in themselves precipitate depression. If they did, all women, rather than a small but significant minority, would be depressed. Scientists have found few, if any, differences in absolute levels of reproductive hormones between depressed and nondepressed women. However, some women— for reasons that may have to do with heredity, life stress, or underlying physiology—seem especially sensitive, either to their own hormones or to the changes in them that occur during puberty, the menstrual cycle, at childbirth, or during perimenopause.

"A woman who develops one hormonal depression, whether it's triggered by birth control pills or premenstrual changes, is more likely to have another," says Stewart. "We don't know why some women develop this sensitivity and others don't, but it is real, and it is important to recognize its existence." Identifying vulnerable women could lead to interventions that might prevent a depression or catch it early—a crucial advantage, because a depressive episode, if unrecognized, can persist and worsen for months, often becoming more difficult to treat and increasing the risk of recurrence. The reason may be a phenomenon called "kindling." According to this theory, any episode of depression, whether its trigger is psychological, sociological, or physiological, alters brain chemistry, leaving behind highly combustible remnants that can reignite, often for no discernible reason.

While some reproductive events increase susceptibility, others, including some long considered fodder for female depression, do not. Neither menopause nor hysterectomy—once assumed, though without scientific proof, to be surefire precipitants of psychic trauma—plunges women into depression. As noted in Chapter 10, women are most likely to develop a first episode of depression in their late twenties and their late forties.

The hypothalamus and pituitary—the all-important conductor and concertmaster of a woman's reproductive life—may also play roles in stress-related depression. Preliminary research shows significant differences in the responsiveness of stress hormones across the menstrual cycle. At certain phases they seem blunted, as if to buffer the impact of external stressors, while at others a woman may be more likely to feel their full brunt. As mentioned above, the alternating current of reproductive hormones, which fluctuate over a much larger range than those of men, may foster greater vulnerability to the impact of stressful events.

Gender-specific differences in brain functioning (described in Chapters 11 and 12) may also be contributing factors. According to brain-imaging studies, women experience sadness much more intensely than men. If their neuronal circuits, located in the emotional brain, become activated repeatedly or for long periods of time, they may burn out and cease to react at all—one of the neurological signs associated with depression.

Another type of sensitivity, to changes in light and temperature, may explain why women are at least four times more likely than men to develop seasonal affective disorder (SAD) and to become depressed in the dark winter months. Like those with other forms of major depression, women with SAD feel helpless, guilt-ridden, and hopeless and have difficulty thinking and making decisions. Rather than eating less and losing weight—as typically happens during an episode of depression—many crave rich carbohydrates, eat more, and gain weight. Rather than sleeping less, they spend many more hours asleep, yet feel chronically exhausted.

Most women with SAD first develop seasonal depressions in their twenties; many improve with phototherapy, daily exposure to specially designed bright lights, sometimes in combination with antidepressants.

It is tempting, in surveying these studies and statistics, to conclude that women are biologically primed for sadness. Yet the reality of vulnerability,which must be recognized, should not overshadow other facts of female life: The overwhelming majority of women do not become depressed, and those who do can, with recognition and treatment, fully recover and lead fulfilling, high-functioning lives.

Risk and Resilience

Carly, the little girl who stared somberly from her childhood photos, had reason not to smile. Her first memory is of running toward her house as a toddler, only to see the kitchen window shatter as her father thrust her mother's head through it. Whatever her biological disposition to depression, Carly's childhood experiences—a horrific mix of abuse, abandonment, neglect, and insecurity—provided a more than adequate breeding ground for psychological trauma.

Therapists asked the causes of depression in women almost always mention biological predisposition first. A very close second is childhood abuse, an all-too-common component of many girlhoods. By current estimates, more than a third of all women are physically or sexually abused before age twenty-one. The psychological scars can linger long after any physical ones heal.

A frightened, beaten child learns early to abandon hope. In epidemiological studies, 60 percent of women diagnosed with depression—compared with 39 percent of men—have been abused as children. "When you're small and your parents slap you around, you try to make sense of it," says a woman who grew up in a home where beatings were business as usual. "But the only thing you can think of is that you're bad and you deserve to be hit." Repeated abuse not only strips a child of any sense of self-worth but inculcates a terrible message: that, regardless of what she does or says, regardless of how very good she tries to be, nothing will change.

Sexual abuse adds to this sense of betrayal and loss of control. In a three-year study of working-class mothers in London, British researchers found that among those diagnosed with depression, 64 percent had experienced sexual abuse before age seventeen, compared with 29 percent of those with no history of abuse. When they looked into the severity of abuse, there was a direct correlation. All of the women who had had sexual intercourse as girls became depressed, as did 70 percent of those who'd been molested repeatedly without intercourse and 30 percent of those whose abuse was limited to a single incident that did not involve intercourse.

"The violation is always there," a therapist explains, "but it also makes a difference if the abuser was someone the child should have been able to trust or had to rely on—a father, stepfather, teacher, grandfather. And if the girl's mother knows but does nothing or refuses to believe her daughter, the betrayal is total."

Other forms of childhood trauma—a parent's death or abandonment, life-threatening illness, natural disasters, exposure to violence—can set a girl up for depression either in youth or later in life. Some studies suggest that females of all ages actually experience a greater number of traumatic events than males; others, that it's not the quantity but the subjective impact of the trauma that makes women more vulnerable to depression.

"How much trauma is enough?" asks a woman whose father walked out on the family when she was four. "We survived. We managed. Eventually my mother remarried, and I grew up in a blended family that wasn't like the Brady Bunch but wasn't a house of horrors. But even though I tell myself that a lot of people have had it a lot worse, I still have that hole in my heart that I've never been able to fill."

Other risk factors for female depression extend beyond the family. Throughout the world, certain groups of women are at higher risk of depression: minorities, adolescents, lesbians, poor women, women with eating or substance abuse disorders, unemployed mothers with very young children. The reasons sometimes involve not just gender but ethnicity.

"Many ethnic groups live in 'high-context' cultures," explains psychiatrist Freda Lewis-Hall, director of women's health at Eli Lilly and Company. "Rather than experiencing the egocentric phenomenon of feeling guilty about what 'I-me' did—which happens among whites—they're more likely to feel shame over letting anyone down. African-American women often believe that it is our responsibility to bear the world on our shoulders—all of it, every single piece of it, every day, all the time. Should we 'weaken' and either shirk even a little tiny bit of that responsibility or complain about the burden, we think we have done a significant injustice not just to ourselves but to the entire community."

Despite their high-context culture, the frequency of depression among African-American women is often lower than among white women. In comparison, Latina women, who may feel confined in a traditionally male-dominated culture, have high rates of this disorder. Yet what is often forgotten in the long list of women at risk is that most women, regardless of race, ethnicity, or life circumstances and despite trauma, poverty, discrimination, or lack of opportunity, forge on. Why, then, do some falter?

Traditional psychoanalytic thinking blamed women for bringing themselves down. It's just like a woman, the argument went, to be so passive, so self-critical, so willing to serve as an emotional doormat that she ends up depressed. "There's a popular belief that women's psychological structure predisposes them to depression," says psychiatrist Kathleen Pajer. "Women are thought to be more dependent and less able to take control of their lives, more likely to internalize stress and to blame themselves rather than looking toward others as a source of stress. Yet there's relatively little hard evidence to prove that any of these premises actually leads to depression."

There also is little scientific proof for the classic view of depression, especially female depression, as anger turned inward. According to this theory, women internalize their negative feelings and blame themselves for setbacks in life, while men, blaming others, lash out in anger. Others contend that women's tendency to ruminate about problems rather than take action to solve them (as men seem more likely to do) may make them more prone to depression. The same has been said for the great emotional investment that women make in relationships. Because they derive so much of their self-esteem from others, some speculate, women make themselves vulnerable to upheavals not just in their own lives but in those of their extended network of family and friends.

No one denies the key role relationships play in women's lives. Oriented outward from birth, sensitive to every nuance in the ebb and flow of their interactions, attuned to others' needs and wants, women form such deep attachments that it may seem plausible that any threat to them would jeopardize their sense of identity and self-worth. Nonetheless, while it's difficult to accumulate hard data for such subjective experiences, there is no proof that the female tendency to value relationships increases a woman's risk of depression.

In fact, the converse may be true. Women's friendships, the remarkable latticework of caring and compassion that forms the underpinning of their lives, do indeed offer solace and support when they need it most. Women with at least one "confiding relationship," as researchers put it, are physically and psychologically less vulnerable. In one review of studies of thirty-seven thousand people in the United States, Finland, and Sweden, the more isolated women were up to three times more likely to die at an earlier age than those who reported having one or more close relationships. Their risk of the death of hope—a poetic description of depression—is even higher.

Relationships have proved downright beneficial for mental health, in males as well as females, and the more intimate the union, the greater the rewards. Interestingly, at least on a statistical level, marriage—the closest of relationships—provides more benefits for men than women. Married men consistently report lower rates of depression than single, separated, or divorced ones; the same is true only of women in happy unions. Overall, women without mates are not at significantly greater risk of depression than married ones. And while happily married women report the most robust sense of psychological well-being, wives with troubled marriages experience depression at three times the rate of either married men or unmarried women.

However, if a marriage ends, women are not at higher risk. After divorce or the death of a spouse, men are as likely or more likely than women to suffer depression. The reason may be that women rarely rely on their spouses alone (as men often do) for emotional support, and their strong social network may act as a buffer against depression when they lose a spouse to divorce or death.

Black Hole Time

"How does it feel?" It's the classic question of tabloid journalism, of obnoxious television reporters thrusting a microphone into the faces of tearful survivors, fearful victims, dazed bystanders. But when it comes to depression, even the most articulate fail to find the words. "Miserable," say some of the women I interview, searching for a synonym for their suffering. "Empty," say others. Many simply sigh.

"I saw the world through dark-tinted glasses—my house was a wreck, my children monsters, my marriage in trouble, my body fat, my wardrobe ugly, my work without merit, and on and on," recalls Kathy Cronkite in *On the Edge of Darkness*. " 'I can't stand this, I can't stand feeling this way,' I thought a million times, but I would have been unable to define what 'this way' was. I labeled myself 'irritable,' 'cranky,' 'bitchy,' but the feeling was 'out of control.' "

On an Internet chat site, one woman described her depressions as "black hole time." Plagued by hypochondriacal symptoms, she found that her memory and concentration were shot. "I couldn't retain anything I read. I lay in bed every morning trying to think up a reason to get up and go to work. When I wasn't at work, the only thing I had the energy to do was watch TV." One morning, after hearing her boyfriend drive off, she started screaming and couldn't stop. That was the day she finally arranged to see a psychiatrist.

Far too often women and health care professionals chalk symptoms of depression up to an of-course-she's-depressed explanation. After all, the argument goes, if your husband ran away with his personal trainer, if you had three fussy, feuding children under age four, if you'd put on thirty pounds or hadn't had a date in four years, wouldn't you be depressed? Not necessarily. Angry, sad, tearful, frustrated, discouraged? Yes. But a cold gray fog that settles over you for weeks or months, disrupting sleep and sapping your very will to live? No.

Depression may indeed feel different in women than men. "How could it not?" asks Lewis-Hall. "Women hear things, see things, read things, understand things, process information differently from men when we're not depressed, and these differences don't go away when women become depressed." Women typically report more symptoms of depression than men and experience symptoms at an earlier age than men (in their mid-teens rather than their mid-twenties).

Just like gender, race can affect depression's impact. Of all the diagnostic symptoms that are considered characteristic of this disorder, says Lewis-Hall, African-American women are most likely to report appetite change and least likely to report a sad mood. "If therapists sit around waiting for African-American women to come in and say how depressed they feel, I tell them they'll have to keep waiting," she says. "They aren't coming." In her experience, she's also seen more increases than decreases in appetite among African-American women. "I used to see young overweight African-American women and think that they were depressed because they were obese. Now I've come to wonder if perhaps they're obese because they are depressed."

Women also experience more of what psychiatrists call "comorbidity," that is, depression along with another physical or mental disorder such as chronic fatigue, an eating disorder, abuse of alcohol or drugs, migraines, rheumatologic illnesses, or pain disorders. Usually this means a poorer prognosis and a longer stint of suffering compared with those whose sole diagnosis is depression.

Whatever its cause, a woman's depression can spread to those she loves most. A depressed mother cannot care for her children with the same energy and tenderness as when she's healthy. As a result, her youngsters face three times the risk of becoming depressed themselves, and they're more likely to develop symptoms early in life. "Particularly when I'm treating depression in a pregnant woman or a mother of young children," says Burt, "I realize that what's at stake is not just her own health but her family's."

Beyond Worry:
The Anxiety Disorders

The largest person I ever interviewed was a massively muscled exprofessional football player with hands the size of snow shovels. I wasn't talking to him about his physical prowess or brilliant athletic career, but about a problem that had brought his postretirement life to a bewildering halt. For months he suffered from mysterious attacks that would make his heart pound, his chest muscles tighten, his hands shake, his lungs gasp for air. Nothing he had ever encountered on the football field had ever filled him with greater dread.

After medical tests could pinpoint nothing wrong, he found himself staying close to home and family for fear of these unpredictable episodes of psychological and physiological terror. Finally, a knowledgeable friend suggested that he might be suffering from panic attacks; a psychiatric evaluation confirmed the diagnosis and led to effective treatment. When my story about him ran in a national magazine, a friend's husband commented that he was stunned to learn that one of his football heroes had an anxiety disorder. "I thought that was chick stuff," he said.

Despite the obvious sexism in his remark, I could understand why he said what he did. As Chapter 12 describes, women have long been seen as the "sensitive" sex, more prone to fretting and fearing for ourselves and others. But worry is one thing; anxiety—whether in the form of endless obsessing, heart-pounding fear, or sleep-robbing edginess—is another. When these problems become so intense and persistent that they interfere with normal functioning, they qualify as mental disorders. The anxiety disorders are, in fact, the most prevalent of all psychological illnesses—and women are indeed more vulnerable.

According to the National Comorbidity Survey, 30 percent of women develop an anxiety disorder over the course of a lifetime. Compared with men, they are three to four times more likely to develop a phobia, an inordinate fear of a specific object or situation; are two to three times more prone to a panic disorder, with frequent attacks of dread and fear; and have twice the risk of generalized anxiety disorder, a state of chronic distress, or post-traumatic stress disorder (PTSD), a persistent psychological reaction to a traumatic experience. Women also are more vulnerable to the double whammy of mixed anxiety and depression.

Only one anxiety disorder, obsessive-compulsive disorder (OCD), strikes both sexes equally. This problem, characterized by upsetting, invasive thoughts or images and repetitive behaviors, is believed to stem from a malfunction of information-relaying mechanisms within the brain. Women usually develop OCD somewhat later in life, between the ages of twenty and twenty-nine, while males may show symptoms as early as age six to fifteen.

As with depression, biological factors, including heredity and neurobiology, seem to set the stage for anxiety disorders. Among individuals, female or male, with a close relative with panic disorder, about 25 percent may develop the same problem, compared with only 2 or 3 percent of the general population. Certain phobias, such as those involving injury or blood, also seem to have a genetic component, as do generalized anxiety disorder and obsessive-compulsive disorder. Brain chemistry may also be involved. During a panic attack, for instance, the brain's alarm system seems to misfire, signaling danger even though none exists. The fine-tuned, highly adaptive, externally focused female brain may be especially sensitive to such glitches.

Some biological events, such as giving birth, may also make women vulnerable. The period after delivery is a time of increased risk not just for depression but for anxiety disorders, including OCD. Most new mothers, eager to keep their helpless babies safe in a world of potential dangers, do their share of worrying. We tiptoe into the nursery at night just to make sure the baby is breathing. We test and retest the temperature of bottles, scrub everything in reach, fret over every cough or sniffle. In some women, these ordinary anxieties grow into relentless fears, and mundane cleaning turns into ceaseless scouring. Sleep deprivation, which can extend for weeks or even months after delivery, may exacerbate the problem.

In women with panic attacks, hormonal fluctuations may explain why such attacks increase premenstrually, when estrogen and progesterone are low, rather than at other times in their cycle. Other risk factors include frightening experiences in early childhood, discomfort with aggression, low self-esteem, and life stressors that trigger frustration or resentment. While none of these is an out-of-the-ordinary phenomenon in women's lives, they can trigger a problem in those with an inborn susceptibility to fearfulness.

Social conditioning undoubtedly contributes. As girls, we listen to a steady barrage of cautionary commands: Be careful, don't touch, you'll get hurt, that's too dangerous. Even today, when girls are encouraged to be physically active and have more opportunities in athletics and competition than ever before, they may still grow up thinking that there's plenty to be anxious about in an undeniably perilous world. They're right. Sexual assault is indeed a real danger, and warnings about it—though justified—can themselves generate anxiety.

Another long-held theory suggests that women trapped by dependency in unhappy marriages are most vulnerable to anxiety disorders. However, epidemiological research has shown that half of such problems begin before age fifteen and 70 percent start before age twenty-five—well before most women's wedding days. Nonetheless, dependency can perpetuate anxiety. In one study of men married to phobic wives, the husbands were no more—and often significantly less—unhappy in their unions than other men. Indeed, some seem to enjoy their protective or controlling role in a marriage so much that they may not want their wives to become less dependent.

In PTSD, the trigger of anxiety is always external: a traumatic event that has threatened a person's life or safety. Perhaps because of complex chemical and hormonal reasons, women seem more vulnerable to such stressors. According to researchers' estimates, more women than men (31 percent versus 19 percent) exposed to major trauma develop symptoms of PTSD, and women's symptoms are more likely to persist for more than a year.

For women, a rape or brutal assault is the most frequent trigger of PTSD. While any woman may be extremely distressed and require time to work through such terrible events, some repeatedly reexperience their fear and helplessness in their dreams or thoughts. To block this psychic pain, they may enter a state of emotional numbness or become so anxious and fearful that they cannot venture out by themselves. Women who have experienced previous traumas (such as childhood abuse) may be especially vulnerable.

Depression is common in PTSD, as is a state of emotional anesthesia in which women feel cut off from others, uninterested in activities they once enjoyed, and incapable of intimacy, tenderness, and sexuality. They may not be able to fall asleep or stay asleep, in part because of recurrent nightmares in which they relive the trauma. They jump at the slightest sound. During the day, they are always on guard and may have difficulty remembering, concentrating, or completing tasks.

"I used to hate waking up because the memory would come right back to me," says a woman who was raped on her way home from work on a wintry evening. "And I hated falling asleep because I'd wake up screaming from yet another nightmare." She stayed up later and later, hoping to get so tired that she wouldn't dream at all. Then the flashbacks started. She'd be sitting at her desk, reading a newspaper, or walking down the street, and something—a scene, a sound, a smell—would trigger a flood of memories of the rape. Finally a rape counselor referred her to a therapist with extensive experience in helping trauma victims. In therapy she was able to face her memories, put them in perspective, and, after several months, leave them behind. "I'll never forget what happened," she says. "But I've been able to put the past in the past so it no longer has such power over me."

Women Under the Influence

In recent decades, drinking has become more acceptable for women. Particularly among those under age thirty-five, more women use alcohol regularly—a potentially dangerous trend because drinking can be a more insidious problem for them than it is for men. Because of differences in body fat, fluids, size, digestive enzymes, and metabolism, women absorb alcohol more quickly, and the amount of alcohol in their blood rises faster and stays higher longer.

Although some studies suggest that very light drinking—about three drinks a week—may provide benefits not just for men but also for postmenopausal women (who face increased risk of heart disease as they age), medical experts believe that, in general, anything more than moderate drinking—which they define as seven or fewer drinks a week, half the amount allotted for men—may be hazardous to a woman's health. Women who consistently exceed this limit increase their risk of breast cancer, damage to the brain, liver, heart, reproductive organs, and digestive system, and alcoholism.

According to the National Institute on Alcohol and Alcohol Abuse, at least five million women are alcoholics—chronic, compulsive drinkers who cannot control how much they drink and suffer withdrawal symptoms, such as shaking hands, if they quit. For men, it usually takes ten years of chronic heavy drinking (twenty drinks or more a week) for alcohol to cause significant damage to internal organs and for alcoholism to develop. In women drinking half as much, this process telescopes into a period as short as five years. They become dependent on alcohol more quickly, and its toll on their bodies is high. Female alcoholics develop cirrhosis of the liver and a life-threatening heart condition called cardio-myopathy at an earlier age than men, and are twice as likely to die prematurely. On average, they lose an average of fifteen years of life expectancy.

Although scientists have not identified any specific "alcoholism" genes, they believe that genetics may account for 50 to 60 percent of the factors that determine vulnerability in both women and men. Psychological factors, including a history of abuse or depression, also increase a woman's risk. Alcoholism is about three times more common in women with a history of childhood sexual abuse than in the general population.

For every female alcoholic, another three or four women drink in a way that could be harmful to their emotional or physical well-being. They do not tend to drink—or lose control of their drinking—in the same ways as men, who typically drink because they want to blow off steam, blot out problems, or have a good time. In men, hard, heavy drinking increases their risk of depression. In women, it works the other way around: When they become depressed, they reach for a drink to feel better. However, since alcohol is a mood depressant, they end up feeling worse. They may drink more or also take prescription drugs, such as sedatives, and become dependent on them as well.

In a pioneering fifteen-year study involving about 1,100 women, psychologist Sharon Wilsnack, of the University of North Dakota, found that most women use alcohol "as a kind of ego glue, something that holds them together when they feel depressed or anxious or stressed." Women don't see alcohol as a problem because they use it like medicine, she explains, something they need to help them cope, relax, feel less anxious, get to sleep, feel comfortable at parties. As long as they're taking alcohol for a reason, they see it as acceptable.

Contrary to popular assumptions, busy women juggling a variety of responsibilities do not drink more than others. The more roles women play—as wives, mothers, and employees—the less likely they are to have drinking problems, perhaps because they have less time, higher self-esteem, and more sources of emotional support. The exceptions are women in occupations still dominated by men, such as engineering, science, law enforcement, and top corporate management. "Often women in these fields drink as a way of fitting in," observes Wilsnack. "Drinking takes on symbolic value. It's a way of signaling power, equality, status."

While both men and women may reach for the bottle after a marriage breaks up, for some women the loss of any important role can trigger heavy drinking. Such women turn to alcohol to fill up, at least temporarily, the emptiness they feel when they lose a job, a partner, or a way of life they'd once loved. If they find themselves drinking too much, they face a special burden: intense social disapproval. Nice girls, good wives, responsible mothers aren't supposed to have drinking problems. Because of this stigma, women are especially likely to push themselves to function as normally as possible despite heavy alcohol use. The more competent and in control women appear (or convince themselves that they appear), the easier it is for them—and those close to them—to deny any problem. As one counselor puts it, "Women think, 'As long as I get dinner on the table for the kids, my drinking doesn't count.'"

Every woman who's finally sought professional help for a drinking problem describes a different turning point. A thirty-year-old waitress who used to chug bottle after bottle of beer with her hard-drinking husband swore off alcohol when she saw a sonogram of their unborn child. A divorced secretary in her late thirties decided to seek help after she woke up in a hotel room with no idea of how she'd gotten there or what happened the night before. A forty-year-old artist developed pancreatitis, an alcohol-induced inflammation, and realized her drinking could literally kill her.

Fortunately, treatment options, once based entirely on male models of alcoholism, have become more female-friendly. Rather than spending a month or more in a hospital or a specialized treatment facility, growing numbers of problem drinkers and alcoholics are getting outpatient substance abuse treatment in their own communities—a definite advantage for women with young children. Some facilities provide day care. Many offer all-women group therapy, along with individual counseling and training in specific coping skills, such as assertiveness. At the Betty Ford Center in Rancho Mirage, California, counselors have found that women often feel safer talking about issues like abuse in a single-sex group. In mixed groups, they often end up comforting the men rather than dealing with their own emotional issues.

Around the world women make up 40 percent of members of Alcoholics Anonymous, and many communities offer women-only AA meetings. For individuals who dislike AA's spirituality, there is Women for Sobriety (WFS), an all-female support network that emphasizes moving toward the future rather than dredging up the past. Like AA, WFS holds confidential meetings, views recovery as a one-day-at-a-time process, and believes in a goal of complete abstinence.

"In twelve-step programs, they say that a drinking problem is like an elevator that only moves in one direction: down," says a woman who's made the trip. "But it stops at every floor, and you can get off at any time. In the past, people, especially women, used to wait until they hit the bottom. Now I see more and more women getting off a lot earlier, finding help, and moving on with their lives."

Coming into the Light

"The house was always dark," recalls Janice, whose mother, midway through her forty-ninth year, quietly and uncomplainingly "pulled all the shades and took to her bed." Her children away at college, her husband busy at work, she no longer rose with the dawn to prepare breakfast or tidy the house. "When I came home to visit, my father used to say, 'Mother is reading in her room,' but I don't remember seeing any books. The first thing I'd do is fling open the drapes, but my mother would try to stop me. She'd say, 'It hurts too much.' I didn't know what she meant at the time. Now I do."

Janice doesn't recall exactly when the light started dimming in her own life. There had been a hasty, unhappy marriage in her twenties, a series of personal and professional dead-ends in her thirties. Yet just as things were looking up—after a blissful romance, an elegant wedding, and a just-in-time pregnancy—Janice sensed something fading inside her.

"I'd look at my son, this treasure whom I adored, and it was as if I were on the outside of a nursery window looking in. I'd think, 'What a gorgeous creature!' but I just didn't connect. With my husband, I felt that same sort of distance, as if I were alone even when I was lying next to him. Oddly enough, it didn't really bother me until he came home one day and found me sitting in the dark. When he asked why I hadn't opened the shades, I suddenly thought of my mother, and I knew it wasn't fair—to me, to my husband, to our son—to let that happen to me."

At first Janice's therapist thought her depression was purely seasonal and suggested phototherapy. When her symptoms lingered into late spring, Janice tried an antidepressant medication. "I was like Goldilocks," she recalls. "The first seemed too big, and I felt on edge all the time. The second seemed too small, and I still was dragging around. But the third was just right. I didn't feel different. I felt like the me I used to be."

Janice's greatest regret is that her mother never got the help that would have brought the light back to her life. However, the treatments she would likely have been given then might not have been very helpful. Even though women have always received the great majority of prescriptions for psychiatric drugs, most medications, as noted in Chapter 5, were tested only on men. The first generation of antidepressant drugs, the tricyclic antidepressants, which were the mainstay of treatment for many years, usually worked better for men and caused many more side effects in women.

Not too long ago, women complaining of almost any emotional upset were routinely given tranquilizers—often without warnings that certain of these medications could be addicting. Fortunately, both the medications and the way psychiatric drugs are prescribed have changed. More than anything else, the advent of serotonin-boosting drugs—the SSRIs (selective serotonin receptor inhibitors), which include Prozac (fluoxetine), Zoloft (sertraline), and Paxil (paroxetine), and other agents such as Serzone (nefazadone) and Luvox (fluvoxamine)—has revolutionized psychiatric treatment for women. These serotonin enhancers cause far fewer side effects in both sexes and are much safer and easier to use. They have proven especially beneficial for women—not only for depression but for phobias, panic disorder, OCD, premenstrual mood disorders, bulimia, and impulse disorders.

Serotonin-boosting drugs seem to be, if not the answer, at least *an* answer. "What's happened is that we've found medications that work in women, and now we're backpedaling like crazy to explain why," says psychiatrist Pajer, who believes we are just at the beginning of a new era of medications more precisely tailored to female physiology as well as psychology. Some of the discoveries discussed earlier—such as the fact that women produce less serotonin than men and that estrogen and serotonin are intricately connected—are sure to help in fine-tuning future therapies.

Many questions remain—about gender and drug metabolism, about the impact of the menstrual cycle and menopause, about interactions with birth control pills and hormone replacement therapy. Yet what is clear is that overall success rates for treating depressive and anxiety disorders are high, an estimated 75 to 80 percent. And new options are being developed for the women who now are slowest to recover—those with comorbid physical or psychological disorders, a family history of mental disorders, or long-standing marital problems, and those whose prior episodes of depression or anxiety were never adequately treated.

Just as psychiatric medications are at last being fine-tuned to meet women's unique needs, the same has occurred with psychotherapy. Open-ended psychoanalysis—once a standard approach for both sexes—has proven more effective in men. In depressed women, rehashing the past may actually be counterproductive. Ruminating over the whys and wherefores of depression may actually extend a woman's suffering and interfere with her recovery.

One approach that does work for women is goal-oriented cognitive-behavioral therapy, which confronts negative thinking and teaches women to reframe issues in their lives and respond to them differently. Interpersonal therapy, which focuses on relationship issues as factors that precipitate or exacerbate depression and on improving the dynamics of relationships, is also effective. Many therapists combine these approaches with other techniques, such as assertiveness training, and with medication. All-female group therapy also may offer special benefits, and not just in recovery from substance abuse. According to researchers at Wellesley College, women talking with women don't censor themselves as they do in the company of men—nor do they feel a need to defer to or take care of men.

With the advent of treatments specifically designed to address women's needs, the prospects for better tomorrows have brightened. In the past, "outcome" studies had shown that women with depression tended to have longer episodes and a greater risk of recurrences than men. Although there is an inevitable research lag in gauging the efficacy of the newest approaches, this seems to be changing. In a follow-up study of 188 depressed adults—70 percent female and 30 percent male—Brown University researchers tried to tease out the extent to which gender, types of treatment, life events, social support, and negative attitudes predicted the severity of symptoms six, twelve, and eighteen months after treatment began. At the end of the study, women and men were doing equally well, and gender alone did not determine who fared best. Interestingly, factors that were, theoretically, particularly beneficial to women—such as close friendships and positive social support—turned out to be just as important to men's recovery.

Given biological predisposition, stubborn societal inequities, and the inherent strains of modern life, psychological disorders are likely to continue to shadow women's lives. Sadly, too many women still remain in the dark. Of the seven million women in the United States who are estimated to suffer from a diagnosable depression, only 37 percent seek treatment. Those who do typically express one regret: that they didn't get help sooner.

"If you think you're depressed or anxious, if you're doing self-destructive things, if you're just going through the motions of living, get help," says a woman who, as she puts it, "lost a decade" to depression. "If there weren't so many misconceptions about mental illness, I would have gone to a therapist long, long ago. If I knew how effective today's treatments are, I never would have wasted so many precious years and so many chances to be happy. For me, medication opened the door to a new life, and therapy helped me move through it."

CHAPTER 14

Sensuous
Spirits

"Notice the face," the art history professor says as a slide of a baroque sculpture appears on the screen. "The eyes are closed; the lips are parted. This is a real woman." "Yeah," a voice from the vast lecture hall rings out, "a real woman having an orgasm."

Giggles sweep across the auditorium as the college freshmen realize that this is exactly what they are beholding—although it is no ordinary climax. Bernini's creamy marble statue of Teresa of Avila captures the saint in a state of ecstasy that obscures any distinction between sacred and sensual. "If that is divine love," an eighteenth-century French observer commented at its sight, "I know all about it." So did Teresa herself, a sixteenth-century Spanish mystic who described her union with God as so passionate that it left her "prone, into the very arms of Love."

When I first saw the actual sculpture, in an ornate chapel of Rome's Santa Maria Vittoria that seems more stage than altar, my childhood readings of the lives of the saints hadn't prepared me for such a nakedly erotic interpretation of mystical experience. Then I remembered a line from another lecture: All ecstasy is sensual because we experience it in the body, and all sensuality is ecstatic when it touches the soul. Bernini had gotten it absolutely right. A woman experiences fulfillment—religious or romantic—inside and out, physically and spiritually, body and soul. With our sensitive psyches and holistic brains, female passion may quite literally know neither bounds nor boundaries.

Perhaps this is why, in the Greek myth, Tiresias, who had spent much of his life as a woman, stated that females experience greater sexual pleasure than males. Perhaps this is also why, throughout history, men have so often feared and condemned what they saw as woman's insatiable carnality. This too, for very different reasons, may be why women in different cultures and religions have reported more experiences of bodily transformation, whether of transcendence or of trance.

Just as a woman's physiology and psychology are distinctive, so too are female sexuality and spirituality. Neither quite fits the paradigms created by and for men—which may be why men so long reviled, dismissed, or even doubted whether women were capable of either. In a church council in 585, a bishop questioned whether women were "men" at all—that is, human beings with immortal souls—or the devil's designates, disguised in dangerously appealing ways. As recently as the early twentieth century, many people, including medical experts, believed that "the majority of women are not very much troubled with sexual feelings of any kind," as the widely quoted physician William Acton put it.

While women today are acknowledged as spiritual and sexual beings, the nature of both female piety and passion has been understudied and undervalued. From the traditional—that is, male—perspective, sex is primarily a biological propulsion, while religion is something else entirely: a construct of the brain questing for greater meaning for the immortal soul. This is not the way women, with our tendency toward the "and-but" rather than the "either-or," see it. For women, the sexual often resonates into the realm of the spiritual, and vice versa.

The famed female "relationality" also comes into play. Our bodies are designed for connection and inclusion. In making love with a man, we receive him into our very depths. In giving life to a child, we carry another being beneath our hearts. And whether our lovers are female or male, whether we ever become pregnant or give birth, we remain the gender that embraces possibility. Ours is an openness that draws us inexorably into relationships. Some of these connections are physical unions; others are not. We connect by touch and sight and sound; we reach out to strangers as well as friends; we relate not just to people but to nature and life itself.

"To a woman, spirituality, or a life of the Spirit, implies relationship in its very essence," writes Irene Claremont de Castillejo in *Knowing Woman*, noting that a woman becomes aware of her relationship to God by means of any experience that "does not separate and divide but connects and brings together spirit and flesh, humanity and nature, God and matter."

Contemporary female theologians have applied this perspective to one of the oldest religious concepts, viewing the Christian belief in a divine trinity of Father, Son, and Holy Spirit not as a symbolic hierarchy but as the prototypical relationship. The essence of God, from this perspective, is relationship, and it is through our relationships that we come to understand and unite with the divine.

Women may always have sensed the enormous significance of context and connection, but with our tendency to look outward for affirmation, we may not have trusted the lessons our bodies were trying to teach us. Even today many women see sexual gratification and spiritual grace as opposing forces, particularly in young adulthood, when the sheer heat and force of sexual desire may hold us completely in its thrall. Only as youthful passion moderates do many women begin to search for wholeness of another sort.

"It works out great," exclaims anthropologist Martha Ward, of the University of New Orleans. "A woman can have the joys of the flesh in the first half of her life and the fulfillment of the soul in the second." Yet these two pursuits need not be mutually exclusive. Although the juxtaposition of sacred and profane may seem improbable, it is not an impossible stretch. And appreciation of the link between body and soul may ultimately free women from one of their oldest and most pernicious burdens: a deep mistrust of their bodies, the dwelling place where senses and souls abide.

"I know no woman—virgin, mother, lesbian, married, celibate," Adrienne Rich observed in *Of Woman Born*, "whether she earns her keep as a housewife, a cocktail waitress, or a scanner of brain waves—for whom her body is not a fundamental problem: its clouded meaning, its fertility, its desire, its so-called frigidity, its bloody speech, its silences, its changes and mutilations, its rapes and ripenings." Yet, as she noted, this need not remain so, because "there is for the first time today a possibility of converting our physicality into knowledge and power."

Rather than letting revulsion or hatred of our bodies cripple our souls and blight our brains, we can learn to appreciate the flesh in which our spirits dwell. By honoring the physical, we can come to know the spiritual. And by getting in touch with the spiritual, we can free ourselves to celebrate the physical. As this chapter shows, a woman's most satisfying sexual encounters and most uplifting experiences take root in her body and fill up her senses as well as her soul.

Virtual Virginity

When a magazine editor asked me to do an article on why women don't enjoy sex more, I protested that it was an idea whose time had gone. Yes, way back in the days of Puritans and prudes, before Kinsey, Masters and Johnson, and the other modern cartographers of passion's possibilities, women may have been shortchanged on sexual enjoyment. But that was then. This is now, a time when sex sizzles everywhere and women, no less than men, seem to be turning up the heat.

I was wrong. As sex therapists around the nation confirmed, many women of all ages—although they hate to admit it—don't get a lot of physical pleasure from sex. For all the outspokenness that followed the sexual revolution, the physiological and emotional elements of sexuality that are essential parts of what it means to be a woman often remain unknown or unexpressed. Hoping for the intensity of a sexual bonfire, many women end up with the sensual equivalent of a Bunsen burner. And they wonder: Is this normal? Is this the way other women feel?

In a surprising number of cases, the answer is yes. "In my sexuality workshops, I see a lot of women I think of as middle-aged virgins," says Lana Holstein, the physician who heads the women's health program at the Canyon Ranch in Tucson, Arizona. "They may have had sex thousands of times and given birth to several children, but they've never gotten to know who they really are as sexual beings." Despite their experience, these women remain curiously innocent, their innate sensuality tucked away like a fabulous dress, cut low and slit high, that they fantasize about wearing but leave in the closet. It seems a bit too daring, far too revealing for public display or private enjoyment. After a while, they even forget it's there.

This is not unexpected. Through most of history, men controlled women's sexuality. A girl's father bartered her innocence for a husband of means. A woman's spouse so zealously prized her fidelity that men in many nations—and still today in certain fundamentalist societies—could beat, desert, or even kill an adulterous wife without legal reproach. Women were taught that sex is dangerous for the unmarried and a duty for the married, a pleasure to offer their partners, not to partake of themselves.

The female body itself was viewed as an occasion of sin, the means of Eve's temptation and the reason for God's condemnation. The very earliest legal codes spelled out strict regulations for female sexual conduct and dire penalties for any violations. "The power of the sensual is so strong that religions and societal institutions long demeaned, deprecated, and made it sinful and dirty," observes Holstein. "And since women carry the sensual, since we are so connected with the life force, we too have been demeaned, deprecated, and made sinful."

Today's women may no longer view sex as "bad," yet it often doesn't feel as good as they think it could and should. In a surprising number of cases, ignorance as well as conditioning is at least partly to blame. "Twenty percent of the female patients I see don't know where their clitoris is," a sex therapist tells me. "I've seen physicians, nurses, and college professors who didn't know how to find their own clitoris. People with M.D.'s, Ph.D.'s, all kinds of D's, have no accurate knowledge of female sexual anatomy."

Women and men know even less about normal female sexual response. A lot of women, for instance, think there's something wrong with them if they don't climax during intercourse. However, many experts estimate that only one third of women do so. Nor do many women and their partners realize that it generally takes a woman an average of thirteen or fourteen minutes to climax from the beginning of genital stimulation—four times as long as it takes the average man to go from erection to ejaculation.

Physicians aren't likely to be of much help in educating women about their sexual potential. When it comes to sex, most doctors don't ask and most women don't tell. With little more than a lecture or two on human sexuality (if that) as part of their training, health professionals generally are no more at ease talking about sex than their patients. This uneasiness pervades medical research as well as practice. Although sexuality is a basic human concern, only in recent decades has it become the subject of serious scientific investigation. Even then, the focus—as in other fields of medical research—has been on pathology rather than normalcy, and mostly on men.

A sex therapist once tried to justify his profession's preoccupation with the penis and its problems by noting that if a man can't get an erection, then "a woman can't have sex, so it's her problem, too." When I repeat this comment to women, they roll their eyes. It is indeed something only a man would say (and something that made Viagra, the impotence pill, the fastest-selling new drug in pharmaceutical history).

The almost total emphasis on erection reflects not only an erroneous assumption that it is the sine qua non of gratification for both genders but also a fundamental lack of appreciation of what turns women on. Intercourse, although not without undeniable appeal to women, is a guy's game. Boys in the United States still compare sex to baseball—you try to get to first base with a girl, then second, then third. Finally you go all the way and score. Most women would opt for more time on the infield, the outfield, and other pleasurable detours on the way to home plate.

Yet female passion and pleasure remain largely unexplored. When Viagra was released in 1998, urologists weren't the only ones beseiged by calls from their patients. Gynecologists reported that they were hearing from their female patients, who were asking not what the new medication could do for their sex partners but what it could do for them.

Once again there were few answers. While much about male sexuality remains unknown, science knows even less about women. A recent study in the *British Medical Journal* reported that regular sex reduced the risk of death by roughly half in about a thousand men in a Welsh village. No one looked at its impact on women.

"Even basic questions about female sexuality, as opposed to reproduction—such as nerve function in the pelvic area or details of clitoral responsiveness—remain unasked and unanswered," says Beverly Whipple, president of the American Association of Sex Education Counselors and Therapists. In her laboratory at Rutgers University, Whipple and her colleagues have challenged many conventional notions about female sexual response. Her research, which, like most investigations into female sexuality, has provoked ire and fire from all sides, has shown that women can achieve orgasm through force of fantasy alone, confirmed the location of the "G spot" felt through the vaginal wall documented the existence of female ejaculation, and demonstrated that even women who've suffered spinal cord injuries can achieve orgasm.

"Women have a variety of sexual responses, and not all fit in with the monolithic pattern described by Masters and Johnson," says Whipple. "Female sexual response may be much more complex than anyone ever guessed." Men, she notes, tend to view sex—like many other things—in a linear way. To them, a sexual encounter is like ascending a staircase that leads step by step to only one endpoint: ejaculation. Women's sexuality, like our ways of taking in and thinking about the world, is more holistic.

"I see female sexual response as a circle, with every aspect of sexual interaction—touching, kissing, hugging—as a pleasurable endpoint in itself," Whipple says. For women, the process of making love—the holding and the hugging and the tenderness—can be as emotionally gratifying as orgasm itself, and sometimes even more so. This view can be liberating for a woman's soul as well as her sexuality. When women experience sex not as a ten-nine-eight countdown to climax, not as quest or test, but in terms of sensing, knowing, and feeling what one poet calls "the song of life singing" through them, then eros offers more than mere physical gratification. This may indeed be what sex was meant to be—an experience that touches the essence of who we are in ways not unlike a spiritual revelation.

"For full enjoyment of sex, for true completeness," the writer Maya Angelou observes, "one does the same thing one does with God. One says, 'I am Thine' to that force of energy that has created us. It's only when you can give over the concern about everything else—whether the bills are paid or the phone is ringing—and join that moment, join that other body, that you can have total completeness in sex. So it is the same as the development of true spirituality. You must admit to yourself that you are a part of everything, and then there is total enjoyment. In eating, in sex, in laughter, in crying—complete enjoyment, a complete joining and joy with the other. And why shouldn't we enjoy it? It's all God's gift."

Female Eros

In a private screening room at the University of Amsterdam, female volunteers watched two sexually explicit clips from pornographic movies as sensors of vaginal vasocongestion, or increased blood flow, monitored this telltale sign of physiological arousal. One film, made by a male director, presented a more-or-less-standard brothel scene in which a woman "services" a man with no foreplay and no sign of enjoyment. The other, directed by a woman, offered a more romantic context for its hard-core sex: A rather ordinary-looking woman (compared to the life-size Barbies who appear in many pornographic films) and man meet in an elevator. They glance at each other; she takes the initiative; they stroke, kiss, and undress each other. In their graphic sexual encounter, she seems to be enjoying herself immensely.

When asked, the forty-seven women who participated in this experiment said they were aroused only by the second, woman-directed video, not by the first film, which they described as gross, repulsive, and disgusting. Yet despite these very different appraisals, increases in vaginal vasocongestion revealed that the women's physiological responses to both movies were equally intense.

What does this discrepancy between subjective appraisal and objective reaction mean? Can a woman's body be turned on even when she is intellectually and psychologically turned off? Yes, says sex researcher Ellen T. M. Laan, of the University of Amsterdam, who theorizes that a woman's sexual response, unlike a man's, does not rest on biology alone. "Men listen to their bodies," she explains. "They say, 'Oh, I have an erection; I must be aroused.' " Women are different.

Just as with the other physiological processes discussed in Chapter 12, women don't tune in to internal cues to the same extent that men do. Even if their vaginal lubrication and blood flow increase—probably a biological reaction that evolved over time to protect women from injury during rough or forced sex—women are not aware of this response or, if they are, don't experience it as a form of pleasure. The fact that their genitals respond to intense erotic stimulation does not mean their hearts and minds necessarily follow.

The science is new; the insight is not. In 1876 the pseudonymous

Mrs. E. B. Duffey, author of the most popular sex manual of the time, *The Relations of the Sexes*, observed that "women are not like men in sensual matters. They—most of them at least—do not love lust for lust's sake. Passion must come to them accompanied not only with love, but with the tender graces of kindness and consideration." More recently the late Audre Lorde, the black feminist poet and activist, made a similar observation: "The erotic is not a question of what we do. It is a question of how acutely and fully we can feel in the doing."

Using far more prosaic language, scientists have come to similar conclusions about the significance of sexual context. In interviews with thousands of Americans, researchers at the National Opinion Research Center at the University of Chicago have found that women who were married or living with a partner reported more sex, more orgasms, and more sexual satisfaction than uncommitted singles of every age. And even though men were far more likely than women to climax during intercourse, the percentage of women who were extremely emotionally and physically satisfied with their sex lives was about as high as for men. Orgasm itself, the researchers concluded, does not determine a woman's sexual satisfaction.

What does? When University of Arkansas researchers attempted to discover the answer by studying the sex lives of married couples, the number-one factor for women was satisfaction with the nonsexual aspects of the relationship. In other words, what happened outside the bedroom had the greatest impact on how satisfied the wives were with what happened in it. "The quality of a relationship," as one sex therapist observed, "always has a lot more to do with how satisfied women are than whether they'd rate their orgasm a ten or an eight."

This realization was a hard-won revelation for many members of my generation, the baby boomers who made love not war, defied the double standard, and redefined female sexuality. Even before the ultimate morning-after concerns of failed contraception and sexually transmitted diseases, the sexual revolution—like most social and political upheavals throughout history—turned out to be far less liberating for women than for men. Although the purported demise of the double standard and the availability of the birth control pill freed a woman to make love just like a man—that is, without fear of social or reproductive consequences—most of us still prefer to make love just like a woman, in a context of love, trust, and commitment.

These values do more than enhance sexual experiences; they transform eros, as Lorde observed, into "a spiritual instinct" that urges us "toward relationship on every level of our being." And when sex is a means of connecting with someone we cherish, the way we view our bodies changes. We become not so much a vessel, a passive entity that takes in what it is given, but a messenger, a conduit for both giving and receiving pleasure. But the relationship is not just with a lover; it is with life itself.

Nonetheless, the lover, the person with whom we share pleasure, always matters more than any techniques of pleasuring. What ultimately makes us heterosexual or homosexual, as researchers into sexual orientation have discovered, is not any molecular marker or specific sexual interaction, but the gender of the person we love. "I had sex with a lot of men over the years, and I always felt that something was missing," says one woman. "It wasn't until I fell in love for the very first time—with a woman—that I realized what." Living and loving as a lesbian, she rediscovered her body. "I used to think a woman's body would be wasted without a man. Why do you need a vagina if your lover doesn't have a penis? What good is the uterus if you're not going to make a baby? What I learned from my female lovers is that every part of the body is erotic. Now I think that it's when she's with a man that a woman's body is wasted."

Men too are discovering the importance of intimacy to sex. In 1984, in a large survey of a representative sample of Americans sponsored by *Parade* magazine, 59 percent of the men and 86 percent of the women said they found it difficult to engage in sex without love. Ten years later, in a 1994 follow-up survey, the percentage of women feeling this way remained the same, but considerably more men—71 percent—found it difficult to relate sexually to someone they didn't love.

This way of thinking is taking hold even in the most sexually liberal lands, the Scandinavian countries. University of Helsinki sociologists have described a dramatic change in sexual values since the "silken revolution" of the 1960s. In the mid-1990s younger Scandinavians of both sexes began to express much greater sexual caution and ambivalence. One-

night stands seemed too risky to them, and casual sex, though not uncommon, was no longer idealized. Commitment had come into favor, with
more young people reporting fidelity and a belief in serial monogamy.
Rather than the love-the-one-you're-with morality of previous decades,
the new generation, born into an era of sexual ambivalence, now believes
in responsible sexuality and a "love ideology" built on values like caring
and tenderness. As many a woman would say, it's about time.

Reclaiming the Body

From head to toe, a woman's body has always been her number-one
self-improvement project, something to be molded, folded, pressed, and
prodded to suit standards of beauty that changed with every age. The
medieval ideal possessed small breasts and narrow hips; the Renaissance
favored a full-breasted, wide-hipped figure. A beautiful woman of the six-
teenth century, according to an Italian treatise, possessed thirty-three
perfections, including three long: hair, hands, and legs; three short: teeth,
ears, and breasts; three wide: forehead, chest, and hips; and three narrow:
waist, knees, and "where nature places all that is sweet."

Rarely did standards of female beauty bear much resemblance, if
any, to the biological realities of the female form. This hasn't changed.
Today, in a time of unprecedented health, nourishment, and opportunity
for adult women, fashion's ideal is an emaciated, breastless, hipless girl.
Glancing from magazine advertisements and television screens into their
own full-length mirrors, women may again feel the disconcerting gap
between the ideal and the real. It is thus not surprising that as many as
two thirds of American women say they dislike their bodies.

Perhaps, a friend of mine suggests, women would be happier in a
world without mirrors. There may be a more practical alternative: a
change in the way we look at our bodies, a switch from peering in from
the outside to appreciating them, as suggested earlier, from the entirely
different direction of the inside out.

This is what individuals in two very different—and some would say
diametrically opposed—areas, sexuality and spirituality, are urging women
to do. By rediscovering the tangible pleasures of inhabiting a human

form, say these "body mystics," women can move from appreciation of the physical toward fulfillment of the spiritual.

As human beings, we don't simply *have* bodies, they note; we *are* bodies—and this is indeed a joyous thing. It is what makes babies chirp with delight at the discovery of their toes, why laughing children spin and spin until they spiral breathlessly to the ground, what athletes savor when their hard-trained muscles propel them higher, farther, faster.

Throughout the day, even ordinary bodies ground us in the eros of the here and now, the vitality of the immediate second. As the antennae of the body, our senses are in constant communication with the world around us. They take in the mundane: the crunch of gravel underfoot, the slippery skin of a squealing child lifted from the bath, the bracing aroma of morning coffee. And they delight in the marvelous—a rainbow spilling across the sky, the sound of rain drumming on the roof, the buttery warmth of the sun on chilled flesh. Without our bodies, we do not exist; without our senses, existence loses its exhilaration.

The new "theology of embodiment," rooted in the tangibles of the flesh, holds special meaning for women, since we so often use our senses to tune in to the external, to the sounds, sights, smells, and tastes of the outside world. But there is another direction in which we can turn: inward and downward, into the vital flow that we sometimes sense when we make love, nurse a baby, comfort a child, hug a friend, lose ourselves in prayer or meditation.

For some women, awareness of this subterranean energy begins when they give birth. With the delivery of her first child, one therapist recalls an "embodied revelation . . . a knowing of the sacred through my body." Participating in the miracle of creation shifted her consciousness, changing her forever. Other women recall different situations in which boundaries melted away, leaving no distinctions between themselves and another being, or nature, or life itself.

Such awareness, felt in the body as well as the soul, is profoundly female. Some call it our magic, our ability to transform, to take what we find, even scraps of food, fabric, flowers, or fables, and make something new and wondrous—be it a pot of soup, a patchwork quilt, a table center-piece, a lullaby, or a bedtime tale. As we do these things, we work our magic, with sensing, sensual, sensuous bodies as well as questing souls and curious minds.

All These Things, and More

In a circle of women dancing around a bonfire in the woods of Wisconsin, Rosemary Bray, a divinity trainee and author of *Unafraid of the Dark*, sensed a Presence, "suddenly there, in me. I felt it from the soles of my feet to the top of my head." Then she heard "the Voice," neither male nor female, not even human, but "absolutely clear and supportive." As she wordlessly poured out her heart's many desires, she sighed, "It's just that I want so many things." And the Voice said, "All these things, and more."

The search for the elusive "more" is leading a growing number both to mainstream churches and synagogues and to more female-friendly alternatives. Traditionally, patriarchal religions, with their rigid hierarchies and ironclad (and often mossy) rules, have not been particularly welcoming to women. An Orthodox Jew begins his day by thanking God he has not been born a woman. The Muslim religion literally keeps women under wraps. Christian tradition views women as Eve's sinful and sinning daughters. As recently as 1998 the Southern Baptist coalition— one of the largest Protestant groups in the United States—declared that wives should "submit" to their husbands.

Not surprisingly, long shut out of roles as rabbis, priests, or shamans, many women have never felt quite at home in the traditional houses of the Lord. In some denominations this is changing, and more women are joining what some call the "theological chorus." The language of many religious prayerbooks, texts, and hymnals is becoming gender-free. Women now make up more than 20 percent of students enrolled in the five largest divinity schools. And more women ministers are rising into leadership roles (one in five of Episcopalian bishops, priests, and deacons is female).

Many women, though, have followed their quest for more in different directions—to weekend retreats, courses in miracles, New Age circles on mountaintops and beaches. All of these alternatives are sometimes lumped together under the heading of "feminist spirituality," a movement that has been described as "unorganized and decentralized to the point of anarchy," with no recognized leaders, no designated rituals, not even a universal belief in a single deity or higher power.

"Spiritual feminists," notes theologian Cynthia Eller, "remain determinedly eclectic, borrowing deities, meditation techniques, and magical recipes from whatever cultures appeal to them." Some prefer circles to altars and personal testimonies to rote liturgy. Rather than awaiting a savior, many acclaim the saving grace that comes from within. Rather than worshiping one God in one way, they talk of "honoring what is personally true." Some engage in prayer dances and walking meditations; some chant and clap and sing; some prepare huge communal feasts; many hold hands, laugh, hug, and celebrate the sheer energy of the female life force.

Within spiritual homes of their own, women pay homage not to a forbidding Father but to a compassionate Mother, the female force who gave birth to the cosmos and all of creation. Expanding the concept of God into a more androgynous image, they have developed special liturgies for women's unique life experiences, such as abortion or miscarriage.

"In women's religions, motherhood is the pivotal motif or metaphor, the quintessential experience," says anthropologist Martha Ward. This translates not into worship of fecund earth mothers, she adds, but into an emphasis on connection, on women in relation to children, to each other, to ancestors, to an eternal source of life energy. Often, as one theologian puts it, women "find the holy through the body," espousing principles they know in their gut, feel in their heart, sense with hands, ears, and eyes.

"The soul is capable of much more than we can imagine," St. Teresa once wrote, adding that it is very important for any soul that practices prayer "not to hold itself back and stay in one corner. Let it walk through those dwelling places which are up above, down below, and to the sides." Today relatively few women (or men) experience the nothing-held-back ecstatic communion with the divine that Bernini captured in his sculpture of Teresa. In other cultures and times, however, states of bodily transformation have often been more common, especially among women.

This may be because women have always been more open to visitations by otherworldly beings. "After all, if men and babies enter or inhabit our bodies, then spirits can, too," observes Ward, who contends that women, more comfortable with relationships of every sort, are less likely to shut off any part of themselves—body or soul—from the forces and feelings that give meaning to life.

The Return of the Goddess

Anthropologists call them "Venus figures," dozens of carvings of stone and ivory found in archaeological digs throughout Europe. Dating back to the end of the last Ice Age, some 20,000 to 25,000 years ago, they differ somewhat in style and form, but all represent big women with ample breasts, pillowy buttocks, and mounded bellies. No one knows if these primitive Venuses were objects of worship or magical charms used by early healers to cure infertility or ease the pain of childbirth. Whatever their purpose, they reveal something timeless: awe at the splendid female essence that could miraculously bring life into the world. Whoever carved them—women or men living in a time before the written word—captured with their hands the tremendous energy that emanates from the strong and sensual female body.

According to legends, the very first civilizations of "old Europe" venerated a "great goddess" who represented this life force. Archaeologists have never been able to document the existence of these matriarchal societies, but we do know from written records that later cultures— including those of ancient Egypt, Greece, Rome, and India—included goddesses in their pantheons. Half of the original twelve deities of Mount Olympus were female. The Japanese Shinto tradition included major female deities; ancient Hindus viewed women as keepers of the life force.

In the Western world, goddesses disappeared with the emergence of the Judeo-Christian tradition, which honored the one, true God as the quintessential patriarch. However, in recent years women seeking greater relevance in their quests for sensual, spiritual, and psychological meaning have resurrected the legends of goddesses past.

Even though modern women may never envision "goddess" as one of their career aspirations, many identify with the mythic Olympians. The reason, explains psychiatrist Jean Bolen, author of *Goddesses in Everywoman*, is that the ancient goddesses represent archetypes, or powerful inner patterns, that counter society's often stultifying stereotypes about women and that resonate within the female psyche. Goddesses—be they domestic, home-loving Hera or fearless, assertive Athena—are complex and multidimensional, with vulnerabilities as well as strengths, flaws as well as virtues. They compete and sometimes lose; they become jealous and rage against those who defy their wishes. With their all-too-human yearnings of the heart, goddesses open up to mortal women new ways of thinking about their own personalities, relationships, conflicts, and life goals.

The goddesses also offer women, so long ignored by history and orphaned by man-made traditions, a new respect for the oft-maligned female body as the tangible stuff of which a goddess, or a would-be goddess, is made. As reincarnated today, goddesses represent the female embodiment of the life force, of nature's power and beauty, of an untamed and untamable spirit that glows like a flame within us.

Goddesses remind us that we too are miraculous creatures—and the reason lies in both our bodies and our souls. All human life, after all, begins in the female body, the first home any of us knows. In some ways we all, female and male, yearn to return to this special haven. We cannot, but as women, we can reach deep within our body to connect with a timeless source of wisdom and serenity, with what one writer describes as the rivers of connection that flow from all mothers into us.

This poetic truth has a physiological basis. "Our bodies contain information that is beyond our intellectual mind's capacity to understand," notes women's health specialist Christiane Northrup, author of *Women's Bodies, Women's Wisdom*, who traces this deep bodily wisdom to mitochondrial DNA, the genetic legacy (discussed in Chapters 2 and 3) that has been passed from every mother to every daughter for more than 100,000 years. Because of its presence, ancient memories quite literally live in our cells. "We are much more than we think we are," Northrup observes. "Our bodies are the conduits through which we connect with the earth"—and, as spiritual feminists might add, with the heavens, too.

Although I've always taken pride in having my feet planted solidly on the ground, something about the goddess path, as some call it, appeals to me. Perhaps it's because I am named for a goddess—Diana, the free-spirited goddess of the hunt and the moon. Before my baptism, the priest at our neighborhood Catholic church expressed misgivings about such a pagan name. And so my parents chose Mary, after the mother of Jesus, for my middle name. At confirmation, I tacked on Ann—Mary's mother's name—for extra good measure.

Given Diana's independence, Mary's compassion, and Ann's wisdom and patience, I cannot think of a more impressive trio of female idols and ideals to guide my life. And if otherworldly beings can indeed help women encompass passion as well as piety, if they teach us to celebrate the sensual rather than castigating the sinful, if they affirm the joys of the physical and fill the yearnings for the spiritual, we have ample reason to welcome them into our earthly lives. They too, as Maya Angelou reminds us, are God's gift, and as such, they enrich us in body and soul.

C H A P T E R   1 5

Tomorrow's Woman

"I am going to interview a professor about the life of Italian women," I explain to the curious Roman taxi driver as we swerve through the maze of ancient city streets.

"*È buona,*" he assures me. "It's good. For Italian women today, life is very, very good." He pauses a moment and adds: "Maybe it's too good. They go to the universities. They have their own jobs. They have their own money. They have their own houses. They drive their own cars. They can do whatever they want."

"And Italian men—how do they feel about this?" I ask.

"*Signora,*" he says, rolling his eyes upward as if invoking divine intercession, "*abbiamo paura!*"—a phrase that literally translates as "we have fear."

Whenever I repeat this story, women laugh heartily and men smile edgily (except in Italy, where men solemnly exclaim, "*È vero!*"—it's true). Women are changing, everywhere, seemingly in every way, and men are watching with a mix of awe and apprehension. Such anxiety is not new, especially in Rome. More than two thousand years ago, in 195 B.C., Cato complained that "women have become so powerful that our independence has been lost in our homes and is now being trampled and stamped underfoot in public." The reason for his concern: Roman women had sought repeal of a law that forbade their sex from riding in chariots and wearing multicolored dresses.

In the last quarter century, women around the world have changed far more than colors, clothes, and modes of transportation. In a paradigm shift as dramatic as any since the industrial revolution, women have rewritten the roles they live in and the rules we all live by. Women now learn more, earn more, do more, spend more, wield more influence in more places and ways than women of the recent past, let alone antiquity, ever dreamed possible. They also have demonstrated, beyond doubt, that a woman's uniquely female biology—the form of her skeleton, the functioning of her organs, the flux of her hormones, the intricacies of her psyche—is neither a limitation nor a liability.

"We have crossed a great divide," states one corporate demographic analyst, noting a slowing, but no reversal, in the breakneck pace of the recent upheavals. In 1950, one in three American women of working age had a paid job; now almost three in four do. At some point in their lives, 99 percent of women in the United States will work for pay. The same is true for most Nordic countries, and the percentage of working women throughout Europe continues to increase.

From 1970 to 1990 the proportion of American households made up of married couples with children fell from 40 to 26 percent; from 1990 to 1997 the decline was just 1 percent. The divorce rate, once up to 55 percent in the United States, has dropped, and the Census Bureau now estimates that most new marriages will endure, with a mere (at least relatively) 40 percent predicted to fail. While more households are headed by single mothers (18 percent in 1997) and single fathers (5 percent), their numbers are rising more slowly than in previous years. The percentage of working married women who also have school-age children—now 77 percent—is expected to grow, but more gradually, to an estimated 80 percent within the next decade.

Unquestionably, the world is a different place than it was not very long ago. Some call the silent revolution that has restructured modern culture "feminization"; others see it as a long-overdue normalization. I think of it as humanization, the stretching of a man-sized world into a universe large and deep enough to accommodate the perspectives and potential of two similar but distinct sexes. Whatever the name, it's taking some getting used to.

On a flight across the United States, Wendy Reid Crisp, of the National Association of Female Executives, sits next to a man who echoes the Roman cabbie's anxieties. "Women don't need men anymore," he laments. "They can support themselves. For sex, they have vibrators. For babies, they have sperm banks. If something breaks, they hire plumbers and electricians." She and I chuckle over this backhanded tribute to the newfound self-sufficiency of our sex, but then I ask, "So why *do* women still want men in our lives?" "Because," says Crisp, "it's no fun doing it all by yourself."

Ah, yes. At the dawn of a brand-new century, we—women and men—are still figuring it out as we go, feeling our way into the future. In some ways, female and male lives overlap more than ever before. More women are fighting fires or serving as soldiers; more men are teaching in primary schools or nursing the ill. Women are kick-boxing; men are meditating. Board a plane, and the pilot in the cockpit may well be female. Drop by a preschool, and the parent clapping and singing at morning circle may be a father or a mother. Stroll through an office on a dress-down Friday, and female and male employees are wearing unisex combinations of khakis, T-shirts, and athletic shoes. But under the veneer of casual androgyny runs an undercurrent of vague unease.

What's behind it? Revolutions, even silent ones, topple the powerful. Men—particularly the elite of mainly white, middle- and upper-class men—have had to share once-exclusive prerogatives and power with women. And at every socioeconomic level, men have had to confront a jarring new reality: Women no longer need them to provide provisions and protection.

This is not a trivial change. In tracking social attitudes across the United States over the course of two decades, the Yankelovitch Monitor Survey annually asked women and men to define masculinity. The most common answer, from both sexes, had nothing to do with male biology, athletic ability, or sexual prowess; it was being a good provider for his family. This standard has become moot. These days married women are likely to be equal or primary breadwinners. In two of every five American families, women are the sole earners; one in four makes more than her husband.

No longer defined by their paychecks, men are struggling to figure out who they are and what they want to become—something women have been doing for years. "Women are developing a new belief system; a new way of viewing life is coalescing," one accomplished man tells Gail Sheehy in *Understanding Men's Passages.* "Most men don't know what's happening to them. . . . It's a time when men are very, very uncertain." The reason is not simply that women are changing, but that men realize they too must change. "Generally speaking, they associate change with loss, giving up, being overtaken, failing," Sheehy observes. "It is not seen as a positive part of inner growth and the road to a new kind of power."

Women too are still sorting out options. We know what we are not; we have a good idea of what we don't want to be. But our concepts of who we truly are or want to become are still evolving. On the one hand, we yearn to see ourselves and to be seen as people, detached from gender and free of female tethers. On the other, we don't want to stop being women or exploring all the dimensions of our womanly natures.

From Neverland to Critical Mass

At age five Denilha Jackson watched a man blast concrete with a jackhammer near her home in Oakland, California, and said, "I want to do that when I grow up." He leaned over and said, "Little girl, you'll never be able to use one of these." He was wrong. Today, working for a utility company, she routinely pulverizes asphalt with a ninety-pound jackhammer.

When Dot Richardson was eleven, a baseball scout told her that she'd never get a chance to use her great pitching arm—the best he'd ever seen—unless she cut her hair and pretended to be a boy. She refused. Defying his prediction, she grew up to win an Olympic gold medal in women's softball in 1996.

"It's too bad you were born a girl," her brother once told Marian Diamond. "You'll never amount to anything." He underestimated her. Determined to learn, delighted to teach, she became a professor, a world-renowned brain researcher, a museum director, and the first female associate dean of the College of Arts and Sciences at the University of California, Berkeley.

"Never" used to be part of the "spin" on women: They never could, never would be big, fast, smart, or tough enough to make it in a man's world, a man's game, or a man's job. So declared the conventional wisdom—often justified by standards that seemed reasonable and fair, yet were anything but.

Consider one of the most apparently objective of those standards: height. Whenever this single criterion was used as a basis for selection, women almost inevitably came up short. For years many police departments, among other institutions, set minimum height as a prerequisite for all applicants—in effect, disqualifying women (and a good number of men). When the height standard was challenged and eliminated, many predicted that the women who joined inner-city forces would never measure up, literally or figuratively. Instead, they proved remarkably effective at defusing domestic violence situations and at relating to certain groups, particularly tough-talking young men, in a nonconfrontational way. Over time, the contributions of women in law enforcement changed the definition of what makes a good officer, shifting the emphasis from size to skills such as conflict management and negotiation.

Other women, shut out by traditional barriers, found completely new alternatives. One of these was Mary Louise Cleave, who as a girl loved flying and hoped to become a flight attendant. Barely five feet two inches tall, she never qualified for any of the airlines' training programs. Instead—in my favorite example of a creative career switch— she applied to NASA. As an astronaut, Cleave flew two missions aboard the space shuttle and logged an impressive 262 hours in space, soaring higher than she had ever dreamed she could or would go.

Throughout the 1980s many other women like Cleave went places where few women had ever gone before. They became mayors and federal marshals, admirals and ambassadors, rabbis and race car drivers. In the 1990s the era of fabulous firsts gave way to a different stage: critical mass. In a 1998 review of the major industrial nations, *Newsweek* surveyed the state of their economies and concluded, "It's a woman's world."

The declaration strikes me as premature, but trends do favor tomorrow's woman. Education is the primary reason. In the European Union, 110 women have college degrees for every 100 men who do. In the United States, women now receive 37 percent of MBAs, 43 percent of medical degrees, and 41 percent of law school diplomas.

In the global workforce, the ranks of women have soared. More than 40 percent of the women in the European Union now work (the exception is Italy, where the figure is 37 percent). In Russia, Great Britain,

Germany, and the United States, more than 60 percent of women hold paying jobs. The shift from heavy industry to knowledge and information industries—computers, electronics, health care, financial services—continues to open up more opportunities for women. In Great Britain, economists predict that women will win 1 million of the 1.4 million jobs created in the next ten years. In the United States, women and minorities are expected to fill the majority of new positions.

Most women, though, still make less money than men in comparable jobs. American women earn about three quarters of what men do; in France, Italy, and Great Britain, women do somewhat better, earning 79 to 81 percent of male income. In certain areas the income gap is narrowing—for instance, in entry-level positions, particularly in science and technology, where college-educated women age twenty-four to thirty-three earn 98 percent of what their male counterparts do. However, as women advance, salary discrepancies remain entrenched.

At the very top, the glass ceiling, though raised to new heights, has proved frustratingly difficult to shatter. Some analysts now advise women to look for glass "skylights" and squeeze through one at a time. Others are calling for reinforcements. Psychiatrist Leah Dickstein, a former president of the American Medical Women's Association, carries a square of virtually impenetrable clear plastic in her purse. "When I give talks, I pass it around to show women what the glass ceiling is really made of. There's no way a woman can break through it on her own." Only a few have managed to do so. Among the Fortune 500 companies, just 11 percent of corporate officers are women; the total number of female chief executive officers in 1998 was two. A survey of the 70,000 largest companies in Germany found that women fill only 1 to 3 percent of top executive and board positions. Great Britain reports only one female chief executive officer—an American woman who heads Pearson, the media giant.

For women in academia, advancement has also been slow—in large part because of pervasive gender bias. Researchers in Sweden, the nation that leads the world in providing equal opportunities for the sexes, recently documented such discrimination in an in-depth analysis of the selection process for postdoctoral fellowships. In order to be rated the equal of a male candidate, a woman had to be more than twice as good.

For every paper a male candidate published in the most prestigious general science journals, for instance, she had to publish at least three. For every paper a man wrote for a top publication in a specific field, she had to publish twenty. If such bias could happen in Sweden, the researchers concluded, "it is not too far-fetched to assume that gender-based discrimination may occur elsewhere."

Unfortunately, it does, but critical mass may improve the situation. Experts in gender equity explain that a woman applicant doesn't have a chance at a fair evaluation unless at least 25 percent of the candidates for a job are female. With fewer women in the running, the position—consciously or not—is seen as a man's job and a woman has to exceed the qualifications of the male candidates simply to appear equally competent.

As the percentage of women in any particular occupation pushes beyond 40 percent, the playing field truly levels out—and this is happening in more and more arenas. In the United States, women fill 48 percent of corporate managerial and professional slots, and make up 43 percent of enlisted soldiers, 43 percent of economists, and 33 percent of those at a decision-making level in government. In other fields, however, they still lag far behind. Moreover, women continue to work in a much narrower range of occupations than men. In the European Union, half of employed women work in sales, clerical work, nursing, or teaching; less than a third of high-tech workers are women. Only 8 percent of American engineers, 10 percent of apprentices in the trades, 12 percent of military officers, and 15 percent of architects are female.

As long as these numbers remain so low, women—as has happened in middle management in the past—may find themselves isolated from the male majority and vying with each other for the next higher "female" opportunity. In such settings, some victors turn into imperious Queen Bees who do nothing to help other women advance. Again, critical mass can change this dynamic. With more women above, below, and at her side, an individual woman is less likely to see female coworkers as threats and more likely to work with them to achieve common goals.

Beyond Men in Skirts

When, at age twenty-five, I became editor of a national magazine for medical students, I decided to dress the part. The first time one of my friends saw me in my professional garb—pinstriped power suit, padded shoulders, floppy tie—she burst out laughing: "You look like a midget man," she said.

At times I did indeed feel like a male impostor, especially when smiling at sexist jokes I didn't find funny or struggling not to blush at vulgarities meant to tease or taunt. It never occurred to me that the men I worked for and with might change their behavior. Back in the 1970s, we women thought we had only one choice: to become one of the boys.

Lord knows we tried. A sports reporter covering the local football team learned to outcurse the athletes in the locker room and the editors in the newsroom. A junior faculty member at an Ivy League university, determined to show how tough she was, went into labor in the middle of an important lecture. "I took off my watch and laid it on the podium so I could time the contractions. Every time one hit, my knees would buckle and I'd grab on to the sides of the lectern." By the time she finished, the contractions were seven minutes apart, and she scurried—as best she could—for a taxi to get to the hospital.

Other women adopted the style of the only management role models they saw. "My bosses had all been warriors whose idea of success was bringing back the bloody head of the enemy on a spear," says one woman who rose swiftly through the ranks of a multinational corporation. "I thought I had to be just as intimidating, so I screamed and bullied. But it was so draining that afterward I'd go back to my office, put my head on the desk, and think, 'There has to be a better way.'"

There was, but it took women a long time not just to find it but to feel confident enough to try it. "We were damned whatever we did," observes Carolyn Duff in *When Women Work Together*. "If we acted like men, men often felt threatened by our directness and competitiveness, and many women found us alienating and difficult to work with. On the other hand, if we acted like women—seeming reluctant to play power politics and insisting on bringing relationship-based values into an objective, competitive 'male' workplace—men found our feminine behavior a sign of weakness."

The toll of such conflicting pressures can be seen in the experience of the women entering the University of Pennsylvania's distinguished law school in the late 1980s. "Before you can become an attorney," a professor told them in an orientation address, "you must first become a gentleman." The women in the audience bristled. Academically, they were virtually identical to their male peers, with stellar scores on their LSATs, near-perfect GPAs, multiple honors, and degrees from distinguished colleges. In their first year of law school, the women found much more to object to, including the ubiquitous use of *he* in lectures, the lack of personal attention from professors, and the hostile baiting from male students.

Over the course of their three years of law school, these women voiced fewer complaints. In fact, they became quieter and quieter. Initially the academic equals of their male peers, they fell behind. By graduation, the men were much more likely to be in the top 10 percent of the class, to make law review, and to win prestigious clerkships. The women scored higher primarily in psychological distress, including depression, insomnia, and diminished self-esteem. By their final year, only 15 percent of the women—compared with 68 percent of the men—said they had never cried during law school; 35 percent of the women—and 4 percent of the men—cried at least once a month.

"What was in the air-conditioning that changed these women?" asks psychologist Michelle Fine, who along with law professor Lani Guinier studied the psychological impact of legal education on women. Was it the adversarial teaching style? The indifference of an almost all-white male faculty? The peer hazing that branded any woman who spoke up a "bitch" or "feminazi"?

"There are ways in which institutions teach you your place, even if they look neutral," says Fine. "You end up losing your voice, losing your politics, losing yourself, and becoming stupid. It's not peculiar to law school, and it's not true that all white males thrived in this school. But the price of success seemed higher for women." The underlying reason, she believes, was not the intellectual challenge of learning law, but the pressures on women to become something they never could be—men.

With more female students and more diverse faculties, law schools are changing. Even the classic adversarial teaching model has come under fire from critics who charge that it neglects the skills most valuable in a legal career: negotiation, thoughtful analysis, and creative problem solving, areas in which women often excel. But such abilities, at least so far, have not translated into career advancement for female attorneys. A 1996 report by the American Bar Association found a gender gap in income at every level of experience and far fewer opportunities for women to advance to the rank of partner or judge.

In other fields, though, women have developed distinctive and effective ways of working and leading. As described by management professor Judy Rosener, of the University of California, Irvine, a "female" approach (neither used by all women nor eschewed by all men) differs from the traditional "male" hierarchical command-and-control model in several ways: flexibility, an emphasis on cooperation, team building, decision making by consensus, and motivation by encouraging individual growth. In the last decade, as companies have "flattened" their organizations to compete in the global workplace, this innovative style has become pervasive.

At the same time, growing numbers of women have created another mold-breaking model as entrepreneurs. In one of the most remarkable economic trends of the last decade, women have gone into business for themselves at twice the rate of men. Some of the newly self-employed were downsized out of their jobs; others became disillusioned with the bottom-line focus of big business; many want greater flexibility, more autonomy, less of the pressure of the rat race (even if they end up racing just as hard on their own), greater independence in decision making, less office politicking, plus the rewards of being one's own boss—and not having to answer to anyone but investors.

A lot of new women-owned ventures are modest—retail shops, online marketplaces, personal services businesses—but their cumulative clout is impressive. According to the National Foundation of Women Business Owners, women-owned businesses increased 78 percent in less than a decade (from 1987 to 1996) to nearly eight million, generating some $2.3 trillion in annual revenues and employing one in four American workers. Female entrepreneurs, as top government officials have proclaimed, are "changing the face of the American and global economy."

Starting businesses isn't the only way women are doing so. With more women bringing home the bacon (or a major chunk of it), they're deciding how it's spent. Economic analysts estimate that American women, as previously noted, control or influence the spending of 80 percent of consumer dollars, make 75 percent of health care decisions, purchase most household appliances, and buy about half of all cars and a quarter of all light trucks. With such formidable financial clout, women have become the consumers most worth wooing.

To attract female buyers, auto manufacturers are adding keyless locks and more of the safety features women want to their vehicles. Architects are changing blueprints to meet women's design preferences (bigger bathrooms are one). Food manufacturers are developing an expanded array of heat-and-eat "meal replacements." Movie and television producers are commissioning scripts that feature meaningful relationships. Even the rigid corporate world is beginning to offer flextime, telecommuting, on-site day care, and other innovations that acknowledge the existence of priorities other than those that come with the job. A world once custom-designed to fit its male residents is becoming more female-friendly.

Some complain that what we're seeing are changes in style, not substance. Women are still fighting for equal pay, better benefits, quality day care, more opportunity for advancement. Even so, they are optimistic about the future. A recent international poll found that two thirds of American women, along with half of European women, expect the next twenty years to usher in more improvements for women. Younger women, between the ages of eighteen and twenty-four, are most optimistic of all. And why shouldn't they be? The financial force some call "womenomics" is with them.

The New Collaborators

I was dashing out of the house to interview a celebrity author when I realized my tape recorder had jammed. Frantically I seized the only recording device I was sure worked—my then-baby daughter's Sesame Street cassette player. When I set the garish yellow-and-green device, decorated with Big Bird and pals, down on the author's elegant coffee table, both of us burst out laughing. "It was the best ice-breaker I ever saw," she says. It also got the job done.

This is the bottom line today's mothers focus on as we speed-dial through our busy days. Forget the supermoms of the eighties, who were expected to do it all, or the "jugglers" of the nineties, always struggling to keep all the balls in the air. "Say hello to the new millennium woman," says *Working Mother* magazine. "Meet Improv Mom."

It's a natural fit. Females have always had to adapt, to react quickly, to be flexible enough to handle ever-changing situations. These days what works best for many women is improvising, moving to the ever-changing rhythms of their lives with the virtuosity of a musician playing a jazz riff, going with the flow, adapting creatively but always coming back to a basic theme. Undeniably stressed, often sleep-deprived, improv moms survive by setting priorities. Children rank at the very top. Jobs get their share of attention and energy. Last on most lists is housework, which Lenin, hardly a feminist hero, once described as "the most unproductive, savage, and most arduous work a woman can do."

American women started liberating themselves from this oppressor decades ago. From 1965 to 1985, demographers have calculated, married mothers reduced the time they devoted to housework by ten hours a week (from thirty hours to twenty); husbands doubled theirs (from five to ten). Couples who could afford them hired cleaning services. Those who couldn't lowered their standards from the spic-and-span perfection of a generation ago. But as recently as the 1980s, many women were still putting in a second shift of domestic toil, and "chore wars" were erupting in sticky-countered kitchens across the land.

In the last decade something happened—at first I assumed it was only in my house. Overwhelmed by deadlines to meet, homework to check, and a dozen daily emergencies, I simply stopped doing things I always had, like cooking dinner from scratch or constantly monitoring refrigerator and pantry supplies. As I did less, my husband did more—not just the weekly grocery shopping (a survival strategy, since our cupboards so often resembled Mother Hubbard's) but more hands-on fathering as well. And he did it without a single pitched battle (though there were many not-so-veiled hints). Little did either of us realize that he was part of a trend. A new breed of collaborative dads, as it turns out, is joining forces with improv moms to do what needs to be done in their daily lives.

Like my husband, one in four men now does most of the grocery shopping, up from 15 percent of men in 1986, according to *American Demographics*. In an eye-opening (and eyebrow-raising) report released in 1998, the Family and Work Institute of New York calculated that American husbands put in 75 percent as much time as wives on workday chores—a dramatic rise from 30 percent in 1977. Now the gender difference in domestic "scutwork" amounts to just forty-five minutes a day.

Plenty of sociologists—and lots of weary women still doing the lioness's share of chores—doubt whether all men in all income groups are doing as much as those in the survey (and even they may have overstated their contributions). However, the trend toward greater husbandly involvement is real and likely to continue as more Generation X–ers form households of their own. "Younger men don't even think twice about pitching in," says a woman in her mid-thirties with a spouse almost ten years her junior. "They have working mothers who raised them differently—thank God."

Every family's arrangement may be a little different, but the pattern is similar. Mom drops the kids off at day care; Dad picks them up. She does the laundry; he handles the dry cleaning. She pays the bills; he gets the cars serviced. And when he's on deadline or she's out of town, they pinch-hit for each other. "Does it work all the time?" says a friend in one of these makeshift marital arrangements. "Of course not—but nothing does. And as long as each of us feels that the other is trying, we don't get bogged down in fights over who did or didn't take out the garbage last."

The basis of the new collaboration goes beyond shared chores to shared values. In a study of three hundred dual-earner couples in the Boston area, women and men showed remarkable similarities in how they felt about their relationship with each other and with their children. Contrary to the old assumption that family problems were female concerns and work issues male, both spouses showed equal sensitivity to stress at home, problems in the marital relationship, and job concerns. Another study found that gender has virtually no bearing on how parents respond, physically or psychologically, to situations in which work interferes with family life or family life interferes with work. Mothers *and* fathers care—and care deeply—about both.

Will husbands and fathers—as wives and mothers so often have— put their families ahead of their careers? For many, the answer is yes.

According to a survey of more than six thousand Dupont employees, only slightly fewer men than women say they have made career trade-offs to try to balance their work and family life, including turning down relocations or jobs that require extensive travel. In another survey of forty large companies, responses were similar. "There is increasing congruence between men's answers and women's," observes a corporate consultant. "More men are making trade-offs in favor of their families."

What's behind this sea change? My own theory is that today's wives and husbands, rather than remaining stranded on other planets, are coming down to earth. Dealing with similar problems and pressures, sharing similar commitments and ideals, they each "get it." Working wives know the pit-in-the-stomach lurch when sales figures slump for the third quarter in a row. Involved fathers know the helplessness of waiting for the pediatrician's call while a feverish child wails in their arms. We sympathize; we empathize; and, if only for pragmatic reasons, we pitch in. But such cooperation—still not the norm in many marriages, especially when both spouses are putting in too many hours for too little money—is just one aspect of what truly synergistic relationships can become.

Synergy and Soul Mates

Like many long-married couples, neuroscientists Raquel and Ruben Gur, of the University of Pennsylvania, often couldn't understand why their spouse did the things he or she did. Why did he react to a crisis by rushing into action? Why did she spend endless hours mulling over the same old problem? Why was he so preoccupied with numbers and details? Why was she so focused on feelings?

"At times it almost feels like Raquel and I are two different species trying to deal with the same problem," says Ruben Gur. "Ours is a fundamental difference in the way we approach life. I see a lot of things from the perspective of territory. My reaction is, 'I won't let that son-of-a-bitch take over.' Raquel competes more against her own standards, without paying too much attention to what others are doing, and she naturally considers personal commitment, feelings, and issues. I have to force myself to look at things that way."

The Gurs (whose work is described in previous chapters) decided to look for answers by comparing and contrasting female and male brains. What they found were fundamental differences—subtle but potentially significant—in the way the sexes process information, respond to provocation, and interpret emotion. Why should such differences exist? "It makes sense evolutionarily," Ruben Gur speculates. "It's more adaptive for the species to have two different angles on reality that are not entirely overlapping but complementary. As long as there is cooperation among males and females, the variability becomes a strength."

It's a strength we've rarely taken advantage of. Most of what we know about ourselves as humans is a story seen by one eye, heard by one ear, conceived by one part of the brain—all male or modeled on the male. I am not suggesting we have lived in the reign of a cyclops. But we certainly haven't availed ourselves of dimensions that might be grasped only by binocular vision and stereophonic hearing.

Imagine the possibilities such a combination might create: strength working in tandem with stamina, the male's laserlike focus expanding to take in the female's embrace of big-picture context, the female's quest for meaningful connections enriching the male's determination to get things done. In theology, business, education, and communications, there is an emerging recognition of a different vision, a different voice, a different viewpoint—a female one, neither inferior nor superior, neither right nor wrong, neither better nor worse, but one that may open up new and unexplored possibilities for both sexes.

Recently I listened as a broadcast interviewer asked a group of teenagers what they would look for in a mate. Thinking of the evolutionary theories discussed in Chapter 3, I waited for a modern variation on the male's allegedly age-old desire for an attractive, fertile, narrow-waisted woman and the female's preference for a resource-rich, willing-to-commit man. Instead, girls and boys all said the same thing: They want to marry their soul mates. Don't we all?

By my definition, a soul mate isn't a clone or even a reverse-image mirror reflection of who we are, but a person who complements and completes, who takes the hidden best part of us and burnishes it till it glows. What one soul mate brings to and does for the other isn't defined by gender—even though that's the traditional assumption.

"Quite a few years back I figured out what that piece in Corinthians that starts out, 'Wives, be subject to your husbands' was all about—at least for me," comments a lector in the Catholic Church. "Everybody needs a wife sometimes—a wife who will be subject to the needs of a sometimes demanding spouse. My thirty-four years of happy marriage taught me that sometimes, when I came staggering home from law school or from the office, I needed Richard to set aside his needs for the moment and see to mine. I had plenty of opportunities to do the same for him as well, picking him up in the wee hours after marathon film-editing sessions, cheering him on through lean spots in the freelance career that was so dear to his heart. I cooked for the first twelve years or so, then I went to law school and he took over the cooking. We nurtured each other and the children, as any wife would do. St. Paul also enjoins husbands to love their wives, and we loved each other, vigorously and passionately and right up until the end."

Now widowed, this woman remains "grateful for having had both a husband and a wife, and for having had the opportunity to be both. St. Paul's text is wonderful in that it doesn't attach any gender to the roles of husband and wife; it just describes their essential qualities. I pity the stiff-necked folks who read in cultural constraints that just aren't there and narrow their lives accordingly."

I do, too. The synergy of mutual commitment dissolves gender's tethers—to the benefit not just of the soul but of the body. As researchers have consistently confirmed, loving, supportive relationships nourish emotional well-being and robust physical health. Initially everyone assumed this would be primarily true of women, but it turns out to be even more relevant for men. A University of California, San Francisco, study of men between the ages of forty-five and sixty-four found that those who lived with wives were twice as likely to live ten years longer than their unmarried age peers—regardless of income, education, and risk factors such as smoking and obesity. Curiously, live-in lady friends did not have the same beneficial effect, nor did grown children or other relatives.

Longevity is just one of the dividends men derive from marriage. "Men often tell me in interviews, 'My wife has helped me to discover aspects of myself I never knew were there,'" observes Gail Sheehy, who has described wives as "sensibility specialists." Some women may object to this designation or duty; I do not. To touch and be touched by another soul, to reach beyond self-interest or need, is an experience enriching to both partners. It is the essence of the synergy that binds soul mates together, that keeps both alive and shining through all the years they share.

Although this may sound like new-millennium philosophizing, the idea, like many a utopian vision, is hardly new. Peering into the twentieth century, the pioneering feminist Susan B. Anthony expressed a similar vision: "The day will come," she predicted, "when man will recognize woman as his peer, not only at the fireside but in the councils of the nation. Then, and not until then, will there be perfect comradeship, the ideal union between the sexes that shall result in the highest development of the race." At long last we may be moving at least a little closer to this goal.

Stretching into the Future

I saw tomorrow's woman today—one of them, anyway. She was looking into a mirror and grinning at something she considers a personal triumph: the fact that, at age twelve, she already towers over me, her mother. In the years in which I was working on this book, my daughter grew four inches. She also shot ahead of me in other ways, learning to speak Spanish, play basketball, ride horses—all things I cannot do.

"Well," I tell her, "I'm still taller than Grandma." I also do plenty of things my mother never did—drive a car, use a computer, jog five miles a day. Isn't this the way it's supposed to be? Each generation reaches upward, stretches taller, learns new things, creates more opportunities for those who will come next.

My generation of baby boomers has certainly done its share of stretching—if only because we've been so determined to have it all. Did we succeed? You wouldn't know from the headlines. Daughters of careerist women, I read, are rejecting their driven mothers' ambitions—yet never have there been more young women in colleges and universities. Working women, the glum headlines note, are stressed to the max—yet on surveys of happiness they consistently outscore all comers. Aging women, newscasters report, are melting down in menopausal funks—yet record numbers of fifty-plus women are forging into classrooms, competing in master's-level sports, taking to sea kayaks and snowshoes to explore the world. Teenage girls supposedly are self-destructing—but I see them banding together and cheering each other on with "you go, girl" enthusiasm. In 1998 the *New York Times* dedicated a special issue of its Sunday magazine to the subject "Mothers Can't Win"—as if winning had something to do with mothering. But there wasn't a loser among the mothers featured inside—just complex, busy, questioning women who loved their kids, their jobs, and, yes, their complicated, hectic, exhausting, but enormously gratifying lives.

The women I know are like that. While we may not have it all, we have a lot. What do we want for the future? More—for ourselves and for our daughters. And I think we're going to get it. In the last quarter century, time and again, women have repeatedly defied predictions of failure—that they'd wimp out in crises, wear out in crunches, break down in courtrooms, cry under fire. Rather than heeding the alarmists or wasting energy arguing with them, they pressed on, identifying what they wanted and going after it.

What women want, however, isn't necessarily the same as what many men seek. Some of the successful women I talked with—many of whom had never expected to run their own departments, head their own staffs, or earn hefty six-figure salaries—are feeling the pangs of what I think of as the Peggy Lee syndrome, a vague sense that if this is all there is, it's not what it was cracked up to be. "I'm definitely in the top one percent of women in my field—in pay, security, prestige," one chief operating officer told me. "But the rewards don't seem like enough. A corner office and a big expense account just don't do it for me."

Disillusioned, downsized, battered by the brutal realities of business, more men are having similar misgivings—not just about the symbols of success but about the sacrifices it demands. However, the ones who are taking the lead in creating more varied and fulfilling lives—by starting their own businesses, by cultivating personal interests, by exploring their spirituality, by pursuing passionate quests of every type—are women. The trails they blaze may open up new territory for everyone.

Some of tomorrow's women, no doubt, will soar into new realms of achievement in politics, government, business, industry, law, science. For others, a career will be not a life, but an enriching part of a multifaceted existence. Most will marry and have children, though a growing minority will not. Some will do noble and ennobling things; others will be petty, mean-spirited, and downright malicious. Some will work tirelessly to help the less fortunate; others will never look out for anyone but themselves. In all these ways, the lives of tomorrow's women will resemble those of tomorrow's men.

Yet even as opportunities for the two sexes become more equal, even as women and men grow closer as they work and love together, they will never be the same. Female biology will sweep our daughters and grand-daughters into its cycles and rhythms, awakening in them a sense of growth and renewal. The genetic legacy of our foremothers will live in their cells, serving as reservoirs of ancient wisdom. They will share our complexity, our flexibility, our flair for weaving the rich tapestry threads of profound emotional attachments into our lives, and the abiding affection for the other gender that most of us feel. Being female will remain an experience at the same time universal to all women and unique to every woman.

A friend of mine, an astute trendwatcher, speculates that we are at the dawn of what will become the women's millennium. Thinking of all the inequities, injustices, and discrimination still to be overcome, I rue-fully tell him that we'd settle for a decent century or two. Nonetheless, I do think we are moving to a better place and time, one that is taking shape in the minds and hearts of today's women.

In researching this book, I posted numerous queries on the Internet. A poet responded to one. "I liked the title: just like a woman," she wrote, then continued in verse:

> after all, we, most of us, are only Just Like
> we appear,
> and did not yet learn to BE.

More and more of us are moving beyond the limits of "like." When people ask me where I see women heading, I say we are becoming our-selves. We are not defying or denying our bodies; we are fighting—and slaying—stereotypes about female biology. We are not compromising our innermost being; we are discovering new aspects of our identity. We are not striving to meet male standards for success; we are setting our own agendas. We are making choices today that, for all the tomorrows to come, will allow women to stretch beyond any single notion of what being "just like a woman" must or might mean. And the more that all of us learn about our possibilities—as women, as men, as human beings—the less that any of us will have to fear.

ACKNOWLEDGMENTS

My greatest debt, in ways that go far beyond this book, is to a trio of remarkable individuals, all named Harris. This is the third book I have written for Ann Harris, editor, mentor, collaborator, and friend. Over many years, she has guided my growth as a writer more than any other individual, always encouraging me to push beyond my limits, ever helpful in steering me away from cliff edges. This book is infinitely better because of her countless contributions to it. I am deeply grateful for her expertise, wisdom, and inspiration.

My agent Joy Harris also has been a partner, advocate, friend, and—when I needed it most—unflagging cheerleader. Her belief in me has sustained me through the very long gestations all my books seem to require. I value immensely her judgment, insight, humor, and tremendous loyalty.

Another friend and mentor, the editor-extraordinaire T George Harris, has lit up my life ever since I first worked for him on the launch of *American Health* almost twenty years ago. On this project, George was there to help every time I bumped into a creative block or a wall of discouragement. And at his side has been another great lady and new ally, Jeannie Pinkerton Harris.

Many others contributed greatly to the preparation of this book. I am especially grateful to Marianne Legato, who repeatedly made time to help, talk, review drafts, and illuminate my understanding of gender medicine. I owe special thanks to Ruth McClendon for allowing me to sit in on her extraordinary women's retreat, and to the women in the group for their fierce honesty.

In addition to these two women, I want to thank the following individuals for their review of various parts of the manuscript: Vivien Burt, Barbara Parry, Lynn Ponton, Carol Tavris, Carol Wade, and Beverly Whipple. Their comments saved me from many a careless statement or foolish mistake. (The errors that remain are wholly my own.)

I also am most appreciative of those who made time for personal interviews, including: Myrna Blyth, Mark Breedlove, Louann Brizendine, Thomas Crook, Marian Diamond, Leah Dickstein, Chris Essex, Leah Fisher, Pier Maria Furlan, Deborah Gale, Mark George, Judith Gold, Raquel and Ruben Gur, Judith Hall, Alexander Harcourt, Sharon Harvey, Robin Hayden, Chris Hayward, Lana Holstein, Nina Jablonski, Nancy Kaltreider, Liz Kramer, Joan Leiman, Mary Clare Lennon, Ellen Levine, Franca Lolli, Felice Lieh Mak, Norma McCoy, Robin McFarland, Myriam Van Moffaert, Monique Borgerhof Mulder, Amelia Mussacchio, Carol Nadelson, Barbara Parry, James Pennebaker, Ethel Person, Elisabetta Rasy, Lusanda Rataemane, Jane Reese, Gail Robinson, Ruth Rosen, Alexis Rubin, Lynsey Rubin, Virginia Sadock, Sofia Salamovich, Diane Schechter, Juliana Schiesari, Sally Shaywitz, Barbara Sherwin, Barbara Sommer, Donna Stewart, Susan Sussman, Wenda Trevathan, Martha Ward, Beverly Whipple, Gary Wright, and Adrienne Zihlman.

I also thank the following for supplying me with invaluable research materials: American Anthropological Association; American Association of University Women; American College of Obstetrics and Gynecology; American Engineering Society; American Psychiatric Association; American Psychological Association; Beatrice Bain Research Group at the University of California, Berkeley; Susan Blumenthal; Joan Carter; Catalyst; Commonwealth Fund; Jean Endicott; Endocrine Society; Carolyn Tucker Halpern; Institute for the Study of Gender at Stanford University; Jacobs Institute of Women's Health; Jeanne Leventhal; Ellen Mercer; Ms. Foundation; Murray Research Institute at Radcliffe College; Museum of Menstruation; National Association of Female Executives; National Black

Women's Health Project; National Center for Infertility; National Institute of Mental Health; News Office at the University of California, San Francisco; North American Menopause Society; Obstetrics and Gynecology Research and Education Foundation; Office of Women's Health Research; Partnership for Women's Health at Columbia University; Vivien Pin; Procter & Gamble Business Information Services; Mona Lisa Schulz; Stephanie Shields; SIECUS; Society for Menstrual Research; Society for Neuroscience; Society for the Advancement of Health Research in Women; Myrna Weissman; Women's Center and Library at the University of California, Davis; Women's History Project.

As always, I am profoundly thankful for my husband Bob and daughter Julia, the joys of my life. During the years in which this project engulfed my time and attention, they were constantly supportive and encouraging. In a thousand ways, they made writing this book possible.

To all these individuals and organizations, and so many others who have expanded my understanding and appreciation of women, thank you.

N O T E S

Chapter 1: What Is a Woman?

Page 3. "Just like a woman, I can act like a lady . . . ": This observation comes from Marilyn Martin, "The Stressless Woman: An Oxymoron," presentation at the Jacobs Institute of Women's Health, Washington, DC, October 10, 1996.

Page 4. "A head too small for intellect": The obstetrical textbook by Charles Meigs is quoted in Estelle Ramey, "How Female and Male Biology Differ," in Florence Haseltine (editor), *Women's Health Research: A Medical and Policy Primer* (Washington, DC: American Psychiatric Press, 1997), p. 47.

Page 4. Women receive the majority of baccalaureate degrees: Steven Holmes, "Women Surpass Men in Educational Achievement, Census Reports," *New York Times*, June 30, 1998, p. A18.

Page 4. Women's marital and fertility rates: These data come from the U.S. Census Bureau and other sources, including Jean-Claude Chesnais, "Fertility, Family and Social Policy in Contemporary Western Europe," *Population and Development Review*, vol. 22, no. 4 (December 1996), p. 729.

Page 5. Survey on which sex has an easier time in life: These results were reported in "Easy Sex," *Psychology Today*, vol. 29, no. 5 (September–October 1996), p. 22.

Page 6. "Just like a woman" misses the essential point: Paola Bono and Sandra Kemp (editors), *Italian Feminist Thought: A Reader* (Oxford: Basil Blackwell, 1991), p. 15.

Page 8. "Neither women nor men can be considered superior":

David Buss, "Psychological Sex Differences," *American Psychologist*, vol. 50, no. 3 (March 1995), p. 164.

Page 9. Biological sex differences: Sources for these observations include Marianne Legato, *Gender-Specific Aspects of Human Biology for the Practicing Physician* (Armonk, NY: Futura Publishing, 1997); Miriam Stoppard, *Woman's Body: A Manual for Life* (London: Dorling Kindersley, 1994); Edward Dolnick, "Super Women," *In Health*, July–August 1991, p. 42; Carol Rinzler, "Gender Differences Quiz," *American Health*, September 1995, p. 13; "Women and Men: Biologically the Same?" fact sheet prepared by the Partnership for Women's Health at Columbia University, February 1997; Robert Pool, *Eve's Rib: Searching for the Biological Roots of Sex Differences* (New York: Crown, 1994); Diane McGuiness, "Away from a Unisex Psychology: Individual Differences in Visual Perception," *Perception*, vol. 5 (1976), p. 375.

Page 9. Women's troubling propensity for dizzy spells: Clelia Mosher reported her findings in her book *Women's Physical Freedom* (New York: The Woman's Press, 1923).

Page 12. Anxiety and depression effects: The anxiety research is reported in Daniel Pine et al., "Emotional Problems During Youth as Predictors of Stature During Early Adulthood: Results from a Prospective Epidemiologic Study," *Pediatrics*, vol. 97, no. 6 (June 1996), p. 1; the depression study is Ulrich Schweiger et al., "Low Lumbar Bone Mineral Density in Patients with Major Depression," *American Journal of Psychiatry*, vol. 151, no. 11 (November 1994), p. 1691.

Page 14. Cross-cultural studies of women and depression: These are summarized in Frances Culbertson, "Depression and Gender: An International Review," *American Psychologist*, vol. 52, no. 1 (January 1997), p. 25.

Page 15. Martha Ward's quote. Her textbook on women, *A World Full of Women* (Boston: Allyn and Bacon, 1996), was a rich source of information and inspiration throughout this book.

Page 16. Lou Andreas-Salome's quote: This appears in Genevieve Fraisse and Michelle Perrot, "Lou Andreas-Salome: 'The Humanity of Woman,' " in *Emerging Feminism from Revolution to World War*, vol. 4 in Georges Duby and Michelle Perrot (series editors), *A History of Women in the West* (Cambridge: Harvard University Press, 1993), pp. 542–45.

Page 18. "Spiritual feminist": This quote is from Meinrad Craighead, in Ruth Anderson and Patricia Hopkins, *The Feminine Face of God: The Unfolding of the Sacred in Women* (New York: Bantam Books, 1992), p. 192.

Chapter 2: The Female of the Species

Page 21. Afternoon at the seashore: This description was derived from observations in Beverly McLeod, "Life History, Females, and Evolution: A Commentary," in Mary Ellen Morbeck, Alison Galloway, and Adrienne Zihlman (editors), *The Evolving Female* (Princeton: Princeton University Press, 1997), pp. 270–71.

Page 22. Female diversity: Many of the examples of females of other species throughout this chapter come from Irene Elia, *The Female Animal* (New York: Henry Holt, 1988).

Page 24. The beginning of sex: Biologist Lynn Margulis, of the University of Massachusetts at Amherst, has traced animal sex back to a group of single-cell organisms some 1.5 billion years ago. During periods of starvation, one was driven to devour another, and if not completely digested, the nuclei of prey and predator fused.

Page 24. Size difference in egg and sperm: Richard Dawkins's provocative views on this subject can be found in *The Selfish Gene* (Oxford: Oxford University Press, 1976).

Page 26. The egg's "rehabilitation" of the sperm: Scientists vary in their perspective on this process. In a presentation at the American Society for Cell Biology in January 1996, Cambridge University biologist Laurence Hurst described conception as setting off a tiny war, in which the egg destroys some of the sperm's defective genes, and argued that this competition may be why two sexes evolved in the first place. Psychologist Joan Borysenko sees this process as a nurturing one and comments that women "appear to be programmed at a cellular level to fix the wounds of men" in *A Woman's Book of Life* (New York: Riverhead Books, 1996).

Page 27–28. Competition among female elephant seals: These observations come from Joanne Reiter, "Life History and Reproductive Success of Female Northern Elephant Seals," in Mary Ellen Morbeck, Alison Galloway, and Adrienne Zihlman (editors), *The Evolving Female* (Princeton: Princeton University Press, 1997), pp. 44–52.

Page 29. Courting behaviors: The sexual strategies included here are described in greater depth in David Buss, "The Evolution of Human Intrasexual Competition: Tactics of Mate Attraction," *Journal of Personality and Social Psychology*, vol. 54, no. 4 (1993), p. 616; David Buss, *The Evolution of Desire* (New York: HarperCollins, 1994), and Helen Fisher, *Anatomy of Love* (New York: Fawcett Columbine, 1992).

Page 30. Sexual selection: The importance of feather length and symmetry in sexual selection in birds is documented in Rufus Johnstone et al., "Mutual Mate Choice and Sex Differences in Choosiness," *Evolution*, vol. 50, no. 4 (August 1996), p. 1382; and Rufus Johnstone, "Sexual Selection, Honest Advertisement and the Handicap Principle: Reviewing the Evidence," *Biological Reviews of the Cambridge Philosophical Society*, vol. 70, no. 1 (February 1995), p. 1.

Page 31. Pheromones and major histocompatibility complex (MHC): Sources include Claus Wedekind et al., "MHC-dependent Mate Preferences in Humans," *Proceedings of the Royal Society of London*, vol. 160 (1995), p. 245; Claus Wedekind and Ivar Folstad, "Adaptive or Nonadaptive Immunosuppression by Sex Hormones?" *American Naturalist*, vol. 143, no. 5 (May 1994), p. 936; and David Berreby, "Studies Explore Love and the Sweaty T-shirt," *New York Times*, June 9, 1998, p. B14.

Page 33. Female redback spider: Sex among these spiders is described in Natalie Angier, "For an Australian Spider, Love Really Is to Die For," *New York Times*, January 9, 1996, p. B9.

Page 33. Sexual strategies: For a fascinating review, see Meredith Small, *What's Love Got to Do with It?: The Evolution of Human Mating* (New York: Anchor Books, 1995).

Page 33. Fruit flies: The research cited is from William Rice et al., "Sexually Antagonistic

Male Adaptation Triggered by Experimental Arrest of Female Evolution," *Nature*, vol. 384 (May 16, 1996), p. 232.

Page 34. Sexual infidelity: Observations challenging the notion that females are "naturally" monogamous are summed up in Meredith Small, *Female Choices: Sexual Behavior of Female Primates* (Ithaca, NY: Cornell University Press, 1993).

Page 35. Pregnancy termination: For further discussion, see Sarah Blaffer Hrdy et al., "Infanticide: Let's Not Throw out the Baby with the Bath Water," *Evolutionary Anthropology*, vol. 3, no. 5 (1994–95), p. 151, and Sarah Blaffer Hrdy, *The Woman that Never Evolved* (Cambridge: Harvard University Press, 1981).

Page 36. Cannibalization: The research on guppies, conducted by C. M. Breder of the American Museum of Natural History, is described by Irene Elia in *The Female Animal* (New York: Henry Holt, 1988), p. 64.

Page 39. Primate mothers: Sources for this discussion include Karen Wright, "Babies, Bonds and Brains," *Discover*, vol. 18, no. 10 (October 1997), p. 74; and Stephen Suomi, "Adolescent Depression and Depressive Symptoms: Insights from Longitudinal Studies with Rhesus Monkeys," *Journal of Youth and Adolescence*, vol. 20, no. 2 (April 1991), p. 273.

Page 41. Similarities with nonhuman primate females: The sources I primarily drew on are Barbara Smuts, "Social Relationships and Life Histories of Primates," in *The Evolving Female* (cited above), pp. 62–68; Mariko Hiraiwa-Hasegawa, "Development of Sex Differences in Nonhuman Primates," in *The Evolving Female*, pp. 69–75; Adrienne Zihlman, "Natural History of Apes: Life-History Features in Females and Males," in *The Evolving Female*, pp. 86–103; and Susan Sperling, "Baboons with Briefcases: Feminism, Functionalism and Sociobiology in the Evolution of Primate Gender," *Signs*, vol. 17, no. 1 (autumn 1991), p. 1.

Page 42. Jane Goodall: She is quoted in Stephen Schwartz, "Exploring Our Kinship with the Apes," *San Francisco Examiner*, December 15, 1996, p. 3.

Chapter 3: Lucy's Daughters

Page 43. Lucy: Estimates of Lucy's age range from 3.2 million to as old as 4 million years. My primary sources of the descriptions of Lucy, her discovery, and her life are the books by her discoverer, Donald Johanson: *Lucy, The Beginnings of Humankind*, with Maitland Edey (New York: Simon and Schuster, 1981); *Lucy's Child: The Discovery of a Human Ancestor*, with James Shreeve (New York: Morrow, 1989); *From Lucy to Language*, with Blake Edgar (New York: Simon and Schuster, 1996).

Page 44. Adrienne Zihlman's remarks: In addition to a personal interview I drew on her "Human Bodies, Women's Bodies: An Evolutionary Perspective," presentation, American Anthropological Association annual meeting, San Francisco, November 1996, and "Women's Bodies, Women's Lives: An Evolutionary Perspective," in *The Evolving Female* (cited above), pp. 185–97.

Page 45. Origins of bipedalism: George Chaplin, Nina Jablonski, N. Timothy Cable, "Physiology, Thermoregulation and Bipedalism," *Journal of Human Evolution*

(1994), p. 497; and Nina Jablonski and George Chaplin, "Origin of Habitual Terrestrial Bipedalism in the Ancestor of the Hominidae," *Journal of Human Evolution*, vol. 24 (1993), p. 259.

Page 46. Female body fat: In addition to a personal interview with Robin McFarland, I drew on her presentation "What Good Is Body Fat? Functional Evolutionary Perspectives from Comparative Studies" at the American Anthropological Association annual meeting, San Francisco, November 1996, and "Female Primates: Fat or Fit?" in *The Evolving Female* (cited above), pp. 163–75.

Page 46. Body fat differences in girls and boys: The study cited is R. W. Taylor et al., "Gender Differences in Body Fat Content Are Present Well Before Puberty," *International Journal of Obesity and Related Metabolic Disorders*, vol. 21 (November 1997).

Page 46. Reduced fertility of nursing mothers: The correlation between body fat, nursing, and fertility is discussed in Rose Frisch, "Body Weight, Body Fat, and Ovulation," *Trends in Endocrinology and Metabolism*, vol. 2, no. 5 (1991), pp. 191–97.

Page 47. Hips: Sources include a presentation by Lori Hager, "The Female Pelvis in Evolutionary Perspective," at the American Anthropological Association annual meeting, San Francisco, November 1996, and Adrienne Zihlman, "Locomotion as a Life History Character: The Contribution of Anatomy," *Journal of Human Evolution*, vol. 22 (1992), p. 315.

Page 48. Waist-hip ratio: This research has been reported in several articles by Devendra Singh, including "Body Weight, Waist-to-Hip Ratio, Breasts, and Hips: Role in Judgments of Female Attractiveness and Desirability for Relationships," *Ethology and Sociobiology*, vol. 16, no. 6 (1995), p. 483; "Female Health, Attractiveness, and Desirability for Relationships," *Ethology and Sociobiology*, vol. 16, no. 6 (1995), p. 465; and "Is Thin Really Beautiful and Good? Relationship Between Waist-to-Hip Ratio (WHR) and Female Attractiveness," *Personality and Individual Differences*, vol. 16, no. 1 (January 1994), p. 123.

Page 48. Male-female size difference: The rethinking of the evolution of sex differences in size was reported in John Noble Wilford, "New Clues to History of Male and Female," *New York Times*, August 26, 1997, p. B7.

Page 49. Male symmetry: Randy Thornhill has done extensive research into this subject, as reported in "Fluctuating Asymmetry and Sexual Selection," *Trends in Ecology and Evolution*, vol. 9, no. 1 (January 1994), p. 21; and "The Allure of Symmetry," *Natural History*, vol. 102, no. 9 (September 1993), p. 30.

Page 50. Evolutionary advantages of female orgasm: Robin Baker and Mark Bellis, *Human Sperm Competition: Copulation, Masturbation and Infidelity* (London: Chapman and Hall, 1995).

Page 50. Testicle size: A good summation of this research can be found in Jared Diamond, *The Third Chimpanzee: The Evolution and Future of the Human Animal* (New York: HarperCollins, 1992), p. 72.

Page 51. Paternity: Robin Baker, *Sperm Wars: The Science of Sex* (New York: Basic Books, 1996).

Page 51. Male interest in female looks: Among the sources used are Alan Feingold,

"Sex Differences in the Effects of Similarity and Physical Attractiveness," *Basic and Applied Social Psychology*, vol. 12 (September 1991), p. 357, and "Gender Differences in Effects of Physical Attractiveness on Romantic Attraction," *Journal of Personality and Social Psychology*, vol. 57, no. 5 (November 1990), p. 981.

Page 52. Courtship behaviors: This discussion draws upon the extensive research of David Buss, including "The Strategies of Human Mating," *American Scientist*, vol. 82 (May–June 1994), p. 238; and with David Schmitt, "Sexual Strategies Theory: An Evolutionary Perspective on Human Mating," *Psychological Review*, vol. 100, no. 2 (1993), p. 204.

Page 52. Female interest in male assets. William Allman summarizes research on this subject in *The Stone Age Present* (New York: Simon and Schuster, 1994).

Page 53. Older fathers siring sons: The study cited is John Manning and Roger Anderson, "Age Difference Between Husbands and Wives as a Predictor of Rank, Sex of First Child, and Asymmetry of Daughters," *Ethology and Sociobiology*, vol. 19, no. 2 (1998), p. 99.

Page 53. Cad-or-dad theory: Anthropologist Elizabeth Cashdan studied female mating strategies in "Attracting Mates: Effects of Paternal Investment on Mate Attraction Strategies," *Ethology and Sociobiology*, vol. 14 (1993), p. 1.

Page 53. Kipsigis women: Monique Borgerhoff Mulder, "Women's Strategies in Polygynous Marriage," *Human Nature*, vol. 3, no. 1 (1992), p. 45; and "Kipsigis Women's Preferences for Wealthy Men: Evidence for Female Choice in Mammals?" *Behavioral Ecology and Sociobiology*, vol. 27 (1990), p. 255.

Page 55. Lucy as sex doll: Donna Haraway, *Primate Visions: Gender, Race and Nature in the World of Modern Science* (New York: Routledge, 1992).

Page 55. Female awareness of fertility: The topic of concealed estrus is discussed in R. D. Alexander and K. M. Noonan, "Concealment of Ovulation, Parental Care and Human Social Evolution" in N. A. Chagnon and W. Irons (editors), *Evolutionary Biology and Human Social Behavior: An Anthropological Perspective* (North Scituate, MA: Duxbury Press, 1979).

Page 56. Human pair bonds: In "Evolution of Human Serial Pair Bonding," *American Journal of Physical Anthropology*, vol. 78 (1989), p. 331, Helen Fisher calculated that pair bonds of an average four-year duration were part of hominid reproductive strategy.

Page 57. The precise timing of ovulation: reported in Allen Wilcox et al., "Timing of Sexual Intercourse in Relation to Ovulation," *New England Journal of Medicine*, vol. 333, no. 23 (December 7, 1995), p. 1517.

Page 57. Dioramas: Anthropologist Diane Gifford-Gonzalez's study is described in Adrienne Zihlman, "The Paleolithic Glass Ceiling," in *Women in Human Evolution* (London and New York: Routledge, 1997), p. 91.

Page 58. Relative importance of hunting and foraging: An excellent discussion can be found in John Relethford, *The Human Species* (third edition) (Mountain View, CA: Mayfield Publishing, 1997).

Page 58. Clan of female hunters: This discovery was reported in J. Kimball et al., "Warrior Women of the Eurasian Steppes," *Archaeology*, vol. 50, no. 1 (January–February 1997), p. 44. The Center for the Study of the Eurasian Nomads (CSEN) in Berkeley, California, provides updated information on the woman warriors of the Kazakh at its website (http://garnet.Berkeley.edu/~jkimball).

Page 59. Why women didn't hunt: This discussion draws largely from Adrienne Zihlman, "Did the Australopithecines Have a Division of Labor?" (monograph), *The Archaeology of Gender*, University of Calgary Archaeological Association, 1991, p. 64.

Page 59. The string revolution: Elizabeth Wayland Barber, *Women's Work: The First 20,000 Years* (New York: W. W. Norton, 1994), pp. 42–70.

Page 59. Sewing: The popularity of sewing was reported in Mitchell Owens, "Sewing: 30 Million Women Can't Be Wrong," *New York Times*, March 4, 1997, p. B1. Its health benefits were described in "Stress Reduction's Common Thread," *Journal of the American Medical Association*, vol. 274, no. 4 (July 26, 1995).

Page 60. Grandmothers: Kristen Hawkes's papers include "Hadza Women's Time Allocation, Offspring Provisioning, and the Evolution of Long Postmenopausal Life Spans," *Current Anthropology*, vol. 38, no. 4 (August–October 1997), p. 551, and "Hardworking Hadza Grandmothers," in V. Standen and R. Folley (editors), *Comparative Socioecology of Mammals and Man* (London: Blackwell, 1991), pp. 341–66.

Page 61. Mitochondrial Eve: The late biologist Allan Wilson headed the research team that discovered mitochondrial Eve in 1987. Its methods and conclusions have been challenged ever since, particularly the contention that modern humans first lived in Africa. The discovery of a chromosomal Adam, also of African descent, by research teams at Stanford University and the University of Arizona, is described by Ann Gibbons in "Y Chromosome Shows that Adam Was an African," in *Science*, vol. 278 (October 31, 1997), p. 804; she reports on the spread of mtDNA in "The Women's Movement," *Science*, vol. 278 (October 31, 1997), p. 805.

Chapter 4: The Body of a Woman

Page 64. Sex differences: I compiled these examples from a variety of sources, including Marianne Legato, *Gender-Specific Aspects of Human Biology for the Practicing Physician* (Armonk, NY: Futura, 1997); Miriam Stoppard, *Woman's Body: A Manual for Life* (London: Dorling Kindersley, 1994); Edward Dolnick, "Super Women," *In Health*, July–August 1991, p. 42, and Carol Rinzler, "Gender Differences Quiz," *American Health*, September 1995, p. 13.

Page 65. The female liver: Florence Haseltine makes these points in "Conclusion," in her edited volume *Women's Health Research: A Medical and Policy Primer* (Washington, DC: American Psychiatric Press, 1997), pp. 331–36, and "Gender-Based Biology: What Does It Mean and Why Does It Matter?" speech for the Society for the Advancement of Women's Health Research, June 18, 1996.

Page 66. Female hearts: Sources include Marianne Legato and Carol Colman, *The Female Heart* (New York: Avon, 1991), and Judith Hsia, "Gender and the Heart," *Journal of Women's Health*, vol. 4, no. 4 (1995), p. 437.

Page 66. The female immune system: In addition to the books cited in the note to page 64 above, see Michelle Petri, "Gender-Based Differences in Autoimmunity and Autoimmune Disease," *Journal of Women's Health*, vol. 4, no. 4 (1995), p. 433.

Page 66. Pain and pleasure: This discussion draws on presentations at a National Institutes of Health conference on pain and gender in May 1998. The research on pleasure pathways was reported in Barry Komisaruk, Carolyn Gerdes, and Beverly Whipple, "Complete Spinal Cord Injury Does Not Block Perceptual Responses to Genital Self-stimulation in Women," *Archives of Neurology*, vol. 54 (December 1997), p. 1513.

Page 67. Sensory sex differences: In addition to the sources previously cited in Chapter 1, this section drew on Richard Doty, "Gender and Endocrine-Related Influences on Human Olfactory Perception," in Herbert L. Meiselman and Richard Rivlin (editors), *Clinical Measurement of Taste and Smell* (New York: Macmillan, 1986), p. 377, and Richard Doty et al., "Sex Differences in Odor Identification Ability: A Cross-Cultural Analysis," *Neuropsychologia*, vol. 23 (1985), p. 66.

Page 67. Genetic imprinting: Florence Haseltine's speech on this topic for the Society for the Advancement of Women's Health Research, June 18, 1996, provided my introduction to the subject of gametic imprinting and was a key source for this section. Other sources include: Louise Wilkins-Haug, "Genetic Imprinting: Evidence for Parent of Origin Effects on DNA Expression," *Journal of Women's Health*, vol. 4, no. 4 (1995), p. 423; Carmen Sapienza, "Genome Imprinting: An Overview," *Developmental Genetics*, vol. 17, no. 3 (1995), p. 185; Denise Barlow, "Gametic Imprinting in Mammals," *Science*, vol. 270 (December 8, 1995), p. 1610; and H. Sharat Chandra and Vidyanand Nanjundiah, "The Evolution of Genomic Imprinting," *Development* 1990, Supplement (summary of the first major international symposium on genomic imprinting held in April 1990 at Manchester University), p. 47.

Page 68. The gender of parental genes: This topic is discussed in Stephen Day, "Why Genes Have a Gender," *New Scientist*, vol. 138, no. 1874 (May 22, 1993); Steve Jones, "Ys and wherefores," *New Statesman and Society*, vol. 6, no. 256 (June 11, 1993), p. 30; and Judith Hall, "Genomic Imprinting and its Clinical Implications," *New England Journal of Medicine*, vol. 326, no. 12 (March 19, 1992).

Page 70. The Y chromosome: Biologist David Page of the Howard Hughes and Whitehead Institutes in Cambridge, Mass., identified the genes on the Y that direct its operations as a fertility factory. This research is described in Peter Radetsky, "Y?" *Discover*, vol. 18, no. 11 (November 1997), p. 88.

Page 70. Sexual development: An excellent overview can be found in Mark Breedlove, "Sexual Differentiation of the Brain and Behavior," in Jill Becker, Mark Breedlove, and David Crews (editors), *Behavioral Endocrinology* (Cambridge: MIT Press, 1992), pp. 39–68.

Page 72. Prenatal hormonal disorders: In addition to Breedlove's work, cited immediately above, this section draws from Maria New and Perrin White, "Genetic Disorders of Steroid Hormone Synthesis and Metabolism," *Balliere's Clinical Endocrinology and Metabolism*, vol. 90, no. 3 (July 1995), p. 525.

Page 73. Estrogen: Its depiction as the Marilyn Monroe of hormones comes from Theresa Crenshaw, *The Alchemy of Love and Lust* (New York: G. P. Putnam's Sons, 1996). Other sources for this discussion include Elizabeth Vliet, *Screaming to be Heard: Hormonal Connections Women Suspect and Doctors Ignore* (New York: M. Evans, 1995), and Deborah Blum, *Sex on the Brain: The Biological Differences Between Men and Women* (New York: Viking, 1997).

Page 74. Two types of estrogen receptors: This was reported in Michael Fritsch et al., "Two Populations of the Estrogen Receptor Separated and Characterized Using Aqueous Two-phase Partitioning," *Biochemistry*, vol. 36, no. 20 (May 20, 1997).

Page 75. Estrogen in males: The study cited is Rex Hess et al., "A Role for Oestrogens in the Male Reproductive System," *Nature*, vol. 390, no. 6659 (December 4, 1997), p. 509.

Page 76. Estrogen and cognition: This section draws on presentations by Bruce McEwen, Sanjay Asthana, Mary Lou Voytko, Diane Murphy, and C. Dominique Toran-Allerand at a press conference on estrogen and cognition at the annual meeting of the Society for Neuroscience in November 1996. The effects of estrogen on memory are described in Susana Phillips and Barbara Sherwin, "Effects of Estrogen on Memory Function in Surgically Menopausal Women," *Psychoneuroimmunology*, vol. 17, no. 5 (1993), p. 485. (More references on this subject can be found in the notes to Chapters 10 and 11.)

Page 76. Estrogen and mood: This discussion draws on a series of lectures given by psychiatrist Louann Brizendine on mood and hormones at the Langley-Porter Institute of the University of California, San Francisco, in 1996, and on her presentation "Hormonal Influences on Mood, Memory, and Sexual Function," Women's Health 2000 conference, University of California, San Francisco, March 8, 1997.

Page 77. The search for male essence: The search for sex hormones is chronicled in Gail Vines, *Raging Hormones* (Berkeley: University of California Press, 1993), pp. 13–32.

Page 77. Testosterone effects: My sources include David Rubinow and Peter Schmitt, "Androgens, Brain, and Behavior," *American Journal of Psychiatry*, vol. 153, no. 8 (August 1996), p. 974, and Julie Harris et al., "Salivary Testosterone and Self-reported Aggressive and Pro-social Personality Characteristics in Men and Women," *Aggressive Behavior*, vol. 22, no. 5 (1996), p. 321.

Page 77. Testosterone in men: Estelle Ramey, "How Female and Male Biology Differ," in Florence Haseltine (editor), *Women's Health Research: A Medical and Policy Primer* (Washington, DC: American Psychiatric Press, 1997).

Page 77. Inner ear differences: The small study was reported in Dennis McFadden and Edward Pasanen, "Comparison of the Auditory Systems of Heterosexuals and

Homosexuals: Click-evoked Otoacoustic Emissions," *Proceedings of the National Academy of Sciences*, March 1998, p. 2915. Critics charge that this study simply perpetuates the stereotype that lesbians are more masculine and that biology, not psychology, society, or culture, determines sexual orientation.

Page 80. Testosterone deficiencies and supplementation in women: Barbara Sherwin, "Androgen Use in Women," in *Pharmacology, Biology, and Clinical Applications of Androgens* (New York: Wiley Liss, 1996).

Page 81. "The weaker vessel": Antonia Fraser traces the origins of this phrase in *The Weaker Vessel* (New York: Alfred A. Knopf, 1984), pp. 1–6.

Page 81. Women in Olympic competition: The International Amateur Athletic Federation (IAAF) posts record-breaking times in various events at its website (http://www. iaaf.org). The information on Olympic records comes from this source.

Page 81. Female athletic performance: Sources include Lori Miller Kase, "The Weaker Sex," *American Health*, December 1994, p. 64, and Elizabeth Kaufmann, "The New Case for Woman Power," *New York Times Magazine*, April 28, 1991, p. 18.

Page 82. Female athletic advantages: Recent studies in this area are reported in Kim McDonald, "New Research Casts Light on Physiological and Biochemical Differences Between the Sexes," *Chronicle of Higher Education*, vol. 2, no. 25 (June 10, 1997), p. A16; Kim McDonald, "Why Do Female Athletes Outdistance Men in Endurance Sports?" *Chronicle of Higher Education*, vol. 42, no. 25 (June 20, 1997), p. A16; and Ayala Ochert, "Could Women Take a Lead over Men in the Long Run?" *Nature*, vol. 381, no. 6586 (July 4, 1996), p. 15.

Page 84. Ann Trason: Robert Lipsyte, "Running with a Goal of Ultra Equality," *New York Times*, January 7, 1996, and "Narrowing the Gap," *Women's Sports and Fitness*, vol. 14, no. 7 (October 1992), p. 15.

Page 85. Test of female physiological potential: These data come from the U.S. Army Research Institute of Environmental Medicine at Natick, Massachusetts.

Page 86. Sedentary women: The statistic on sedentary women appeared in a federal report, *Health, United States 1995*, which was released in June 1997.

Page 86. Exercise and breast cancer risk: Sources include Rose Frisch et al., "Former Athletes Have a Lower Lifetime Occurrence of Breast Cancer and Cancers of the Reproductive System," *Advances in Experimental Medicine and Biology*, vol. 322 (1992), p. 29; and Larry Katzenstein, "Preventing Breast and Ovarian Cancer," *American Health*, May 1995, p. 8.

Page 87. Bone health: This discussion draws on many sources, including Eric Orwoll, "Gender Differences in the Skeleton: Osteoporosis," *Journal of Women's Health*, vol. 4, no. 4 (1995), p. 429, and Miriam Nelson with Sarah Wernicke, *Strong Women Stay Young* (New York: Bantam Books, 1997).

Chapter 5: The Invisible Patient
Page 90. Women's treatment in health care: The ways in which medicine has neglected women is well documented in Florence Haseltine (editor), *Women's Health*

Research: A Medical and Policy Primer (Washington, DC: American Psychiatric Press, 1997), and in Eileen Nechas and Denise Foley, *Unequal Treatment: What You Don't Know About How Women Are Mistreated by the Medical Community* (New York: Simon and Schuster, 1994).

Page 90. Surveys on women's health fears: "Fear of Cancer Makes Women Ignore Other Killers, Study Says," *San Francisco Chronicle*, November 18, 1997, p. A5.

Page 91. Commonwealth Fund survey: Marilyn Falk and Karen Collins, *Women's Health: The Commonwealth Fund Survey* (Baltimore: Johns Hopkins University Press, 1996).

Page 91. Importance of gender: In addition to the sources on biological sex differences cited in Chapters 1 and 4, I drew on "Gender-Specific Medicine Sets New Direction for Healthcare Future," Partnership for Women's Health at Columbia University, February 1997, and Estelle Ramey, "How Female and Male Biology Differ," in *Women's Health Research: A Medical and Policy Primer* (cited above), pp. 47–62.

Page 92. Life expectancy: The twentieth edition of the Department of Health and Human Services' annual report on the nation's health, *Health, United States, 1995* (Washington, DC: GPO, 1997), featured a special profile on women's health that tracked major trends in women's life expectancy. It is the source of these statistics.

Page 92. Gender differences in longevity: This topic is well covered in Royda Crose, *Why Women Live Longer Than Men: And What Men Can Learn from Them*, (San Francisco: Jossey-Bass, 1997).

Page 93. Women living dangerously: Recent reports on the risks to women include Phyllis Greenberger, "New from the Society for the Advancement of Women's Health Research: Put Out that Light!" *Journal of Women's Health*, vol. 7, no. 3 (1998), p. 297, and Wendy Bjornson et al., "The Growing Problem of Smoking in Women," *Patient Care*, vol. 30, no. 13 (August 15, 1996), p. 142.

Page 94. The toll of disability: Demographer Eileen Crimmins of the University of Southern California calculated years of disability based on data collected by the National Center for Health Statistics. Her work was reported by Lawrence Altman in "Is the Longer Life the Healthier One?" *New York Times*, June 22, 1997.

Page 94. Gender differences in disease: This discussion draws on many sources, including Marianne Legato, *Gender-Specific Aspects of Human Biology for the Practicing Physician* (Armonk, NY: Futura, 1997); Bernardine Healy, *A New Prescription for Women's Health* (New York: Viking, 1995); and Jeane Ann Grisso and Roberta Ness, "Update in Women's Health," *Annals of Internal Medicine*, vol. 125 (1996), p. 213.

Page 95. Interactions of gender and race: The data on breast cancer mortality in African-American women comes from *Health, United States, 1995* (cited above). I also drew on an audiotaped presentation by Freda Lewis-Hall, "The Influence of Race and Culture on Women's Health," sponsored by the Jacobs Institute for Women's Health, in Washington, DC, on May 4, 1994.

Page 96. Lesbian health risks: These observations were made by gynecological oncologist Katherine O'Hanlan of Stanford University in a review article in *Current Problems in Obstetrics, Gynecology and Fertility*, vol. 18, no. 4 (August 21, 1995) and by

Beverly Biddle and Susan Hester in "Lesbian Health Issues: What Is Different?" presentation sponsored by the Jacobs Institute for Women's Health, in Washington, DC, on September 21, 1994.

Page 96. Work and health: See Judith LaRosa, "Executive Women and Health: Perceptions and Practices," *American Journal of Public Health*, vol. 80, no. 12 (December 1990), p. 1450.

Page 97. Health effects of working like a man: Catherine Ross and Chloe Bird, "Sex Stratification and Health Lifestyle: Consequences for Men's and Women's Perceived Health," *Journal of Health and Social Behavior*, vol. 35 (June 1994), p. 161.

Page 98. Exclusion of women from research trials: The history of this exclusion is reported in *Unequal Treatment: What You Don't Know About How Women Are Mistreated by the Medical Community* (cited above) and Ruth Merkatz and Elyse Summers, "Including Women in Clinical Trials: Policy Changes at the Food and Drug Administration," in *Women's Health Research: A Medical and Policy Primer* (cited above), pp. 265–84.

Page 99. Findings related to the menstrual cycle: Among the specific studies cited are G. D'Andrea et al., "Metabolism and Menstrual Cycle Rhythmicity of Serotonin in Primary Headaches," *Headache*, vol. 35, no. 4 (April 1995), p. 216; Merle Goldberg, "Chronobiology," *GW Medicine*, fall 1995, p. 16; G. Mondini et al., "Timing of Surgery Related to Menstrual Cycle and Prognosis of Premenopausal Women with Breast Cancer," *Anticancer Research*, vol. 17, no. 1 (1997), p. 717; Susan Flagg Godbey et al., "Cyclical Breathing: Asthma Flare-ups Tied to Menstrual Cycles," *Prevention*, vol. 49, no. 1 (January 1997), p. 28.

Page 99. Drugs in women: Among my sources are K. A. Yonkers et al., "Gender Differences in Pharmacokinetics and Pharmacodynamics of Psychotropic Medication," *American Journal of Psychiatry*, vol. 149 (1992), p. 587; Elizabeth Stone, "Risky Prescriptions: What Doctors Don't Know About Your Medications," *American Health*, January–February 1997, p. 50; and Steven Dubovsky, "Selected Topics in the Psychopharmacology of Women," unpublished manuscript.

Pages 101–06. Heart disease: Sources for this section include Roberto Malacrida et al., "A Comparison of the Early Outcome of Acute Myocardial Infarction in Women and Men," *New England Journal of Medicine*, vol. 338 (January 1, 1997), p. 8; Pamela Douglas and Geoffrey Ginsburg, "The Evaluation of Chest Pain in Women," *New England Journal of Medicine*, vol. 334, no. 20 (May 16, 1996), p. 1311; Meir Stampfer et al., "Vitamin E Consumption and the Risk of Coronary Disease in Women," *New England Journal of Medicine*, vol. 328, no. 20 (1993), p. 1444; and Thomas Pearson and Merle Myerson, "Treatment of Hypercholesteremia in Women," *Journal of the American Medical Association*, vol. 277, no. 16 (April 23–30, 1997), p. 1320.

Pages 106–09. "All in your head": Sources include Donna Stewart et al., "Vulvodynia and Psychological Distress," *Obstetrics and Gynecology*, vol. 84, no. 4 (October 1994), p. 587; Vicki Ratner et al., "Interstitial Cystitis: A Bladder Disease Finds Legitimacy," *Journal of Women's Health*, vol. 1, no. 1 (1992), p. 63; and Deborah Rubin and H. D.

Day, "Familial Heart Valve Disorder Is Not Related to Autonomy, Social Interaction Style or Family Dynamics," *Perceptual and Motor Skills*, vol. 77, no. 54 (1993), p. 54.

Page 109. University of Amsterdam study: This research was reported in Rebecca Voelker, "A New Agenda for Women's Health," *Journal of the American Medical Association*, vol. 272, no. 1 (July 6, 1994), p. 7.

Page 109. Protest for inserts: Nancy Milliken described this scene in "Women's Voices: Are We Being Heard?" the keynote lecture at Women's Health 2000, a symposium at the University of California, San Francisco, March 9, 1996.

Pages 109–11. Women's health advocacy: The campaign for more research and better health care for women is chronicled in "Women's Health: Taking Action, Getting Results," *Women's Health Advocate*, August 1995, p. 4; Karen Hicks (editor), *Misdiagnosis: Woman as a Disease* (Allentown, PA: People's Medical Society, 1994); and Donna Vogel, "Funding for Research and Training," in *Women's Health Research: A Medical and Policy Primer* (cited above).

Page 111. Sexism in medical school: The sources for this discussion include: Adriane Fugh-Berman, "Man to Man at Georgetown: Tales Out of Medical School," in *Misdiagnosis: Woman as a Disease* (cited immediately above); and Erica Frank et al., "Prevalence and Correlates of Harassment Among U.S. Women Physicians," *Archives of Internal Medicine*, vol. 158 (February 1998), p. 352.

Page 112. Women's health specialty: This is discussed in Janet Henrich, "Needed: A Women's Health Curriculum and Program," in *Women's Health Research: A Medical and Policy Primer* (cited above), pp. 241–64.

Page 113. Do women patients want women doctors: This question was addressed in "Gender-Specific Health Information: What Women Want and What They Need," Partnership for Women's Health at Columbia University, February, 1997; and Janet Elder, "Poll Finds Women Are the Health-Savvier Sex, and the Warier," *New York Times*, June 22, 1997, p. 8.

Chapter 6: Girls in Bloom

Page 118. The truth about girls: Two insightful resources are Lynn Ponton, *The Romance of Risk: Understanding Adolescent Lives* (New York: Basic Books, 1997), and Reed Larson and Maryse Richard, *Divergent Realities: The Emotional Lives of Mothers, Fathers, and Adolescents* (New York: Basic Books, 1994).

Page 118. Girls in history: These observations come from Natalie Zemon Davis and Arlette Farge (editors), *A History of Women: Renaissance and Enlightenment Paradoxes*, volume 3 in Georges Duby and Michelle Perrot (series editors), *A History of Women in the West* (Cambridge: Harvard University Press, 1993).

Page 119. Recognition of adolescence: G. Stanley Hall, *Adolescence and Its Relation to Psychology, Anthropology, Sociology, Sex, Crime, Religion, and Education* (New York: D. Appleton and Company, 1904).

Page 120. Alien sociopaths: Mike Males challenges the assumption that a unique form of dementia underlies adolescent behavior in "Adolescents: Daughters or Alien Sociopaths?" *Lancet*, vol. 349, no. 9052 (March 1, 1997), p. SI–13.

Page 120. Sex differences in childhood: My sources include N. L. Galambos et al., "Masculinity, Femininity and Sex Role: Exploring Gender Intensification," *Child Development*, vol. 61 (1990), p. 1905; and E. Macoby, "Gender and Relationships: A Developmental Account," *American Psychologist*, vol. 45 (1990), p. 513.

Page 122. "Omnipotentiality of the young": The study mentioned is by L. A. Linday, "Maternal Reports of Pregnancy, Genital and Related Fantasies in Preschool and Kindergarten Children," *Journal of the American Academy of Child and Adolescent Psychiatry*, vol. 33 (1994), p. 416.

Page 122. Oedipal issues: Psychiatrist Lois Flaherty discussed this perspective in "New Findings on Female Adolescent Development," a presentation at the Program for Women: Developmental Issues for Adolescent Girls, University of California, San Francisco, May 3, 1997.

Page 123. Girls at play: This section draws on a symposium entitled "Girls in Context" at the American Psychological Association's annual meeting in 1995. Presenters included psychologists Michelle Fine, Zella Luria, Judith Meese, Nada Sankster, and Diane Scott Jones.

Page 123. Atypical gender behavior: A discussion can be found in D. E. Sandberg et al., "The Prevalence of Gender-Atypical Behavior in Elementary School Children," *Journal of the American Academy of Child and Adolescent Psychiatry*, vol. 32 (1993), p. 306.

Page 124: Differences in brain development: The research study cited is B. A. Shaywitz et al., "Sex Differences in the Functional Organization of the Brain for Language," *Nature*, vol. 373 (1995), p. 607.

Page 125. Girls' physical and sexual development: The data on girls' growth is from Marcia Herman-Giddens et al., "Secondary Sexual Characteristics and Menses in Young Girls Seen in Office Practice," *Pediatrics*, vol. 99, no. 4 (April 1997), p. 505.

Page 125. Body fat in girls: Rose Frisch pioneered in studies of body composition in girls. Among her articles are "The Right Weight: Body Fat, Menarche, and Fertility," *Nutrition*, vol. 12, no. 6 (1996), p. 452, and "Critical Metabolic Mass and the Age at Menarche," *Annals of Human Biology*, vol. 3 (1976), p. 489.

Page 126. Adrenarche: Its impact and timing are reported in Martha McClintock and Gilbert Herdt, "Rethinking Puberty: The Development of Sexual Attraction," *Current Directions in Psychological Science*, vol. 5, no. 6 (December 1996), p. 178.

Page 127. Emotional impact of menarche: Louann Brizendine, "Mind, Mood, and Hormones," Women's Health 2000, a symposium at the University of California, San Francisco, March 9, 1996.

Page 129. Age at menarche: In addition to the previously cited material, my sources include J. D. Crawford and D. C. Oslr, "Body Composition at Menarche: The Frisch-Revelle Hypothesis Revisited," *Pediatrics*, vol. 56, no. 3 (1995), p. 440, and Jaakko Kaprio et al., "Common Genetic Influences on BMI and Age at Menarche," *Human Biology*, vol. 67, no. 5 (October 1995), p. 739.

Page 129. Environmental influences on menarche: This research can be found in Gustavo Gonzales and Arturo Villena, "Body Mass Index and Age at Menarche in Peruvian Children Living at High Altitude and at Sea Level," *Human Biology*, vol. 68, no. 2 (April 1996), p. 265; Julia Graber et al., "The Antecedents of Menarchal Age: Heredity, Family Environment and Stressful Life Events," *Child Development*, vol. 66, no. 2 (April 1995), p. 346; and Michelle Wierson et al., "Toward a New Understanding of Early Menarche: The Role of Environmental Stress in Pubertal Timing," *Adolescence*, vol. 28, no. 112 (winter 1993), p. 913.

Page 130. Psychological influences on menarche: Among the sources I drew on are Terrie Moffit et al., "Childhood Experience and the Onset of Menarche: A Test of a Sociobiological Model," *Child Development*, vol. 63 (1992), p. 47; Jay Belsky et al., "Childhood Experience, Interpersonal Development and Reproductive Strategy: An Evolutionary Theory of Socialization," *Child Development*, vol. 62 (1991), p. 647; and Belsky et al., "Further Reflections on an Evolutionary Theory of Socialization," *Child Development*, vol. 62 (1991), p. 682.

Page 131. Girls' reactions to menarche: Their responses are described by Sharon Golub, "Menarche: The Onset of Menstruation," in *Periods: From Menarche to Menopause* (Newbury Park, CA: Sage, 1992), pp. 24–45, and Catherine Rategan, "Rites of Passage from Menarche to Menopause," *Current Health*, vol. 20, no. 7 (March 1994) suppl. 1.

Page 131. Girls' talking about menarche: The ways girls respond to their first periods are described in J. Brookes-Gunn et al., "Physical Similarity of and Disclosure of Menarche Status to Friends: Effects of Age and Pubertal Status," *Journal of Early Adolescence*, vol. 6, no. 1 (1986), p. 3, and Elizabeth Kissling, "Bleeding Out Loud: Communication About Menstruation," *Feminism and Psychology*, vol. 6, no. 4 (1996), p. 481.

Page 132. Teens in Italy: Bruna Zani, "Male and Female Patterns in the Discovery of Sexuality During Adolescence," *Journal of Adolescence*, vol. 14, no. 2 (June 1991), p. 163.

Page 132. What girls want: Sharon Golub's chapter "Menarche: The Onset of Menstruation," in *Periods: From Menarche to Menopause*, was a primary source in describing girls' reactions, changes in body image, and preferences for information. Another was Elisa Koff and Jill Rierdan, "Preparing Girls for Menstruation: Recommendations from Adolescent Girls," *Adolescence*, vol. 30, no. 120 (winter 1995), p. 795.

Page 134. Early maturers: Chris Hayward et al., "Psychiatric Risk Associated with Early Puberty in Adolescent Girls," *Journal of the American Academy of Child and Adolescent Psychiatry*, vol. 36, no. 2 (February 1997), p. 255.

Page 135. New Zealand survey: This research was reported in S. Williams and R. McGee, "Adolescents' Self-perceptions of Their Strength," *Journal of Youth and Adolescence*, vol. 20 (1991), p. 325.

Page 136. African-American girls: This research comes from Debra Schultz, "Risk, Resiliency and Resistance: Current Research on Adolescent Girls," *Ms.* Foundation for Women National Girls Initiative, July 1991.

Page 137. Risk-taking in girls: This topic receives comprehensive discussion in R. J. DiClemente et al. (editors), *Handbook of Adolescent Health Risk Behaviors* (New York: Plenum Press, 1996).

Page 139. Susceptibility to depression: Sources include Carnegie Council on Adolescent Development, *Great Transitions: Preparing Adolescents for a New Century* (New York: Carnegie Corporation, 1995); Jane Brody, "Girls and Puberty: The Crisis Years," *New York Times*, November 4, 1997; and Lynn Ponton, "Issues Unique to Psychotherapy with Adolescent Girls," *American Journal of Psychotherapy*, vol. 47, no. 3 (1993), p. 353. See Chapter 13 for more references on depression in women.

Page 140. Anxiety and growth: The study cited is Daniel Pine et al., "Emotional Problems During Youth as Predictors of Stature During Early Adulthood: Results from a Prospective Epidemiologic Study," *Pediatrics*, vol. 97, no. 6 (June 1996), p. 1.

Page 141. Teen sexual activity: The federal statistics are from various sources, including the National Center for Health Statistics; Alan Guttmacher Institute, *Sex and America's Teenagers* (New York: Alan Guttmacher Institute, 1994); and the Bureau of the Census. Condom use among teens in 1998 was estimated to be 44 percent, up from 11 percent in 1983, according to Dr. Robert Blum, director of adolescent health at the University of Minnesota, as quoted in Pat Wingert, "The Battle over Falling Birthrates," *Newsweek*, May 11, 1998, p. 44. The Child Trends study was reported in "Girls in 2-Parent Homes Less Likely to Have Sex," *Marin Independent Journal*, June 19, 1997, p. A1.

Page 141. "Girls trade sex": See Deborah Tolman and Tracy Higgins, "How Being a Good Girl Can Be Bad for Girls," in Nan Maglin and Donna Perry (editors), *"Bad Girls"/"Good Girls"* (New Brunswick, NJ: Rutgers University Press, 1996).

Page 142. Sexual abstinence and intelligence: Carolyn Tucker Halpern, of the University of North Carolina at Chapel Hill, sent me a draft of her research team's unpublished manuscript, "Why Smart Girls Don't Have Sex (or Kiss Much Either)."

Page 143. Christmas service: "A Parent's Dilemma: An Antiphonal Sermon" was written by Rev. Joan Carter of the Sausalito Presbyterian Church.

Page 143. Teen pregnancy rates: The statistics cited were obtained from the National Center for Health Statistics in May 1998; they report birth rates in 1996.

Pages 143–45. Teenage pregnancy: An important source was Kristin Luker, *Dubious Conceptions* (Cambridge, MA: Harvard University Press, 1996). For a discussion on fathers' age, see "Age Differences Between Minors Who Give Birth and Their Adult Partners," *Family Planning Perspectives*, vol. 29, no. 2 (March–April 1997), p. 61.

Page 146. Parents matter: This finding was reported in M. D. Resnick et al., "Protecting Adolescents from Harm: Findings from the National Longitudinal Study Adolescent Health," *Journal of the American Medical Association*, vol. 278, no. 10 (September 10, 1997), p. 823.

Page 147. Girls and sports: Key sources include the Center for Research on Girls and Women in Sport, *Physical Activity & Sport in the Lives of Girls: A Report from the President's Council on Physical Fitness and Sports* (Washington, DC: Department of Health and Human Services,1997); and "Growing Smart: What's Working for Girls in School, Executive Summary and Action Guide" (Washington, DC: American Association of University Women Educational Foundation, 1996).

Page 147. Media images: The study cited was conducted by Children Now and reported in Dinitia Smith, "Role Models Busy with Love, Hair," *San Francisco Chronicle,* May 1, 1997, p. A8.

Page 148. Influence of parents' careers: The study cited is K. A. Updegraff et al., "Gender Roles in Marriage: What Do They Mean for Girls' and Boys' School Achievement?" *Journal of Youth and Adolescence,* vol. 25 (1996), p. 73.

Page 148. Importance of mothers: Sources include Jan Ehrman, "Stress, Depression Climb in Teenage Girls but Mom Can Intervene," *NIH Healthline,* NIH Office of Communications, October–November 1994, p. 6. The APA symposium, entitled "Girls in Context," was held at its annual meeting in 1995.

Page 149. A girl's perspective: The paper quoted, "Surviving Adolescence," was written by Pilar Rubin for an English course at Kenyon College in spring, 1997.

Chapter 7: Riding the Moon

Page 152. Frequency of menstruation in prehistoric women: Other estimates can be found in John Travis, "Why Do Women Menstruate?" *Science News,* vol. 151 (April 12, 1997), p. 230; and Beverly Strassman, "The Biology of Menstruation in *Homo Sapiens*: Total Lifetime Menses, Fecundity, and Nonsynchrony in a Natural-Fertility Population," *Current Anthropology,* vol. 38, no. 1 (1997), p. 123.

Page 154. "Men, poor old things": This quote appeared in Melinda Beck, "Menopause," *Newsweek,* May 25, 1992, p. 38.

Page 155. Rhythmicity: Sources include: Proceedings, Tenth Conference of the Society for Menstrual Cycle Research: 1993 (Kathleen Hubbs Ulman, editor) *Mind-Body Rhythmicity: A Menstrual Cycle Perspective* Donald Golgert, (editor) Seattle, Washington: Hamilton & Cross, 1995; and Natalie Angier, "Modern Life Suppresses an Ancient Body Rhythm," *New York Times,* p. B7, in which the quote from biological rhythms expert Thomas Wehr of the National Institute of Mental Health appeared.

Page 155. Menstrual synchronization: The research studies cited are: M. K. McClintock, "Menstrual Synchrony and Suppression," *Nature,* vol. 229 (1971), p. 244; M. K. McClintock, "Regulation of Ovulation by Human Pheromones," *Nature,* vol. 392, no. 177 (1998); and Wenda Trevathan et al., "No Evidence for Menstrual Synchrony in Lesbian Couples," *Psychoneuroendocrinology,* vol. 18, nos. 5–6 (1993), p. 425.

Page 157. Myths, taboos, and early theories: These are discussed in depth in *Periods: From Menarche to Menopause* (cited above), pp. 1–23, and Janice Delaney, Mary Jane Lupton, and Emily Toth, *The Curse: A Cultural History of Menstruation* (Urbana: University of Illinois Press, 1988), pp. 243–51.

Page 159. "If men were shaped like most tampons": The newsletter of the Museum of Menstruation, *Catamenia,* Summer 1994, featured this advertisement for Dr. White's Contour Applicator Tampons.

Pages 159–62: Molimina: Hormonal fluctuations in the menstrual cycle are summarized in *Periods: From Menarche to Menopause*, pp. 53–83; John Bancroft, "The Menstrual Cycle and the Well-being of Women," *Social Science and Medicine*, vol. 41, no. 6 (September 15, 1995), p. 78; and Alice Dan (editor), *Menstrual Health in Women's Lives* (Urbana: University of Illinois Press, 1992).

Page 162. Inner flow: Among the sources for this section are: Ellen Eibenluft, Patricia Fiero, and David Rubinow, "Effects of the Menstrual Cycle on Dependent Variables in Mood Disorder Research," *Archives of General Psychiatry*, vol. 51 (October 1994), p. 761; Anne Walker, "Mood and Well-being in Consecutive Menstrual Cycles," *Psychology of Women Quarterly*, vol. 18 (1994), p. 271; and Donna Stewart, "Positive Changes in the Premenstrual Period," *Acta Psychiatry Scandinavica*, vol. 79 (1989), p. 400.

Page 164. Intellectual performance: Barbara Sommer, "Cognitive Performance and the Menstrual Cycle," in John Richardson (editor), *Cognition and the Menstrual Cycle* (New York: Springer-Verlag, 1992), pp. 40–66.

Pages 164–66. Premenstrual puzzle: This discussion draws on many sources, including Mary Brown Parlee, "Psychology of Menstruation and Premenstrual Syndrome," in Florence Denmark and Michelle Paludi (editors), *Psychology of Women* (Westport, CT: Greenwood Press, 1993), pp. 325–77; Kathryn Lee and C. Amanda Rittenhouse, "Prevalence of Perimenstrual Symptoms in Employed Women," *Women and Health*, vol. 17, no. 3 (1991), p. 17; and Angelika Wieck, "Ovarian Hormones, Mood, and Neurotransmitters," *International Review of Psychiatry*, vol. 8, no. 1 (1996), p. 17.

Page 166. Women's self-reports of PMS: These observations are based on interviews with therapists and researchers and on Jean Bailey, "Diagnostic Status of Women Who Present with PMS," presentation at the American Psychiatric Association annual meeting, May 1997.

Page 166. Premenstrual depression: Sources include several presentations at the 1996 annual meeting of the American Psychiatric Association in San Diego, including Susan Kornstein, "Premenstrual Exacerbation of Depression," and John Bancroft and Dilys Rennie, "Perimenstrual Depression," *Psychosomatic Medicine*, vol. 57, no. 5 (September–October 1995), p. 445.

Page 166. Causes of PMS: Sources include John T. E. Richardson, "The Premenstrual Syndrome: A Brief History," *Social Science and Medicine*, vol. 41, no. 6 (September 15, 1995), p. 761; Anne Walker, "Theory and Methodology in Premenstrual Syndrome Research," *Social Science and Medicine*, vol. 41, no. 6 (September 15, 1995), p. 793; Peter Schmidt et al., "Differential Behavioral Effects of Gonadal Steroids in Women With and in Those Without Premenstrual Syndrome," *New England Journal of Medicine*, vol. 338, no. 4 (January 22, 1998), p. 209; Joseph Mortola, "Premenstrual Syndrome—Pathophysiologic Considerations," *New England Journal of Medicine*, vol. 338, no. 4 (January 22, 1998), p. 256; and Susan Girdler et al.,"Thyroid Axis Function

During the Menstrual Cycle in Women with Premenstrual Syndrome," *Psychoneuroendocrinology*, vol. 20, no. 4 (1995), p. 395.

Page 167. Serotonin boosters for PMS: The efficacy of these medications was discussed in Ellen Freeman, "Can Antidepressants Be Used to Tame Psychological Symptoms of PMS?" *Medscape Women's Health*, vol. 1, no. 10 (1996) (online website address: www.medscape.com); and Donna Stewart et al., "Follicular and Late Luteal Phase Serum Fluoxetine Levels in Women Suffering from Late Luteal Phase Disorder," *Biological Psychiatry*, vol. 36 (1994), p. 201.

Page 167. Antianxiety medications: See W. M. Harrison et al., "Treatment of Premenstrual Dysphoria with Alprazolam," *Archives of General Psychiatry*, vol. 47 (1990), p. 270, and Ellen Freeman et al., "A Double-blind Trial of Oral Progesterone, Alprazolam, and Placebo in Treatment of Severe Premenstrual Syndrome," *Journal of the American Medical Association*, vol. 274, no. 1 (July 5, 1995), p. 51.

Page 167. Phototherapy for PMS: Jeffrey Rausch and Barbara Parry, "Treatment of Premenstrual Mood Symptoms," *Psychiatric Clinics of North America*, vol. 16, no. 4 (December 1993), p. 829; and Barbara Parry, "Light Therapy of Late Luteal Phase Dysphoric Disorder: An Extended Study," *American Journal of Psychiatry*, vol. 150, no. 9 (September 1993), p. 1417.

Page 167. Nondrug treatments: These recommendations are based on Jean Endicott et al., "PMS: New Treatments that Really Work," *Patient Care*, vol. 30, no. 7 (April 15, 1996), p. 88; Kathryn Lee and C. Amanda Rittenhouse, "Health and Perimenstrual Symptoms: Health Outcomes for Employed Women Who Experience Perimenstrual Symptoms," *Women and Health*, vol. 19, no. 1 (1992), p. 65; and Myra Hunter et al., "Seeking Help for Premenstrual Syndrome: Women's Self-reports and Treatment Preferences," *Sexual and Marital Therapy*, vol. 10, no. 3 (November 1995), p. 253.

Pages 168–70. Premenstrual dysphoric disorder: A thorough report on PDD can be found in Barbara Parry and J. L. Rausch, "Premenstrual Dysphoric Disorder," in H. I. Kaplan and B. J. Sadock, *Comprehensive Textbook of Psychiatry*, vol. 6 (Baltimore: Williams and Wilkins, 1995), pp. 1707–13.

Page 169. PDD classification: This controversy was reported in Paula Span, "Vicious Cycles: The Politics of Periods," *Washington Post*, July 8, 1993, p. C1.

Chapter 8: The Restless Womb
Page 173. Bonnie Anderson and Judith Zinsser, *A History of Their Own*, vol. 1 (New York: Harper and Row, 1988).

Page 175. The dangers of childbirth: Aline Rouselle, "Body Politics in Ancient Rome," in vol. 1 of Georges Duby and Michelle Perrot (series editors), *A History of Women in the West* (Cambridge, Harvard University Press, 1993), p. 306. The current statistics are from the United Nations and the U.S. Centers for Disease Control and Prevention.

Page 177. Education and fertility: This statistic comes from "Mother's Educational

Level Influences Birth Rate," National Center for Health Statistics news release, April 24, 1997, and T. J. Mathews and Stephanie Ventura, "Birth and Fertility Rates by Educational Attainment: *United States, 1994,* vol. 45, no. 10, supplement (Washington, DC: U.S. Dept. of Health and Human Services), 20 pp.

Page 177. Margaret Sanger: H. G. Wells's comments on Margaret Sanger were quoted by Gloria Steinem in "Margaret Sanger," *Time,* April 13, 1998, p. 93.

Page 177. If not for modern birth control techniques: This estimate comes from Luella Klein, former president of the American College of Obstetricians and Gynecologists, quoted in Christiane Northrup, *Women's Bodies, Women's Wisdom* (Revised Edition) (New York: Bantam, 1998), p. 381.

Page 178. Unplanned pregnancies: These statistics come from the Population Institute, which issued a report on childbearing trends in December 1997, and reports from the Alan Guttmacher Institute and the Pew Global Stewardship Initiative.

Page 181. Survey on responsibility for birth control: The results of this survey, sponsored by the Kaiser Family Foundation, were reported in "Birth Control Survey Faults Men," *San Francisco Chronicle,* May 23, 1995.

Page 182. Popularity of various contraceptives: See Linda Piccinino and William Mosher, "Trends in Contraceptive Use in the United States: 1982–1995," *Family Planning Perspectives,* vol. 30 (January–February 1998), p. 4.

Page 182: Conception and ovulation: The study cited is Allen Wilcox, Clarice Weinberg, and Donna Baird, "Timing of Sexual Intercourse in Relation to Ovulation: Effects on the Probability of Conception, Survival of the Pregnancy, and Sex of the Baby," *New England Journal of Medicine,* vol. 333, no. 23 (December 7, 1995), p. 1517.

Pages 182–83. Oral contraceptives: The recent research on the pill's risks and benefits is summarized in Karen Titus, "Even as New Options Emerge, Gynecologists Urge Women to Find Older Contraceptives User-Friendly," *Journal of the American Medical Association,* vol. 276, no. 6 (August 14, 1996), p. 440.

Page 183. Unwanted pregnancies in industrialized countries: This information comes from Andrew Skolnick, "AMA's Science Reporters Conferences Focus on Contraception and Prevention of Premature Birth," *Journal of the American Medical Association,* vol. 276, no. 19 (November 10, 1996), p. 1538.

Page 184. Japanese ban on the pill: This was reported in "The Pill in Japan," *The Economist,* vol. 344, no. 8042 (November 8, 1997), p. 21.

Page 184: Emergency contraception: This report draws on multiple sources, including Willard Cates, Jr. and Elizabeth Raymond, "Annotation: Emergency Contraception—Parsimony and Prevention in the Medicine Cabinet," *American Journal of Public Health,* vol. 87, no. 6 (June 1997), p. 909; and James Trussell et al., "Preventing Unintended Pregnancy: The Cost Effectiveness of Three Methods of Emergency Contraception," *American Journal of Public Health,* vol. 87, no. 6 (June 1997), p. 932.

Page 185. Birth control pills and sexuality: The report on enhance sexual desire is by

Norma McCoy and Joseph Matyas, "Oral Contraceptives and Sexuality in University Women," *Archives of Sexual Behavior*, vol. 35, no. 1 (February 1996), p. 73.

Page 185. History of abortion: Connecticut passed the first law to regulate abortion in 1821; it prohibited the use of poisons in inducing abortion. Between 1825 and 1841, ten other states enacted criminal statutes punishing persons who performed abortions. The history is summarized in "How We Got Here," *Ms.*, May–June 1995, p. 54.

Page 186. Women who have abortions: These statistics come from various sources, including the U.S. National Center for Health Statistics as well as Nada Stotland, *Abortion: Facts and Feelings* (Washington, DC: American Psychiatric Press, 1998), pp. 19–21.

Page 187. The abortion–breast cancer link: The studies cited include Marlie Gammon et al., "Abortion and the Risk of Breast Cancer," *Journal of the American Medical Association*, vol. 275, no. 4 (January 24–31, 1996), p. 321; J. Brind et al., "Induced Abortion as an Independent Risk Factor for Breast Cancer: A Comprehensive Review and Meta-analysis," *Journal of Epidemiology and Community Mental Health*, vol. 50 (1996), p. 481: Polly Newcomb et al., "Pregnancy Termination in Relation to Risk of Breast Cancer," *Journal of the American Medical Association*, vol. 275, no. 4 (January 24–31, 1996), p. 283; Patricia Hartge, "Abortion, Breast Cancer and Epidemiology," *New England Journal of Medicine*, vol. 336, no. 2 (January 9, 1997), p. 127.

Page 188. Psychological impact of abortion: An excellent discussion of this issue can be found in Nada Stotland, "The Myth of the Abortion Trauma Syndrome," *Journal of the American Medical Association*, vol. 268 (1992), p. 2078, and in Stotland's books, *Abortion: Facts and Feelings* (Washington, DC: American Psychiatric Press, 1998), and *Psychiatric Aspects of Abortion* (Washington, DC: American Psychiatric Press, 1991).

Page 190. Laurie Lisle: Her book is *Without Child: Challenging the Stigma of Childlessness* (New York: Ballantine Books, 1996). Information is also drawn from the ChildFree Network and a seminar at the University of California, San Francisco, "Childfree Women," September 21, 1996.

Chapter 9: To Become a Mother

Page 195. Motherhood mandate: These historical trends are described in Robert Martenson, "Physiology as Destiny: Medicine and Motherhood in the Progressive Era," *Journal of the American Medical Association*, vol. 275, no. 15 (April 17, 1996), p. 1213, and "The Despised Office of Motherhood," originally printed in *Journal of the American Medical Association*, vol. 26 (April 25, 1986), p. 835, and reprinted in *Journal of the American Medical Association*, April 17, 1996, p. 1212.

Page 197. Sisterhood of the infertile: Membership in this sorority is one of the many topics touchingly discussed in Anne Taylor Fleming, *Motherhood Deferred: A Woman's Journey* (New York: Fawcett Columbine, 1994).

Page 198. Estimates of infertility and of successful treatment: These vary, depending on which population is being studied, time frame, and other factors. The sources used include the U.S. Office of Technology and Michael Lemonick, "The New Revolution in Making Babies," *Time,* December 1, 1997.

Page 198. Infertility treatments: This discussion draws on several sources, including Miriam Rosenthal, Ruth Anne Queenan, and Lynne Beauregard, "Diseases that Affect Only Women," in Florence Haseltine (editor), *Women's Health Research: A Medical and Policy Primer* (Washington, DC: American Psychiatric Press, 1997); and Luigi Mastroianni et al., "Helping Infertile Patients," *Patient Care,* vol. 31, no. 16 (October 15, 1997), p. 103.

Page 199. The psychological impact of infertility treatments: This subject is discussed in Patricia Scheiber, "The Emotional Impact of Infertility," *Focus on Fertility,* vol. 1, no. 2 (1995), p. 1; and John Collins, "A Couple with Infertility," *Journal of the American Medical Association,* vol. 274, no. 14 (October 11, 1995), p. 1159.

Page 201. Stress and infertility. The interaction between the two is described in Alice Domar et al., "Psychological Improvement in Infertile Women After Behavioral Treatment: A Replication," *Fertility and Sterility,* vol. 58, no. 1 (July 1992), p. 144, and Alice Domar and Henry Dreher, *Healing Mind, Healthy Woman* (New York: Henry Holt, 1996), pp. 228–65.

Page 201. Pregnancy's transformations: I reported extensively on these in *Intensive Caring* (New York: Crown, 1991) and *New Hope for Problem Pregnancies* (New York: Harper and Row, 1982). The change in foot size is from "Larger Feet Postpregnancy," *Working Mother,* March 1996, p. 16.

Page 202. The effects of an invasive placenta: This view comes from David Haig, "Prenatal Power Plays," *Natural History,* December 1995, p. 39.

Page 204. Depression in pregnancy: This topic is addressed in Vivien Burt and Victoria Hendricks, *Women's Mental Health* (Washington, DC: American Psychiatric Press, 1997), pp. 31–62.

Page 205. Psychiatric drugs in pregnancy: Sources include J. G. Auerbach et al., "Maternal Psychotropic Medication and Neonatal Behavior," *Neurotoxicology and Teratology,* vol. 14 (1992), p. 399; K. L. Wisner et al., "Tricyclic Dose Requirements Across Pregnancy," *American Journal of Psychiatry,* vol. 150 (1993), p. 1541; and Laura Miller, "Treating Pregnant Patients with Psychotropic Drugs," presentation at the ninth annual U.S. Psychiatric and Mental Health Congress, November 1996.

Page 205. Miscarriage: The emotional impact is discussed in Hettie Janssen et al., "Controlled Prospective Study on the Mental Health of Women Following Pregnancy Loss," *American Journal of Psychiatry,* vol. 153, no. 2 (February 1996), p. 226; and Gail Robinson et al., "Psychological Reactions in Women Followed for One Year After Miscarriage," *Journal of Reproductive and Infant Psychology,* vol. 12, no. 1 (January–March 1994), p. 31.

Page 206. Postpartum problems: Among the sources used in this section are Karen Kleiman and Valerie Raskin, *This Isn't What I Expected* (New York: Bantam Books, 1994); Rita Suri and Vivien Burt, "The Assessment and Treatment of Postpartum

Psychiatric Disorders" and "Coping with Postpartum Depression," *Journal of Practical Psychiatry and Behavioral Health*, March 1997, p. 67.

Page 208. Effect on children: Jane Brody, "Depressed Parent's Children at Risk," *New York Times*, March 3, 1998.

Page 209. Primate births: Karen Rosenberg and Wenda Trevathan, "Bipedalism and Human Birth: The Obstetrical Dilemma Revisited," *Evolutionary Anthropology*, vol. 45, no. 5 (1996), p. 161, and Wenda Trevathan, *Human Birth: An Evolutionary Perspective* (New York: Aldine de Gruyter, 1987).

Page 210. Brain changes after birth: Joan Borysenko presents an illuminating account of these biochemical processes in *A Woman's Book of Life* (New York: Riverhead Books, 1996), pp. 94–98.

Page 211. A mother falls in love: The quote is from Anne Roiphe's lyrical *Fruitful: A Real Mother in the Modern World* (New York: Houghton-Mifflin, 1996), p. 4.

Chapter 10: Second Puberty

Page 216. Evolutionary view: For further discussion, see K. Hill and A. M. Hurtado, "The Evolution of Premature Reproductive Senescence and Menopause in Human Females," *Human Nature*, vol. 2 (1991), p. 313, and Jared Diamond, "Why Women Change," *Discover*, July 1996, p. 130.

Page 218. Changing attitudes: These are summarized in Sharon McQuaide, "Baby Boom Women Say Midlife Stereotypes Are Not the Norm," *Fordham University Media Report to Women*, Spring 1997, p. 5, and Teri Randall, "Women Need More and Better Information on Menopause from Their Physicians, Says Survey," *Journal of the American Medical Association*, vol. 270, no. 14 (October 13, 1993), p. 1694.

Page 219. Perimenopause: Among the sources are Vivien Burt and Victoria Hendricks, *Women's Mental Health* (Washington: American Psychiatric Press, 1997), pp. 103–16; William Andrews, "The Transitional Years and Beyond," *Obstetrics and Gynecology*, vol. 85, no. 1 (January 1995), p. 1; and Nancy Giordano and Joanne Singleton, "Managing the Perimenopause," *Menopause Management*, January–February 1995, p. 15.

Page 220. Longitudinal study: Norma McCoy, "Menopause and Sexuality," *Hormone Replacement Therapy*, May 1995, p. 32.

Pages 222–24. Menopausal symptoms and changes: This section draws on many sources, including Lorraine Dennerstein and Julia Shelley (editors), *A Woman's Guide to Menopause and Hormone Replacement Therapy* (Washington, DC: American Psychiatric Press, 1998); David Baram, "Physiology and Symptoms of Menopause," in Donna Stewart and Gail Robinson (editors), *A Clinician's Guide to Menopause* (Washington, DC: American Psychiatric Press, 1997), pp. 9–28; N. Avis and S. McKinlay, "The Massachusetts Women's Health Study: An Epidemiologic Investigation of the Menopause," *Journal of the American Medical Women's Association*, vol. 50 (1995), p. 45; and L. C. Swartzman et al., "The Menopausal Hot Flash: Symptom Reports and

Concomitant Physiological Changes," *Journal of Behavioral Medicine*, vol. 13 (1990), p. 15.

Pages 225–27. Mood changes at menopause: The sources include Leslie Hartley Gise, "Psychosocial Aspects," in *A Clinician's Guide to Menopause* (cited above), pp. 29–44; Barbara Sherwin, "Hormones, Mood, and Cognitive Functioning in Postmenopausal Women," *Obstetrics and Gynecology*, vol. 87 (1996), p. 20S; and Donna Stewart and Katherine Boydell, "Psychologic Distress During Menopause: Associations Across the Reproductive Life Cycle," *International Journal of Psychiatry in Medicine*, vol. 23, no. 2 (1993), p. 157.

Page 225. Menopausal depression: The sources used in this section include Dara Charney and Donna Stewart, "Psychiatric Aspects," in *A Clinician's Guide to Menopause* (cited above); and Leslie Tam, "Prevalence of Depression in Menopause," presentation at the American Psychiatric Association annual meeting, San Diego, May 1997.

Pages 227–30. Midlife sexuality: This section takes its name from a workshop run by Linda Perlin Alperstein at the symposium "Women in Midlife: A Celebration," University of California, San Francisco, Program for Women, May 13, 1995. Other sources include Dianne Hales, "The Joy of Midlife Sex," *American Health for Women*, vol. 16, no. 1 (January–February 1997), p. 78; John Lamont, "Sexuality," in *A Clinician's Guide to Menopause* (cited above), pp. 63–76; Norma McCoy, "The Menopause and Sexuality," in Regine Sitruk-Ware and Wulf Utian, *The Menopause and Hormonal Replacement Therapy* (New York: Marcel Dekker, 1992); and Ronald Young, "Androgens in Postmenopausal Therapy?" *Menopause Management*, May 1993, p. 21.

Page 231. Why women don't use HRT: "Older Women Still Unconvinced of the Benefits of HRT; Here's Why," *Geriatrics*, vol. 51, no. 8 (August 1996), p. 16.

Pages 230–33. Hormone replacement: Among the sources are J. Gallagher et al., "Why HRT Makes Sense," *Patient Care*, vol. 30, no. 13 (August 15, 1996), p. 166; Deborah Grady and Steven Cummings, "Postmenopausal Hormone Therapy," *Menopause*, vol. 2, no. 3 (1995), p. 123; Francine Grodstein et al., "Postmenopausal Hormone Therapy and Mortality," *New England Journal of Medicine*, vol. 336, no. 25 (June 19, 1997), p. 1769; Louise Brinton and Catherine Schairer, "Postmenopausal Hormone Replacement Therapy—Time for a Reappraisal," *New England Journal of Medicine*, vol. 336, no. 25 (June 19, 1997); and Nananda Col et al., "Patient Specific Decisions about Hormone Replacement Therapy in Postmenopausal Women," *Journal of the American Medical Association*, vol. 277, no. 14 (April 9, 1997), p. 1140.

Page 231. HRT and osteoporosis: Sources include D. L. Schneider et al., "Timing of Postmenopausal Estrogen for Optimal Bone Density," *Journal of the American Medical Association*, vol. 277, no. 7 (February 12, 1997), p. 543; and Mortensen Lene et al., "Risedronate Increases Bone Mass in an Early Postmenopausal Population: Two Years of Treatment Plus One Year of Follow-up," *Journal of Clinical Endocrinology and Metabolism*, vol. 83, no. 2 (1998), p. 396.

Page 232. HRT treatment to prevent Alzheimer's: The study calling for more research is Kristine Yaffe et al., "Estrogen Therapy in Postmenopausal Women:

Effects on Cognitive Function and Dementia," *Journal of the American Medical Association*, vol. 179, no. 9 (March 4, 1998), p. 688.

Page 234. Cultural context: Among the sources for this section are Gail Weber, "Cross-Cultural Menopause: A Study in Contrasts," in *A Clinician's Guide to Menopause* (cited above), and Margaret Lock, *Encounters with Aging: Mythologies of Menopause in Japan and North America* (Berkeley: University of California Press, 1993).

Page 236. Germaine Greer: Quoted in Melinda Beck, "Menopause," *Newsweek*, May 25, 1992, p. 38.

Page 236. Women's happiness: The Swedish survey was reported in "Love Your Job," *American Health*, January–February 1997, p. 24.

Chapter 11: Is There a Female Brain?

Page 339. Marie-Sophie Germain: Sources include L. S. Grinstein and P. J. Campbell (editors), *Women of Mathematics* (Westport, CT: 1987), p. 47, and Amanda Swift, who wrote the entry on Germain for the "Biographies of Women Mathematicians" website of Agnes Scott College in Atlanta (www.scottlan.edu//riddle/women/).

Page 240. Charlotte Perkins Gilman: "The brain is not an organ of sex" is from her *Women and Economics: A Study of the Economic Relation Between Men and Women in Social Evolution* (New York: Gordon Press, 1975).

Page 241. Brain research: The evolution of brain research and current methods and limitations of such research are summarized in Ruben Gur and Raquel Gur, "Methods for the Study of Brain-Behavior Relationships," in Alan Frazer et al. (editors), *Biological Bases of Brain Function and Disease* (New York: Raven Press, 1994), pp. 261–79.

Page 241. Sex differences in the brain: Sources include Gillian Einstein, "Sex and the Brain: Are There Consequences for Neurology?" *Journal of Women's Health*, vol. 4, no. 4 (1995), p. 427; C. Pilgrim and I. Resisert, "Difference Between Male and Female Brains—Developmental Mechanisms and Implications," *Hormonal and Metabolic Research*, vol. 24 (1992), p. 353; and Tabitha Powledge, "Ever Different; Research Update from the Annual Meeting in Baltimore of the American Association for the Advancement of Science," *BioScience*, vol. 46, no. 6 (June 1996), p. 394.

Page 241. Gender differences in light and sound sensitivity: Sources include Karl Pribram, Brain Research and Informational Sciences Center at Radford University; and Diane McGuiness, "Away from a Unisex Psychology: Individual Differences in Visual Perception," *Perception*, vol. 5 (1976), p. 375.

Page 243. Ioana Dumitriu's quotation: From Karen Arenson, "A: One, from Romania, Q: How Many Women Have Won the Ultimate Math Contest?" *New York Times*, May 1, 1997, p. A19.

Page 243. Brain size alone: There is a detailed discussion of this research in Deborah Blum, *Sex on the Brain: The Biological Differences Between Men and Women* (New York: Viking, 1997). Other sources include C. Davison Ankney, "Sex Differences in Relative Brain Size: The Mismeasure of Woman, Too?" *Intelligence*, vol. 16, nos. 3–4

(July–December 1992), p. 329; and M.-C. de Lacoste et al., "Measures of Gender Differences in the Human Brain and Their Relationship to Brain Weight," *Biological Psychiatry*, vol. 28 (1990), p. 931.

Page 243. Neuronal density: Psychologist Sandra Witelson's work is the subject of Mark Nichols, "Boys, Girls and Brainpower: The Sexes Differ in More than Appearance," *Maclean's*, vol. 109, no. 4 (January 22, 1996), p. 49.

Page 244. Cerebral blood flow: Ruben Gur and Raquel Gur, "Gender Differences in Cerebral Blood Flow," *Schizophrenia Bulletin*, vol. 16, no. 2 (1990), p. 247, and Ruben Gur et al., "Sex and Handedness Differences in Cerebral Blood Flow During Rest and Cognitive Activity," *Science*, vol. 217 (August 13, 1982), p. 659.

Page 245. Bilateral use of brain: B. A. Shaywitz et al., "Sex Differences in the Functional Organization of the Brain for Language," *Nature*, vol. 373 (1995), p. 607; Roland Erwin et al., "Effects of Task and Gender on EEG Indices of Hemispheric Activation," *Neuropsychiatry, Neuropsychology, and Behavioral Neurology*, vol. 2, no. 4 (1989), p. 248; and David Lewis and Marian Diamond, "The Influence of Gonadal Steroids on the Asymmetry of the Cerebral Cortex," in Richard Davidson and Kenneth Hugdahl (editors), *Brain Asymmetry* (Cambridge: MIT Press, 1995), pp. 31–50.

Page 245. Corpus callosum: Among the studies in this controversial area are Alan Beaton, "The Relationship of Planum Temporale Asymmetry and Morphology of the Corpus Callosum to Handedness, Gender and Dyslexia: A Review of the Evidence," *Brain and Language*, vol. 60, no. 2 (November 1997), p. 255; Matthew Hoptman and Richard Davidson, "How and Why Do the Two Cerebral Hemispheres Interact?" *Psychological Bulletin*, vol. 116, no. 2 (September 1994), p. 195; and Ralph Holloway et al., "Sexual Dimorphism of the Human Corpus Callosum from Three Independent Samples: Relative Size of the Corpus Callosum," *American Journal of Physical Anthropology*, vol. 92, no. 4 (December 1993), p. 481.

Page 245. Brain plasticity: Marian Diamond, "The Interaction Between Sex Hormones and Environment," in *Enriching Heredity* (New York: Free Press, 1988), and "How the Brain Grows in Response to Experience," in Robert Ornstein and Charles Swencionis (editors), *The Healing Brain: A Scientific Reader* (New York: Guilford Press, 1990), p. 22.

Page 246. Women underestimate their own intelligence: The research cited is in Mark Bennett, "Self-estimates of Ability in Men and Women," *The Journal of Social Psychology*, vol. 137, no. 4 (August 1997), p. 540; and Mark Bennett, "Self-estimates of Intelligence in Men and Women," *The Journal of Social Psychology*, vol. 136 (1996), p. 411.

Page 247. Sex differences in math and verbal skills: Virginia Valian provides an excellent overview of the controversial and often contradictory research in "Biology and Cognition" in her book *Why So Slow? The Advancement of Women* (Cambridge: MIT Press, 1998), pp. 81–101.

Page 247. Sex differences in various tasks: Doreen Kimura summarizes many of these variations between women and men in "Sex, Sexual Orientation and Sex Hormones Influence Human Cognitive Function" in *Current Opinion in Neurobiology*, vol. 6, no. 2 (1996), p. 259, and "Sex Differences in the Brain," *Scientific American*, September 1992, p. 119.

Page 248. Factors influencing test scores: Matthew Sharps et al., "Gender and Task in the Determination of Spatial Cognitive Performance," *Psychology of Women Quarterly*, vol. 17, no. 1 (1993), p. 71.

Page 250. Cultural variations: The data on Great Britain come from Linda Grant, "The Smarter Sex? (Gender Learning Differences in British Education)," *World Press Review*, vol. 42, no. 1 (January 1995), p. 45, and "Not Working" (editorial on British education), *Times Educational Supplement*, no. 4159 (March 15, 1996), p. A18.

Page 251. Gender differences in learning styles: The evidence for these differences is reported in a growing number of studies, including Ann Pollina, "Gender Balance: Lessons from Girls in Science and Mathematics," *Educational Leadership*, September 1995; and Martha Carr and Donna Jessup, "Gender Differences in First Grade Mathematics Strategy Use: Social and Metacognitive Influences," *Journal of Educational Psychology*, vol. 89, no. 2 (1996), p. 318.

Page 251. Single-sex education: This discussion draws on Tamar Lewin, "All-Girl Schools Questioned as a Way to Attain Equity; Study Finds No Proof Programs Are Better" (American Association of University Women study), *New York Times*, March 12, 1998, p. A1; and Richard Durost, "Single Sex Math Classes: What and for Whom?" *NASSP Bulletin*, vol. 80, no. 577 (February 1996), p. 27.

Page 252. Aging and brain shrinkage: The many sources for this content include Ruben Gur et al., "Gender Differences in Age Effect on Brain Atrophy Measured by Magnetic Resonance Imaging," *Proceedings of the National Academy of Science*, vol. 88 (1991), page 2845; C. Edward Coffey, "Sex Differences in Brain Aging: A Quantitative Magnetic Resonance Imaging Study," *Archives of Neurology*, vol. 55, (1998), p. 169; and Patricia Cowell et al., "Sex Differences in Aging of the Human Frontal and Temporal Lobes," *Journal of Neuroscience*, vol. 14, no. 8 (August 1994), p. 4748.

Page 253. Theories about aging brains: Materials that inform this section include Brian Henry, "Reduced Reactivity of Brain Blood Vessels May Explain Greater Risk of Stroke by Older Women," American Heart Association news release, July 2, 1998. Ruben Gur presented his theories on glucose metabolism rates and their impact on aging at the American Association for the Advancement of Science annual meeting, February 1996, in Baltimore.

Page 253. Sex differences in memory: Sources include Thomas Crook, "Diagnosis and Treatment of Memory Loss in Older Patients Who Are Not Demented," in R. Levy et al. (editors), *Treatment and Care in Old Age Psychiatry* (Wrightson Biomedical Publishing, 1993), pp. 95–111; and Glen Larrabee and Thomas Crook, "Do Men Show More Rapid Age-Associated Decline in Simulated Everyday Verbal Memory than Do Women?" *Psychology and Aging*, vol. 8, no. 1 (1993), p. 68.

Page 254. Estrogen and the aging brain: Background materials include Doreen Kimura, "Estrogen Replacement Therapy May Protect Against Intellectual Decline in Postmenopausal Women," *Hormones and Behavior*, vol. 29, no. 3 (1995), p. 312; and

Joan Stephenson, Elizabeth Barret-Connor, and Donna Kritz-Silverstein, "Estrogen Replacement Therapy and Cognitive Function in Older Women," *Journal of the American Medical Association*, vol. 269, no. 20 (May 26, 1993), p. 2637.

Page 254. Estrogen and Alzheimer's: This topic is discussed in Rebecca Voelker, "More Evidence Links NSAID, Estrogen Use with Reduced Alzheimer Risk," *Journal of the American Medical Association*, vol. 275, no. 18 (May 8, 1996), p. 1389; Tabitha Powledge, "Estrogen: A Key to Alzheimer's Disease?" *BioScience*, vol. 47, no. 5 (May 1997), p. 273; and Kristine Hoff et al., "Estrogen Therapy in Postmenopausal Women: Effects on Cognitive Function and Dementia," *Journal of the American Medical Association*, vol. 179, no. 9 (March 4, 1998), p. 688.

Page 255. Polly Matzinger: This work is profiled in Claudia Dreifus, "Blazing an Unconventional Trail to a New Theory of Immunity," *New York Times*, June 16, 1998, p. B15.

Page 256. Women's creative thinking: See Evelyn Fox Keller and Helen Longino (editors), *Feminism and Science* (Oxford: Oxford University Press, 1996), pp. 264–79.

Page 257. Helen Taussig: In addition to standard biographical sources, I drew on Bernardine Healy's account of her conversations with Dr. Taussig in *A New Prescription for Women's Health* (New York: Viking, 1995), pp. 4–5.

Chapter 12: Gender and Emotion

Page 259. Grey Rock Harbour: Ethnographer Dona Lee Davis reported on "women's nerves" in "The Variable Character of Nerves in a Newfoundland Fishing Village," *Medical Anthropology*, vol. 11 (1989), p. 63, and "When Men Became 'Women': Gender Antagonism and the Changing Sexual Geography of Work in Newfoundland," *Sex Roles*, vol. 29, nos. 7–8 (1993), p. 457.

Page 260. Jacquelyn James: Her articles include "His and Hers," *Boston Globe*, May 25, 1995, and "What Are the Social Issues Involved in Focusing on Difference in the Study of Gender?" *Journal of Social Issues*, vol. 53, no. 2 (1997), p. 213.

Page 260. Emotional intelligence: Daniel Goleman, *Emotional Intelligence* (New York: Bantam Books, 1995) and personal interview.

Page 261. Doing emotion: Sources include Claudia Geer and Stephanie Shields, "Women and Emotion: Stereotypes and the Double Bind," in J. Chrisler, P. Rozee, and C. Golden (editors), *Lectures on the Psychology of Women* (New York: McGraw-Hill, 1995), p. 63; and Stephanie Shields, "Gender in the Psychology of Emotion: A Selective Research Review," in K. T. Strongman (editor), *International Review of Studies on Emotion*, vol. 2 (Chichester, England: Wiley, 1991), pp. 227–45.

Page 262. Gender stereotype: Leslie Brody challenges this assumption in "Gender and Emotion: Beyond Stereotypes," *Journal of Social Issues*, vol. 53, no. 2 (summer 1997), p. 369, and Leslie Brody, Gretchen Lovas, and Deborah Hay, "Gender Differences in Anger and Fear as a Function of Situational Context," *Sex Roles*, vol. 32, nos. 1–2 (January 1995), p. 47.

Page 262. Emotional expressivity: Along with previously cited sources, see Michele Grossman and Wendy Wood, "Sex Differences in Intensity of Emotional Experience," *Journal of Personality and Social Psychology*, vol. 65, no. 5 (November 1993), p. 1010.

Page 262. Crying: Ronald Levant's research into the tough conditioning of little boys is described in "The Real Reason Big Boys Don't Cry," *American Health*, October 1996, p. 19. William H. Frey II of the Dry Eye and Tear Research Center in St. Paul, Minn., reports on the biochemistry of tears in *Crying: The Mystery of Tears* (New York: Harper and Row, 1985).

Page 262. "Schooling" in emotion: Sources include Christi Cervantes and Maureen Callanan, "Labels and Explanations in Mother-Child Emotion Talk: Age and Gender Differentiation," *Developmental Psychology*, vol. 34, no. 1 (January 1998), p. 88; and Pamela Garner et al., "Preschool Children's Emotional Expressions with Peers: The Roles of Gender and Emotional Socialization," *Sex Roles*, vol. 36, nos. 11–12 (June 1997), p. 675.

Page 264. Brain scans: This research is reported in Mark George et al., "Brain Activity During Transient Sadness and Happiness in Healthy Women," *American Journal of Psychiatry*, vol. 152, no. 3 (March 1995), p. 341.

Page 265. Gender difference in reading emotions: Sources include Ruben Gur et al., "Effects of Emotional Discrimination Tasks on Cerebral Blood Flow," *Brain and Cognition*, vol. 25 (1994), p. 271; and Ruben Gur et al., "Facial Emotion Discrimination: II. Behavioral Findings in Depression," *Psychiatry Research*, vol. 42 (1992), p. 241.

Page 266. Externality: James Pennebaker and Tomi-Ann Roberts, "Toward a His and Hers Theory of Emotion: Gender Differences in Visceral Perception," *Journal of Social and Clinical Psychology*, special issue on social psychophysiology, vol. 11, no. 3 (fall 1992), p. 199.

Page 267. Social conditioning: The study cited is Chris Boyatzis, Elizabeth Chazan, and Carol Ting, "Preschool Children's Decoding of Facial Emotions," *Journal of Genetic Psychology*, vol. 154, no. 3 (September 1993), p. 375.

Page 267. Reading emotions: The content on nonverbal communication is largely based on the research of Judith Hall, described in her book *Nonverbal Sex Differences: Accuracy of Communication and Expressive Style* (Baltimore: Johns Hopkins University Press, 1984).

Page 267. Impact of marital arguments: The study cited is Janice Kiecolt-Glaser et al., "Marital Conflict in Older Adults: Endocrinological and Immunological Correlates," *Psychosomatic Medicine*, vol. 59, no. 4 (1997), p. 339.

Page 269. Spoken language differences: Deborah Tannen, *You Just Don't Understand* (New York: Ballantine Books, 1990) and *Talking from 9 to 5* (New York: Avon Books, 1995).

Page 269. Sex differences in communication: Primary sources are Nancy Briton and Judith Hall, "Beliefs About Female and Male Nonverbal Communication," *Sex Roles*, vol. 32, nos. 1–2 (January 1995), p. 79; and Nancy Briton and Judith Hall, "Gender-

Based Expectancies and Observer Judgments of Smiling," *Journal of Nonverbal Behavior*, vol. 19, no. 1 (spring 1995), p. 49.

Page 271. Anger: Anne Campbell et al., "Aggression and Testosterone: Testing a Biosocial Model," *Aggressive Behavior*, vol. 23, no. 4 (1997), p. 229; Anne Campbell and Deborah Richardson, "Men, Women and Aggression," *Psychology of Women Quarterly*, vol. 20, no. 2 (1996), p. 319; Anne Campbell and Kirsti Lagerspetz, "Men, Women and Aggression: From Rage in Marriage to Violence in the Streets—How Gender Affects the Way We Act," *Aggressive Behavior*, vol. 31, no. 2 (1996), p. 149.

Page 272. John Archer reported his study of physical aggressiveness at a meeting of the International Society for Research on Aggression in Mahwah, NJ, in July 1998. Abigail Zuger described this research in "A Fistful of Hostility Is Found in Women," *New York Times*, July 28, 1998, p. B9.

Page 272. Dealing with anger: Sandra Thomas's extensive research includes "Women's Anger: Relationship of Suppression to Blood Pressure," *Nursing Research*, vol. 46, no. 6 (1997), p. 324; "Angry? Let's Talk About It," *Applied Nursing Research*, vol. 10, no. 2 (1997), p. 80; and *Women and Anger* (New York: Springer Publishing, 1993).

Page 273. Women's proneness to guilt: Carol Nadelson sums up psychoanalytic perspectives in "The Psychology of Women," *Canadian Journal of Psychiatry*, vol. 28 (April 1983), p. 210.

Page 274. Emotional happiness: This section draws on many sources, including interviews with therapists and Robin Simon, "Gender, Multiple Roles, Role Meaning, and Mental Health," *Journal of Health and Social Behavior*, vol. 36, no. 2 (June 1995), p. 182.

Page 275. Impact of work: Mary Clare Lennon and Sarah Rosenfield, "Women and Mental Health: The Interaction of Job and Family Conditions," *Journal of Health and Social Behavior*, vol. 33, December 1992, p. 316; and Sharon Lobel et al., "The Impact of Psychological Intimacy between Men and Women at Work," *Organizational Dynamic*, summer 1994, p. 5.

Page 277. "In love the genders . . .": Ethel Person, "Some Differences Between Men and Women: I. The Passionate Quest," *The Atlantic Monthly*, March 1988, p. 71. Dr. Person expands on her theories and insights in *By Force of Fantasy: How We Make Our Lives* (New York: Basic Books, 1995).

Chapter 13: Vulnerable Women

Page 282: Sex differences in mental illness in the United States: The data comes from various sources, including Ronald Kessler et al., "Sex and Depression in the National Comorbidity Survey I: Lifetime Prevalence, Chronicity, and Recurrence," *Journal of Affective Disorders*, vol. 29 (1993), p. 85; Ronald Kessler et al., "Sex and Depression in the National Comorbidity Survey II: Cohort Effects," *Journal of Affective Disorders*, vol. 30 (1994), p. 15; and Myrna Weissman and Mark Olfson, "Depression in Women: Implications for Health Care Research," *Science*, vol. 269 (August 11, 1995), p. 799.

Page 282: Sex differences in mental illness in Europe: The study cited is Birgit Petersson and Marianne Kastrup, "Gender and Mental Health," *Baillière's Clinical Psychiatry*, vol. 1, no. 2 (May 1995), p. 329.

Page 282. Vulnerability to mental disorders in women and men: Sources include Nancy Andreasen, "What Shape Are We In? Gender, Psychopathology, and the Brain," *American Journal of Psychiatry*, vol. 154, no. 12 (December 1997), p. 1637; Mary Seeman, "Psychopathology in Women and Men: Focus on Female Hormones," *American Journal of Psychiatry*, vol. 154, no. 12 (December 1997), p. 1641; Peg Nopoulos, Michael Flaum, and Nancy Andreasen, "Sex Differences in Brain Morphology in Schizophrenia," *American Journal of Psychiatry*, vol. 154, no. 12 (December 1997), p. 1648.

Page 283. Women's greater incidence of depression: In addition to the above-cited sources, I drew on C. Ernest and J. Angst, "The Zurich Study: XII. Sex Differences in Depression. Evidence from Longitudinal Epidemiological Data," European Archives of Practical Psychiatry and Clinical Neuroscience, vol. 241 (1992), p. 222; and Myrna Weissman, "Cross-national Epidemiology of Major Depression and Bipolar Disorder," *Journal of the American Medical Association*, vol. 276, no. 4 (July 24–31, 1996), p. 293.

Page 285. Brain chemistry: Recent findings are reported in George Heninger, "Serotonin, Sex, and Psychiatric Illness," *Proceedings of the National Academy of Sciences*, vol. 94, no. 10 (May 13, 1997), p. 4823, and S. Nishizawa et al., "Differences Between Males and Females in Rates of Serotonin Synthesis in Human Brain," *Proceedings of the National Academy of Sciences*, vol. 94, no. 10 (May 13, 1997), p. 5313.

Pages 286–88. Biological vulnerability: In addition to previously cited works, this discussion is based on the following reports: Mary Blehar and Dan Oren, "Women's Increased Vulnerability to Mood Disorders: Integrating Psychobiology and Epidemiology," *Depression*, vol. 3 (1995), p. 3; "Depression," *Lancet*, vol. 349, no. 9052 (March 1, 1997), p. S117; Barbara Parry, "Women and Depression," *Health in Mind and Body*, vol. 1, no. 1 (1996), p. 1; and Donna Stewart and Katherine Boydell, "Psychologic Distress During Menopause: Associations Across the Reproductive Life Cycle," *International Journal of Psychiatry in Medicine*, vol. 23, no. 2 (1993), p. 157.

Page 288. Risk factors for depression: Sources include American Psychological Association National Task Force on Women and Depression, *Women and Depression: Risk Factors and Treatment* (Washington, DC: American Psychological Association, 1990); and Bruce Link, Mary Clare Lennon, and Bruce Dohrenwened, "Socioeconomic Status and Depression: The Role of Occupations Involving Direction, Control and Planning," *American Journal of Sociology*, vol. 98, no. 6 (May 1993), p. 1351.

Page 289. "Many ethnic groups . . .": Freda Lewis-Hall, audiotaped presentations at the American Psychiatric Association annual meetings.

Page 290. Psychological factors: Additional sources include Susan Blumenthal, "Issues in Women's Mental Health," *Journal of Women's Health*, vol. 3, no. 6 (1994), p. 453, and L. D. Butler and Susan Nolen-Hoeksema, "Gender Differences in Response to Depressed Mood in a College Sample," *Sex Roles*, vol. 30, nos. 5–6 (1994), p. 331.

Page 292. "I saw the world . . .": Kathy Cronkite, *On the Edge of Darkness* (New York: Doubleday, 1994).

Pages 293–96. Anxiety disorders: Women's greater vulnerability is discussed in Mary Seeman, "Psychopathology in Women and Men: Focus on Female Hormones," *American Journal of Psychiatry*, vol. 154, no. 12 (December 1997), p. 1641; and Naomi Breslau et al., "Sex Differences in Posttraumatic Stress Disorder," *Archives of General Psychiatry*, vol. 54 (November 1997), p. 1044.

Page 297. Substance abuse in women: Studies include Sheila Blume, "Sexuality and Stigma: The Alcoholic Woman," *Alcohol Health and Research World*, vol. 15, no. 2 (spring 1991), p. 139; Barbara Lex, "Alcohol and Other Drug Abuse Among Women," *Alcohol Health and Research World*, vol. 18, no. 3 (summer 1994), p. 212; Sharon Wilsnack et al., "How Women Drink: Epidemiology of Women's Drinking and Problem Drinking," *Alcohol Health and Research World*, vol. 18, no. 3 (summer 1994), p. 173; and Edith Gomberg and S. Lisansky, "Risk Factors for Drinking Over a Woman's Lifespan," *Alcohol Health and Research World*, vol. 18, no. 3 (summer 1994), p. 220.

Page 301. Antidepressants and women: Sources include Kathleen Pajer, "New Strategies in the Treatment of Depression in Women," *Journal of Clinical Psychiatry*, vol. 55 (1994); K. Dawkins and W. Z. Potter, "Gender Differences in Pharmacokinetics and Pharmacodynamics of Psychotropics: Focus on Women," *Psychopharmacology Bulletin*, vol. 27 (1991), p. 417; and Kimberly Yonkers et al., "Gender Differences in Pharmacokinetics and Pharmacodynamics of Psychotropic Medication," *American Journal of Psychiatry*, vol. 149, no. 5 (May 1992), p. 587.

Page 302. Psychotherapy for women: In addition to previously cited material, sources include Kathleen Pajer, "Gender Differences in the Psychotherapeutic and Pharmacologic Treatment of Depression in Women," presentation at the symposium "New Advances in the Treatment of Depression," California Pacific Medical Center, March 25, 1995; and Susan Nolen-Hoeksema and J. Morrow, "Effects of Rumination and Distraction on Naturally-occurring Depressed Mood," *Cognition and Emotion*, vol. 7 (1993), p. 561.

Page 302. Improved outlook: One recent study that found that women do just as well as men is H. Blair Simpson et al., "First Episode Major Depression: Few Sex Differences in Course," *Archives of General Psychiatry*, vol. 54 (July 1997), p. 633. The Brown University study cited is Caron Zlotnick et al., "Gender, Type of Treatment, Dysfunctional Attitudes, Social Support, Life Events, and Depressive Symptoms Over Naturalistic Follow-up." *American Journal of Psychiatry*, vol. 153, no. 8 (August 1996), p. 1021.

Chapter 14: Sensuous Spirits

Page 307. "To a woman . . .": Irene Claremont de Castillejo, *Knowing Woman* (Boston: Shambhala Publications, 1997).

Page 307. "I know no woman . . .": Adrienne Rich, *Of Woman Born* (New York: W. W. Norton & Company, 1986).

Page 310. Sex reducing risk of death: The study cited is George Davey Smith, "Sex and Death: Are They Related? Findings from the Caerphilly Cohort Study," *British Medical Journal*, vol. 315 (1997), p. 1641.

Page 310. "Even basic questions . . .": Beverly Whipple's research includes the following: Beverly Whipple et al., "Physiological Correlates of Imagery-Induced Orgasm in Women," *Archives of Sexual Behavior*, vol. 21, no. 2 (1992), page 121; Milan Zaviacic and Beverly Whipple, "Update on the Female Prostate and the Phenomenon of Female Ejaculation," *The Journal of Sex Research*, vol. 30, no. 2 (May 1993), p. 148; and Beverly Whipple and Barry Komisaruk, "Elevation of Pain Threshold by Vaginal Stimulation in Women," *Pain*, vol. 21 (1985), p. 357.

Page 312. Female arousal: The research cited is Ellen Laan et al., "Women's Sexual and Emotional Response to Male- and Female-Produced Erotica," *Archives of Sexual Behavior*, vol. 33, no. 4 (May 1995), p. 441; and Ellen Laan and Walter Everaerd, "Habitation of Female Sexual Arousal to Slides and Film," *Archives of Sexual Behavior*, vol. 24, no. 5 (October 1995), p. 517.

Page 312. "Men listen to their bodies": Laan was quoted in Natalie Angier, "Science Is Finding Out What Women Really Want," *New York Times*, August 13, 1995.

Page 313. "The erotic is not . . .": Audre Lorde, "Uses of the Erotic: The Erotic as Power," in *Sister Outsider* (Trumansburg, NY: Sister Outsider, 1984), p. 55.

Page 313. Sexual context: The major national survey was reported by Robert Michael et al., *Sex in America: A Definitive Survey* (Boston: Little, Brown and Company, 1994).

Page 313. Sexual satisfaction: This topic is discussed in Dianne Hales, "The Joy of Midlife Sex," *American Health for Women*, vol. 16, no. 1 (January–February, 1997), p. 78; Beryl Lieff Benderly, "Secrets of the Bedroom," *American Health*, May 1991, p. 36; Michael Young et al., "Correlates of Sexual Satisfaction in Marriage," unpublished manuscript; and Vern Bullough, *Science in the Bedroom* (New York: Basic Books, 1993).

Page 314. "Silken revolution": Elina Haavio-Mannila et al., "Repression, Revolution and Ambivalence: The Sexual Life of Three Generations," presentation at the symposium "Scientific Study of Sexuality," San Francisco, November 1995.

Page 315. "Body mystics": Virginia Ramet Mollenkott, *Sensuous Spirituality: Out from Fundamentalism* (New York: Crossroad Publishing, 1993), and Elisabeth Moltmann-Wendel, *I Am My Body: A Theology of Embodiment* (New York: Continuum, 1995).

Page 317. "Suddenly there . . .:" The quote is from Rosemary Bray, "A Voice in the Wilderness," *New York Times Magazine*, December 7, 1997, p. 89.

Page 317. Women's quests: The recent developments in female spirituality are reported in Lisa Collier Cool, "Faith and Healing," *American Health*, November 1997, p. 49, and Michael Norman, "Feminists Nurture a More Tolerant Christianity," *New York Times*, April 11, 1998.

Page 319. Goddesses: The classic book on this topic is Jean Shinoda Bolen, *Goddesses in Everywoman: A New Psychology of Women* (New York: HarperPerennial, 1985).

Chapter 15: Tomorrow's Woman

Page 324. "We have crossed a great divide": The demographic data was provided by Gary Wright, "Continuing Change in Women's Roles," Procter and Gamble Business Information Services, June 12, 1996. The statistics on women in the workforce in the United States and Europe are from "Women and Work: For Better, for Worse," *The Economist*, July 18, 1998, p. 3.

Page 325. New providers: The Yankelovitch findings about masculinity were reported in Susan Faludi, *Backlash: The Undeclared War Against American Women* (New York: Doubleday, 1991), p. 65.

Page 326. "Women are developing . . .": Gail Sheehy, *Understanding Men's Passages* (New York: Random House, 1998), p. 5.

Page 327. Height discrimination: This example comes from Lani Guinier, Michelle Fine, and Jean Balin, *Becoming Gentlemen: Women, Law School, and Institutional Change* (Boston: Beacon Press, 1997), p. 18.

Page 327. "It's a woman's world": This was the title of an article by Rana Dogar in *Newsweek*, May 18, 1998, p. 12. Many of the statistics in this section are from "Moving Up in the World," *Newsweek*, May 18, 1998, p. 120; Families and Work Institute, "Women: The New Providers," a study commissioned by Whirlpool Foundation, Benton Harbor, Michigan, 1995.

Page 328. The mix of good news and bad news for working women: This has been the subject of many reports, including Virginia Schein et al., "Think Manager—Think Male: A Global Phenomenon?" *Journal of Organizational Behavior*, vol. 17, no. 1 (January 1996), p. 33; Lisa Mainiero, "The Longest Climb," *Psychology Today*, November–December 1994, p. 40; and Catherine DeAngelis and Michael Johns, "Promotion of Women in Academic Medicine: Shatter the Ceilings, Polish the Floors," *Journal of the American Medical Association*, vol. 273, no. 13 (April 5, 1995), p. 1056.

Page 328. Income gap: Mary Cooper, "Income Inequality," *CQ Researcher*, vol. 8, no. 15 (April 17, 1998), p. 339; Tamar Lewin, "Equal Pay for Equal Work Is No. 1 Goal of Women," *New York Times*, September 5, 1997, p. A13; and Tamar Lewin, "Study Finds Pay Gap Closing for Male and Female Doctors," *New York Times*, April 11, 1996.

Pages 328–29. Gender bias in Sweden: The study cited is Christine Wenneras and Agnes Wold, "Nepotism and Sexism in Peer-Review," *Nature*, vol. 387, no. 6631 (May 22, 1997), p. 341.

Page 329. Gender equity: This analysis comes from Virginia Valian, *Why So Slow?*
The Advancement of Women (Cambridge: MIT Press, 1998).

Page 330. "We were damned whatever we did": From Carolyn Duff and Barbara
Cohen, *When Women Work Together: Using Our Strengths to Overcome Our Challenges*
(Berkeley, CA: Conari Press, 1993).

Page 331. "You must first become a gentleman": Michelle Fine presented these find-
ings in "Whistling Like Teakettles," a presentation at the American Psychological
Association annual meeting in Los Angeles in 1996. This research also is featured in
Becoming Gentlemen: Women, Law School, and Institutional Change (cited above).

Page 331. Female attorneys: Residual problems are reported in Nina Bernstein,
"Equal Opportunity Recedes for Most Female Lawyers," *New York Times*, January 8,
1996, p. A10.

Page 332. Women-owned businesses: Rana Dogar, "The Top 500 Women-Owned
Businesses; In Industries from Software to Ready-to-Wear, Women-Owned Compa-
nies Are Thriving," *Working Woman*, May 1998, p. 35, and Lynne Dumas, "Be Your
Own Boss," *Working Mother*, September 1997, p. 42.

Page 333. Survey of optimism: These data were reported in Marcia Mogelonsky,
"Where Women Do Better," *American Demographics*, vol. 20, no. 3 (March 1998),
p. 35.

Page 334. Improv moms: This description is from Susan Seliger, "The Improv Mom,"
Working Mother, September 1997, p. 34.

Page 334. New breed of collaborative dads: Sources include Mary Clare Lennon and
Sarah Rosenfield, "Relative Fairness and the Division of Housework: The Importance
of Options," *American Journal of Sociology*, vol. 100, no. 2 (September 1994); Tamar
Lewin, "Men Assuming Bigger Share at Home, New Survey Shows," *New York Times*,
April 15, 1998, p. A16; and Sue Shellenbarger, "Work and Family: In Attitude, Sexes
Can Vive La Similarity," *San Francisco Examiner*, April 26,1998, p. CL 25.

Page 335. Shared values: Sources include numerous studies by Rosalind Barnett,
including "Change in Job and Marital Experiences and Change in Psychological Distress: A Longitudinal Study of Dual-Earner Couples," *Journal of Personality and Social
Psychology*, vol. 69, no. 5 (November 1995), p. 839; and "Gender and the Relationship Between Parent Role Quality and Psychological Distress: A Study of Men and
Women in Dual-Earner Couples," *Journal of Family Issues*, vol. 15, no. 2 (June 1994),
p. 229.

Page 337. Interpretation of St. Paul's letter: This commentary appeared in *SPINN*,
the newsletter of the Sausalito Presbyterian Church, June 1998.

Page 338. Benefits of marriage: Maradee Davis and John Neuhasu, "Living Arrangements and Survival Among Middle-aged and Older Adults in the NHANES I Epidemiological Follow-up Study," *American Journal of Public Health*, vol. 82, no. 3 (March
1992).

Page 339. Boomer women: For this section, I drew on a variety of perspectives,
including Joann Lublin, "Family Values: Some Adult Daughters of 'Supermoms' Plan

to Take Another Path," *Wall Street Journal,* December 28, 1995, p. A1; Peter Passell, "Hurdles Are Still High for Women Who Want a Career and a Family," *New York Times,* September 7, 1995, p. D2; Jill Smolowe, "The Stalled Revolution," *Time,* May 6, 1996; and "Mothers Can't Win," special issue, *New York Times Magazine,* April 5, 1998.

SELECTED BIBLIOGRAPHY

Allman, William. *The Stone Age Present*. New York: Simon and Schuster, 1994.

Anderson, Bonnie, and Judith Zinsser. *A History of Their Own*. 2 vols. New York: Harper and Row, 1988.

Anderson, Ruth, and Patricia Hopkins. *The Feminine Face of God: The Unfolding of the Sacred in Women*. New York: Bantam, 1992.

Angier, Natalie. *The Beauty of the Beastly*. Boston: Houghton-Mifflin, 1995.

Baker, Robin. *Sperm Wars: The Science of Sex*. New York: Basic Books, 1996.

Baker, Robin, and Mark Bellis. *Human Sperm Competition: Copulation, Masturbation and Infidelity*. London: Chapman and Hall, 1995.

Barbach, Lonnie. *The Pause*. New York: Signet, 1993.

Barber, Elizabeth Wayland. *Women's Work: The First 20,000 Years*. New York: W. W. Norton, 1994.

Bassoff, Evelyn. *Cherishing Our Daughters: How to Raise a Healthy, Confident Daughter*. New York: Dutton, 1998.

Batten, Mary. *Sexual Strategies: How Females Choose Their Mates*. New York: G. P. Putnam's Sons, 1992.

Beauvoir, Simone de. *The Second Sex*. New York: Vintage, 1989.

Belenky, Mary Field, et al. *Women's Way of Knowing*. New York: Basic Books, 1973.

Blum, Deborah. *Sex on the Brain: The Biological Differences Between Men and Women.* New York: Viking, 1997.

Bolen, Jean Shinoda. *Goddesses in Everywoman: A New Psychology of Women.* New York: HarperPerennial, 1985.

Bono, Paola, and Sandra Kemp (editors). *Italian Feminist Thought: A Reader.* Oxford: Basil Blackwell, 1991.

Borysenko, Joan. *A Woman's Book of Life.* New York: Riverhead, 1996.

Brown, Lyn Mikel, and Carol Gilligan. *Meeting at the Crossroads.* New York: Ballantine, 1992.

Brumberg, Joan Jacobs. *The Body Project: An Intimate History of American Girls.* New York: Random House, 1997.

Burt, Vivien, and Victoria Hendricks. *Women's Mental Health.* Washington: American Psychiatric Press, 1997.

Buss, David. *The Evolution of Desire.* New York: HarperCollins, 1994.

Crenshaw, Theresa. *The Alchemy of Love and Lust.* New York: G. P. Putnam's Sons, 1996.

Cronkite, Kathy. *On the Edge of Darkness.* New York: Doubleday, 1994.

DeBold, Elizabeth, et al. *Mother Daughter Revolution.* Reading, MA: Addison-Wesley, 1993.

Delaney, Janice, Mary Jane Lupton, and Emily Toth. *The Curse: A Cultural History of Menstruation.* Urbana: University of Illinois Press, 1988.

Dennerstein, Lorraine, and Julia Shelley (editors). *A Woman's Guide to Menopause and Hormone Replacement Therapy.* Washington, DC: American Psychiatric Press, 1998.

Diamond, Jared. *The Third Chimpanzee: The Evolution and Future of the Human Animal.* New York: HarperCollins, 1992.

Domar, Alice, and Henry Dreher. *Healing Mind, Healthy Woman.* New York: Henry Holt, 1996.

Duby, Georges, and Michelle Perrot (series editors). *A History of Women in the West.* 4 vols. Cambridge, MA: Harvard University Press, 1993.

Ehrenreich, Barbara, and Deirdre English. *Complaints and Disorders: The Sexual Politics of Sickness.* New York: Feminist Press, 1973.

———. *For Her Own Good: 150 Years of Experts' Advice to Women.* New York: Anchor, 1978.

Elia, Irene. *The Female Animal.* New York: Henry Holt, 1988.

Fausto-Sterling, Anne. *Myths of Gender.* New York: Basic Books, 1985.

Fisher, Helen. *Anatomy of Love.* New York: Fawcett Columbine, 1992.

Fleming, Ann Taylor. *Motherhood Deferred: A Woman's Journey.* New York: Fawcett Columbine, 1994.

Goleman, Daniel. *Emotional Intelligence.* New York: Bantam, 1995.

Golub, Sharon. *Periods: From Menarche to Menopause.* Newbury Park, CA: Sage, 1992.

Hales, Dianne. *Intensive Caring: New Hope for High Risk Pregnancy,* with Timothy R. B. Johnson, M.D. New York: Crown, 1990.

————. *New Hope for Problem Pregnancies,* with Robert K. Creasy, M.D. New York: Harper and Row, 1983; Berkley, 1984.

Hall, G. Stanley. *Adolescence and Its Relation to Psychology, Anthropology, Sociology, Sex, Crime, Religion, and Education.* New York: D. Appleton, 1904.

Hall, Judith. *Nonverbal Sex Differences: Accuracy of Communication and Expressive Style.* Baltimore: Johns Hopkins University Press, 1984.

Haraway, Donna. *Primate Visions: Gender, Race and Nature in the World of Modern Science.* New York: Routledge, 1992.

Haseltine, Florence (editor). *Women's Health Research: A Medical and Policy Primer.* Washington, DC: American Psychiatric Press, 1997.

Haviland, William. *Cultural Anthropology,* 8th ed. Fort Worth: Harcourt Brace, 1996.

Healy, Bernardine. *A New Prescription for Women's Health.* New York: Viking, 1995.

Helgesen, Sally. *The Female Advantage: Women's Way of Leadership.* New York: Doubleday Currency, 1995.

Hrdy, Sarah Blaffer. *The Woman That Never Evolved.* Cambridge: Harvard University Press, 1981.

Johanson, Donald. *Lucy, The Beginnings of Humankind,* with Maitland Edey. New York: Simon and Schuster, 1981.

————. *Lucy's Child: The Discovery of a Human Ancestor,* with James Shreeve. New York: Morrow, 1989.

————. *From Lucy to Language,* with Blake Edgar. New York: Simon and Schuster, 1996.

Keller, Evelyn Fox, and Helen Longino (editors). *Feminism and Science.* Oxford: Oxford University Press, 1996.

Kerns, Virginia, and Judith Brown (editors). *In Her Prime: New Views of Middle-aged Women.* Urbana: University of Illinois Press, 1992.

Kra, Siegfried. *What Every Woman Must Know About Heart Disease.* New York: Warner Books, 1997.

Larson, Reed, and Maryse Richard. *Divergent Realities: The Emotional Lives of Mothers, Fathers, and Adolescents.* New York: Basic Books, 1994.

Legato, Marianne. *Gender-Specific Aspects of Human Biology for the Practicing Physician.* Armonk, NY: Futura, 1997.

Legato, Marianne, and Carol Colman. *The Female Heart.* New York: Avon, 1991.

————. *What Women Need to Know: From Headaches to Heart Disease and Everything in Between.* New York: Simon and Schuster, 1997.

Levinson, Daniel. *The Seasons of a Woman's Life.* New York: Alfred A. Knopf, 1996.

Lisle, Laurie. *Without Child: Challenging the Stigma of Childlessness.* New York: Ballantine, 1996.

Luker, Kristin. *Dubious Conceptions.* Cambridge: Harvard University Press, 1996.

Maglin, Nan, and Donna Perry (editors). *"Bad Girls"/"Good Girls."* New Brunswick, NJ: Rutgers University Press, 1996.

Martin, Emily. *The Woman in the Body.* Boston: Beacon, 1987.

Meader, Jonathan. *In Praise of Women.* Berkeley, CA: Celestial Arts, 1997.

Michael, Robert, et al. *Sex in America: A Definitive Survey.* Boston: Little, Brown, 1994.

Moir, Anne, and David Jessel. *Brain Sex: The Real Difference Between Men and Women.* New York: Lyle Stuart, 1991.

Mollenkott, Virginia Ramet. *Sensuous Spirituality: Out from Fundamentalism.* New York: Crossroad, 1993.

Moltmann-Wendel, Elisabeth. *I Am My Body: A Theology of Embodiment.* New York: Continuum, 1995.

Nechas, Eileen, and Denise Foley. *Unequal Treatment: What You Don't Know About How Women Are Mistreated by the Medical Community.* New York: Simon and Schuster, 1994.

Nelson, Miriam. *Strong Women Stay Young.* New York: Bantam, 1997.

Northrup, Christiane. *Women's Bodies, Women's Wisdom* (Revised Edition). New York: Bantam, 1998.

Notman, Malkah, and Carol Nadelson. *Women and Men: New Perspectives on Gender Differences.* Washington, DC: American Psychiatric Press, 1991.

Pashrow, Fredric, and Charlotte Libow. *The Woman's Heart Book.* New York: Dutton, 1993.

Person, Ethel. *By Force of Fantasy: How We Make Our Lives.* New York: Basic Books, 1995.

Ponton, Lynn. *The Romance of Risk: Understanding Adolescent Lives.* New York: Basic Books, 1997.

Rich, Adrienne. *Of Woman Born.* New York: W. W. Norton, 1986.

Roiphe, Anne. *Fruitful: A Real Mother in the Modern World.* New York: Houghton-Mifflin, 1996.

Rollins, Joan. *Women's Mind, Women's Bodies.* Upper Saddle River, NJ: Prentice Hall, 1996.

Sheehy, Gail. *The Silent Passage.* New York: Random House, 1991.

———. *Understanding Men's Passages.* New York: Random House, 1998.

Small, Meredith. *What's Love Got to Do with It? The Evolution of Human Mating.* New York: Anchor, 1995.

Steinem, Gloria. *Revolution from Within.* Boston: Little, Brown, 1992.

Stewart, Donna, and Gail Robinson (editors). *A Clinician's Guide to Menopause.* Washington, DC: American Psychiatric Press, 1997.

Stewart, Donna, and Nada Stotland (editors). *Psychological Aspects of Women's Health Care.* Washington, DC: American Psychiatric Press, 1993.

Stoppard, Miriam. *Woman's Body: A Manual for Life.* London: Dorling Kindersley, 1994.

Stotland, Nada. *Psychiatric Aspects of Abortion.* Washington, DC: American Psychiatric Press, 1991.

———. *Abortion: Facts and Feelings.* Washington, DC: American Psychiatric Press, 1998.

Tannen, Deborah. *You Just Don't Understand.* New York: Ballantine, 1990.

———. *Talking from 9 to 5.* New York: Avon, 1995.

Tavris, Carol. *The Mismeasure of Woman.* New York: Touchstone, 1992.

Trevathan, Wenda. *Human Birth: An Evolutionary Perspective.* New York: Aldine de Gruyter, 1987.

Valian, Virginia. *Why So Slow? The Advancement of Women.* Cambridge: MIT Press, 1998.

Vines, Gail. *Raging Hormones.* Berkeley: University of California Press, 1993.

Vliet, Elizabeth. *Screaming to Be Heard: Hormonal Connections Women Suspect and Doctors Ignore.* New York: M. Evans, 1995.

Ward, Martha. *A World Full of Women.* Boston: Allyn and Bacon, 1996.

INDEX

Animal species (*cont'd*)
  birth, compared to humans, 209
  courtship behaviors, 27–31, 33
  father as caretaker, 40
  female competitiveness, 27–28
  female cooperation, 29
  Kronism, 37
  mate selection, 29–33
  monogamy and, 34–35
  mothering behaviors in, 38–42
  mother loss in, 39–40
  parenting behaviors, 38–40
  reproductive instinct, 194–95
  reproductive strategies (R and K), 38
  sexual behaviors in, 33
  sexual strategies of, 33–35
  wombed mammals, behaviors in, 174
Anthony, Susan B., 339
Anthropology, traditional focus of, 15
Antidepressants, 167, 227, 301–2
Anxiety disorders, xiv, 283, 293–97
  age of onset, 296
  growth and development influenced by, 12
  incidence of, 294
  menopause and, 224–27
  obsessive-compulsive disorder (OCD), 208–9,
    294
  panic attacks, 208, 294, 295
  postpartum, 208–9
  post-traumatic stress disorder (PTSD), 294, 296
  triggering factors, 294–6
Archer, John, 272
Aromatase, 74
Arthritis, 44, 94
Assisted reproductive technology. *See* Infertility.
Asthma, xii, 74, 93, 95, 161
Athletes, women, xii, 5, 81–84
  advantages in gymnastics and diving, 83
  body fat of, 82, 83, 84
  estrogen and delayed fatigue, 83
  marathon runners, 81
  men, physical and physiological differences in, 82,
    84
  muscle mass, 82
  swimming, physical advantages of, 84
  Title IX legislation and, 84
  ultramarathon runners, 83, 84
Austen, Jane, 15
Authoritative knowledge, xiii
Autoimmune disorders, 74, 161. *See also* Arthritis,
    Lupus erythematosus

Baby boom, 195–6
Baltimore Longitudinal Study of Aging, 98–99
Barbach, Lonnie, 230
Barbados, schools in, 250–51
Bateson, Mary Catherine, 256
Beauvoir, Simone de, 23, 175, 240
Biblical definition of women, 4
Biology of women
  body of woman, 63–67, *See also* Body
  as destiny, xi, 6
  estrogen's role in, 73–77
  links to other species, 21–42
  liver, 65–66
  men's versus, 9, 10, 64, 66, 82
  physiological potential (experiment), 85
Birth control pills (oral contraceptives)
  drug interactions with, 100

effects on cholesterol levels, 103
  fears about, 183–4
  mate selection and, 31–32
  migraines and, 95
  safety and effectiveness of, 182–84
  sexual desire and, 185
  smokers and, 93
Birth defects, 69
Birth rates, 5, 196
Bladder infections, 95
Blood mysteries, 11, 215. *See also* Menarche;
    Menopause; Menstruation
Blum, Deborah, 246
Blyth, Myrna, 276
Body, female, 9–10, 63–67
  form/shape, 45–48
  fat, 46–47
  hips, 47
  media ideal of, 315–16
  mistrust/dislike of, 307–8, 315–16
  physiological processes, 65–7
    tuning into, 266
  sexual maturation of, 125–34
  theology of embodiment, 316
  waist-hip ratio, 47–8
"Body trap," x–xi
Bolen, Jean, 319
Bone density, 87, 95, 224, 231–32
Bone strength
  building, 87–88
  HRT and other treatments, 231–32
  menopause and, 224
Bono, Paola, 6
Brain, 239–58. *See also* Alzheimer's disease
  aging, changes with, 252–55
  empathy, compassion, and intuition and, 12,
    256
  estrogen and, 75–76, 77, 254–55
  evolutionary legacy, and function, 244–45
  gender or sex differences and, xiv, 12, 17, 77,
    124, 241–42, 244, 245, 246–48, 255–57, 264,
    287
  hearing, 241
  HRT and, 232
  imaging techniques, 244–45
  intelligence, cognitive skills, and gender, 240–41,
    243, 246–48, 251–52
  math skills, 249–52
  memory, 253–54
  memory and mental abilities, factors in maintenance
    of, 255
  menopause and, 224
  motherhood and changes in, 210–11
  physiology of, 242–46
  plasticity of, 245, 251–52
  sadness and MRI changes, 264, 287
  size, 241, 243–44, 251
  stroke recovery, men versus women, 245
  testosterone and, 76, 77
  vision, 241
Bray, Rosemary, 317
Breast cancer
  abortion and, 187–88
  advances in treatment, 109–10
  African-American women, in, 96
  alcohol, 94
  birth control pills and, 101
  estrogen and, 74
  exercise and risk reduction, 86

ABOUT THE AUTHOR

DIANNE HALES, one of the most widely published and honored freelance writers in the country, is a contributing editor for *Ladies Home Journal* and *Working Mother*. She has written more than a thousand articles for national publications, including *American Health, Family Circle, Glamour, Good Housekeeping, Mademoiselle, McCall's, The New York Times, Parade, Reader's Digest, Redbook, Seventeen, The Washington Post,* and *Woman's Day*.

Her textbook *Invitation to Health*, now in its eighth edition, is the leading text for college health courses. Her books for a general readership include *Caring for the Mind: The Comprehensive Guide to Mental Health; Intensive Caring: New Hope for High Risk Pregnancy; How to Sleep Like a Baby; The U.S. Army Total Fitness Program: Be All You Can Be; New Hope for Problem Pregnancies;* and *The Complete Book of Sleep*. Her works have been translated into many languages and published around the world.

Dianne Hales is one of the few journalists to have been honored with national magazine-writing awards by both the American Psychiatric Association and the American Psychological Association. She is also the 1998 recipient of the Emma (Exceptional Merit Media Award) for health reporting from the National Women's Political Caucus and Radcliffe College. She has won numerous other writing awards from various organizations, including the National Easter Seal Society, the Arthritis Foundation, CHADD, the Council for the Advancement of Scientific Education, and the New York Public Library.

She lives with her husband, Dr. Robert E. Hales, and their daughter, Julia, in northern California.